OXFORD HISTORICAL MONOGRAPHS

Below
the Magic Mountain

*A Social History of Tuberculosis
in Twentieth-Century Britain*

LINDA BRYDER

CLARENDON PRESS · OXFORD
1988

Oxford University Press, Walton Street, Oxford OX2 6DP

Oxford New York Toronto
Delhi Bombay Calcutta Madras Karachi
Petaling Jaya Singapore Hong Kong Tokyo
Nairobi Dar es Salaam Cape Town
Melbourne Auckland
and associated companies in
Beirut Berlin Ibadan Nicosia

Oxford is a trade mark of Oxford University Press

Published in the United States
by Oxford University Press, New York

British Library Cataloguing in Publication Data
Bryder, Linda
Below the magic mountain: a social history
of tuberculosis in twentieth century
Britain.—(Oxford historical monographs).
1. Tuberculosis—Great Britain—History—20th century
I. Title
616.9'95'00941   RC316.G7
ISBN 0-19-822947-X

Library of Congress Cataloging in Publication Data
Bryder, Linda.
Below the magic mountain.
(Oxford historical monographs)
Bibliography: p.
Includes index.
1. Tuberculosis—Great Britain—History—20th century.
I. Title.   II. Series.
RC316.G7B78 1988   362.1'96995'00941   87-31495
ISBN 0-19-822947-X

Set by Hope Services, Abingdon
Printed in Great Britain by
Biddles Ltd., Guildford and King's Lynn

TO MY PARENTS

ACKNOWLEDGEMENTS

MANY people and institutions have assisted me in producing this book. I am grateful to the following people for passing on to me their personal experiences in the field of tuberculosis—Dr and Mrs Geoffrey Beven, Dr and Mrs J. R. Bignall, Mrs F. C. Carling, Miss Kathleen Colgate, Miss Margaret Coltart, Mrs Goozee, Dr P. D'Arcy Hart, Mrs Kathleen Liddall Hart, Dr and Mrs Peter Heaf, Dr and Mrs John Hurford, Mr and Mrs Harold Huffer, Mr Frank Jordan, Mr and Mrs Norman Langdon, Mrs Joan McCarthy, Drs F. J. W. and S. M. Miller, Dr Walter Pagel, Lady Pedlar, Mr and Mrs Charlie Stockford, Dr and Mrs W. E. Snell, Sir Geoffrey Todd, and Sir Graham Wilson. I am also grateful to the following institutions and organizations for allowing me access to their archives—the British Film Institute, the Brompton Hospital (Frimley Sanatorium), the Cardiothoracic Institute, the Chest, Heart and Stroke Association, Churchill Hospital, Oxford, the King Edward VII Hospital, Midhurst, the Medical Research Council, Papworth Village Settlement, the Royal British Legion Industries (Preston Hall) Incorporated, the Radcliffe Infirmary, Oxford, the Royal Berkshire Hospital, Reading, as well as the Record Offices in London (Kew), Cambridge, East Sussex, and Northumberland. I would like to thank the Chest, Heart and Stroke Association, Papworth Village Settlement (with the kind assistance of Mr Frank Jordan), and the Bodleian Library, Oxford, for permission to reproduce the photographs in this book.

I am indebted to Dr Barry Supple for helpful suggestions in the early stages of the thesis on which this book was based; to Dr Jane Lewis and Janet Howarth, who examined the thesis and made many valuable comments; to Dr Joan Austoker and Margaret Pelling, who read and commented incisively on earlier drafts; and especially to Dr Charles Webster who proved an excellent supervisor for my doctoral thesis, giving me guidance and encouragement throughout. I am grateful to the New Zealand University Grants Committee, Nuffield College, Oxford, and the Queen's College, Oxford, for financial support. Lastly I would like to thank the members of Nuffield College, the Queen's College, and the Wellcome Unit for the History of Medicine, Oxford, for providing me with a congenial and stimulating environment in which to work throughout the time this book was in the making.

CONTENTS

ILLUSTRATIONS

FIGURES

TABLES

ABBREVIATIONS

BJT	*British Journal of Tuberculosis*
BMA	British Medical Association
BMJ	*British Medical Journal*
BTA	British Tuberculosis Association (formerly TA)
CC	County Council
CMO	County Medical Officer
CMOH	Chief Medical Officer of the Ministry of Health
COS	Charity Organisation Society
EMJ	*Edinburgh Medical Journal*
GP	General Practitioner
GMJ	*Glasgow Medical Journal*
Jl. NAPT	*Tuberculosis: the Journal of the National Association for the Prevention of Tuberculosis*
JTC	Joint Tuberculosis Council
LCC	London County Council
LGB	Local Government Board
MAB	Metropolitan Asylums Board
MOH	Medical Officer of Health
MRC	Medical Research Council ('Committee' before 1920)
MRC (SRS)	*Medical Research Council (Special Report Series)*
NAPT	National Association for the Prevention of Tuberculosis
1 NAPT	*Transactions of 1st (etc.) Annual Conference of the NAPT*
NETS	North of England Tuberculosis Society
NTA	National Tuberculosis Association (America)
NWTS	North Western Tuberculosis Society
PRO MH	Public Record Office, Ministry of Health files
RAMC	Royal Army Medical Corp
SMOH	Society of Medical Officers of Health
SSHM	Society for the Social History of Medicine
TA	Tuberculosis Association
TG SMOH	Tuberculosis Group of the Society of Medical Officers of Health
TO	Tuberculosis Officer
TSAC	Tuberculosis Standing Advisory Committee
TT	Tuberculin-tested

WBH   Welsh Board of Health
WNMA   King Edward VII Welsh National Memorial Association

Reports

Astor Committee. Departmental Committee on Tuberculosis, Chairman:
   Lord Astor, *Interim Report*, Cd. 6164 (1912); *Final Report*, i, Cd.
   6641(1913); ibid. ii, Cd. 6654 (1913).
Athlone Report. Inter-departmental Committee on Nursing Services Interim
   Report, Chairman: Earl of Athlone (1939).
Barlow Report. Inter-departmental Committee Appointed to Consider and
   Report upon the Immediate Practical Steps Which Should be Taken for the
   Provision of Residential Treatment for Discharged Soldiers and Sailors
   Suffering from Pulmonary Tuberculosis and for their Re-introduction into
   Employment, Especially on the Land, Final Report, Chairman: Lord
   Astor, Vice-chairman who presided: Sir Montague Barlow, Cmd.
   317 (1919).
Bulstrode Report. LGB, H. Timbrell Bulstrode, *35th Annual Report
   1905–6, Suppl. in Continuation of the Report of the Medical Officer for
   1905–6, On Sanatoria for Consumption, and Certain Other Aspects of the
   Tuberculosis Question*, Cd. 3657 (1908).
Chalke Report. WNMA, H. D. Chalke, Report of an Investigation into
   the Causes of the Continued High Death-Rate from Tuberculosis
   in Certain Parts of North Wales, PRO MH55/1192, Cardiff, 1933.
Clement Davies Report. Ministry of Health, *Report of the Committee of
   Inquiry into the Anti-tuberculosis Service in Wales and Monmouthshire*,
   Chairman: Clement Davies (London, 1939).
Grigg Report. Ministry of Agriculture and Fisheries, *Report of the
   Reorganisation Commission for Milk*, Economic Series 38, Chairman:
   Sir Edward Grigg (London, 1933).
Horder Report. Royal College of Nursing, *Nursing Reconstruction
   Committee Report*, Chairman: Lord Horder, (London, 1943).
Lancet Report. The Lancet Commission on Nursing, Final Report (London,
   1932).
Murray Report. Tuberculosis Grants Committee Final Report,
   Chairman: G. H. Murray, 1920, PRO MH55/169.
Rushcliffe Report. Ministry of Health, *First Report of Nurses' Salaries
   Committee: Salaries and Emoluments of Female Nurses in Hospitals*,
   Chairman: Lord Rushcliffe, Cmd. 6424 (1943).

'I beg your pardon for speaking of it like this, but they seem very jolly over it themselves, your pneumatic friends [tuberculous patients]. The way they were coming along . . .'

Joachim sought for a reply. 'Good Lord,' he said, 'they are so *free*—I mean, they are so young, and time is nothing to them, and they may die—perhaps—why should they make a long face? Sometimes I think being ill and dying aren't serious at all, just a sort of loafing about and wasting time; life is only serious down below. You will get to understand that after a while, but not until you have spent some time up here.'

Thomas Mann, *The Magic Mountain*, trans. H. T. Lowe-Porter, 2 vols. (London, 1927, repr. 1979), 51–2

The obvious despair in the eyes of the patients whose husband or loved one failed to visit, was an acknowledgement of the rejection they felt and the fear that their relationship may never be re-established . . .

Joan McCarthy, '"Tuberculosis" Before and After Waksman', unpublished dissertation, BA (General) Health and Community Studies, Chester College, 1986, 42.

As soon as he knew, Frank Pollitt, soon as he knew she'd got it, he gave her up. . . . She was heart-broken. She'd been going with him three years, but he never came round again, when he heard she'd got TB.

Angela Hewins, *Mary, After the Queen: Memories of a Working Girl* (Oxford, 1986), 35.

Introduction

IN Britain in the first decade of the twentieth century tuberculosis was responsible for approximately 1 death in every 8.[1] It was the single greatest killer of males, causing a death-rate of almost 2 per thousand population per annum in England and Wales at that time. Among females the death-rate from tuberculosis of 1.4 per thousand was exceeded only slightly by heart disease as the major cause of death. Tuberculosis accounted for more than 1 death in 3 among men aged 15–44, one-half of all female deaths in the age group 15–24, and one-quarter of all female deaths in the age group 25–44.

While tuberculosis was primarily a disease of adults, it was not entirely absent among infants and children. The death-rates from tuberculosis in the age group 5–14 were only 0.7 and 0.6 per thousand population respectively among males and females in the first decade of the twentieth century. Nevertheless, tuberculosis was the single greatest cause of death in this age group at the time, causing 24 per cent of male deaths and 20 per cent of female deaths. For infants (under the age of 1 year), other causes of death were far greater killers than tuberculosis, such as infantile convulsions, pneumonia, diarrhoea and enteritis, and prematurity. Tuberculosis was only responsible for 4 per cent of all deaths in this age group in 1901–10. Yet it was causing a high death-rate of 6.8 per thousand population among males and 5.4 among females in this age group and thus contributed to the high infant mortality rates prevailing.

By 1947 tuberculosis among all age groups and both sexes had declined considerably. At this time it was responsible for only 5 per cent of male deaths (with a death-rate of 0.7 per thousand population) and 4 per cent of all female deaths (0.5 per thousand population). As a major cause of death, it was now far exceeded by heart disease and cancer. Among infants the decreasing incidence of tuberculosis contributed to the dramatic decline in mortality which occurred in the

[1] The statistics on tuberculosis cannot be taken as definitive, as will be discussed. The following statistics refer to England and Wales unless otherwise specified. The Scottish rates followed a similar trend though they tended to be slightly higher (see Fig. 1); Registrar-General, *Statistical Review of England and Wales*, and Registrar-General for Scotland, *Annual Reports*, from 1901; W. P. D. Logan, 'Mortality in England and Wales from 1848 to 1947', *Population Studies* (1950), 132–78.

twentieth century, with the tuberculosis death-rate falling from above 5 per thousand population in 1900 to below 0.5 per thousand by 1950. This mortality decline among all age groups was to continue over the following decades, now with the aid of chemotherapy developed in the 1940s, so that the total annual number of deaths from tuberculosis in Britain fell from approximately 15,000 in 1950 to less than 500 by 1985.

The early twentieth century witnessed the launching of an extensive anti-tuberculosis campaign in Britain, which attracted State support and eventually became part of local authority public health services after the First World War. One question addressed in this study is the extent to which the anti-tuberculosis movement in the twentieth century contributed to the decline of the disease. The success (or failure) of the anti-tuberculosis campaign is not, however, the only or even the central concern. An important point of inquiry is why tuberculosis, which had been endemic in the nineteenth century and had indeed been declining over five decades, suddenly attracted widespread interest at the turn of the century. Was the discovery in 1882 of the tubercle bacillus, the causal agent of tuberculosis, the motivating factor in the rise of the movement as has traditionally been assumed, or were other factors more important, such as the concern for 'national efficiency' which was clearly an important influence on other health movements launched at the time, specifically the infant and child health movements?[2] Also under scrutiny is why the campaign, once under way, took the form it did. Was it true, as René and Jean Dubos have asserted in their classic history of tuberculosis, that once the causal agent was discovered, preventive measures 'acquired the compelling strength of common sense'?[3] The extent to which other factors, such as professional interests and current ideologies, played a determining role in the measures adopted will be explored. An attempt will be made to place the campaign in its broader social and political context. The experience of patients will be dis-

---

[2] On the infant and child welfare movements, see A. Davin, 'Imperialism and Motherhood', *History Workshop Journal*, 5 (1978), 9–65; C. Dyhouse, 'Working-class Mothers and Infant Mortality in England, 1895–1914', *Journal of Social History*, 12 (1978), 248–67; J. Lewis, *The Politics of Motherhood* (London, 1980); A. Oakley, *The Captured Womb, A History of the Medical Care of Pregnant Women* (Oxford, 1984); D. Dwork, *War is Good for Babies and Other Young Children: A History of the Infant and Child Welfare Movement in England 1898–1918* (London, 1987).

[3] R. and J. Dubos, *The White Plague: Tuberculosis, Man and Society* (London, 1953), 172.

cussed. A history of tuberculosis is not complete without considering the experience of those who contracted the disease, including the impact of the anti-tuberculosis campaign on their lives.

Present-day understanding of the aetiology of tuberculosis stems largely from the discovery of the tubercle bacillus (*Mycobacterium tuberculosis*) by Robert Koch, a German bacteriologist, in 1882. Following that discovery it was ascertained that tuberculosis was not hereditary as formerly believed but an infectious disease caused by the tubercle bacillus. It was shown that it could affect all parts of the body, although the dominant form was respiratory or pulmonary tuberculosis (formerly known as consumption or phthisis), in which the disease affects the lungs. Approximately 80–85 per cent of all deaths from tuberculosis throughout the twentieth century were caused by the pulmonary form of the disease. Nevertheless, non-pulmonary forms assumed a greater importance than statistically indicated, as these were the forms to which children were susceptible. Almost 85 per cent of all tuberculosis deaths of those under the age of 5 were due to non-pulmonary forms of the disease, and 70 per cent of deaths of those between the ages 5 and 14. The major forms of non-pulmonary tuberculosis included tuberculosis of the bones and joints, the lymph nodes (formerly known as scrofula), the abdomen, the meninges and central nervous system, and the skin (lupus vulgaris).

Five varieties of the tubercle bacillus were discovered, distinguished by their place of origin—human, bovine, avian, murine, and piscine. Only the first two were found to cause disease in humans. Approximately 98 per cent of all pulmonary cases and 70 per cent of all non-pulmonary cases in this period were due to infection with the human type of the bacillus, spread by droplet infection, generally by coughing or sneezing. The remainder was due to infection with the bovine type of the bacillus. Bovine infection could be caused by consuming infected meat, but was more commonly caused by infected milk. Related primarily to non-pulmonary forms of the disease, bovine infection was associated in particular with children and infants. It was estimated in 1931 that over 1,000 children under the age of 15 died of tuberculosis of bovine origin in England and Wales each year.[4]

It was shown in the early twentieth century by the use of newly developed tuberculin skin tests ('von Pirquet', 1907, and 'Mantoux',

[4] Ministry of Health, *A Memorandum on Bovine Tuberculosis in Man with Special Reference to Infection by Milk* (Reports on Public Health and Medical Subjects, 63; London, 1931), 23.

1908), and by biopsies and autopsies, that infection with the tubercle bacillus among the population in an urban community was as high as 90 per cent, but only approximately 1 per cent developed active disease.[5] It has never been determined precisely who was most likely to contract the disease. The question of the influence of a hereditary predisposition remains unresolved; to all appearances environment has been a far more important factor. The historian investigating epidemiology often discovers more about the assumptions and prejudices of the inquirers than about disease patterns themselves. Nevertheless, there appeared to be certain indisputable trends. Such indicators were based on mortality statistics (deaths and death-rates) rather than morbidity statistics (incidence of the disease) as the latter were too unreliable and incomplete in this period to form the basis of a valid study. Studies indicated that the geographical distribution of the disease coincided with less prosperous areas, generally with higher rates in Scotland and Wales than in England (see Figs. 4 and 5). The tabulation of death-rates by class showed higher rates at the bottom of the socio-economic scale (see Table 1). Tuberculosis was commonly

TABLE 1 *Standardized death-rates per 100,000 population from pulmonary tuberculosis among occupied males (aged 20–65) by social class in England and Wales, 1930–2*

Class	No./100,000
I (upper and middle classes)	61
II (intermediate)	70
III (skilled labour)	100
IV (intermediate)	104
V (unskilled labour)	125

Source: Registrar-General, *Decennial Supplement, England and Wales, 1931, Part 2a, Occupational Mortality (1935), 31.*

acknowledged as a disease of poverty; the point of dispute was over which particular aspects in the lives of the poor were responsible for the disease, for example, overcrowding, insanitary conditions, under-nourishment, or 'bad habits'.

Physical symptoms of the disease included fever, sweating at night,

[5] S. Delépine, *Astor Committee Final Report*, ii, Cd. 6654 (1913), 27.

cough and dyspnoea (difficult breathing), haemoptysis (blood-spitting), and loss of weight. None of these was peculiar to tuberculosis, and might be absent from a particular case making diagnosis problematic. Continued ill-health was probably the most constant symptom, but sometimes cases were discovered by chance through X-ray examination. By the mass radiography schemes introduced in the 1940s, an active-case rate of 1 per thousand was discovered among those previously unsuspected of having tuberculosis. Before the effective chemotherapy of the 1950s, the course of the disease was totally unpredictable. Cases which appeared to be advanced might recover spontaneously. The disease might take a fulminating course as was commonly noted among young adults, described in the nineteenth century as 'galloping consumption', or it might linger on for many years, as was commoner among older age groups, causing confusion between tuberculosis and chronic bronchitis. At its final stage, it was often marked by haemoptysis.

Tuberculous meningitis was, before the chemotherapy of the 1950s, invariably fatal, the course of the disease running not more than three to six weeks, with the patient sinking into a deepening coma. Tuberculosis of the bones and joints led to crippling, and tuberculosis of the skin to skin blemishes, often of the face and neck. Children who were sickly-looking in the early twentieth century were frequently diagnosed as 'pre-tuberculous', as cases likely to develop tuberculosis. Many of these children did not suffer from tuberculosis, but from malnutrition or some other deficiency disease such as rickets or anaemia.

Patients with tuberculosis in the twentieth century had more than the physical symptoms of the disease to contend with. With the newly acquired knowledge of the infectiousness of the disease, enthusiastically promulgated by the National Association for the Prevention of Tuberculosis (founded in 1898), and in the absence of effective treatment, tuberculous patients often found themselves cut off from the wider community. Evidence suggests that securing a job following a period in an institution for tuberculosis was difficult, and that tuberculosis patients were even ostracized by friends and family. A short period in an institution did not ensure that patients were no longer infectious, and so ex-patients were stigmatized for the rest of their lives. Moreover, there was also a persistent belief in some form of hereditary predisposition which led some patients to hide their medical histories from their marriage partners and in-laws. For some sufferers from tuberculosis, the social consequences of the disease were far worse than its physical manifestations. In the first half of the twentieth century tuberculosis was not only a major killer, it also became a social problem.

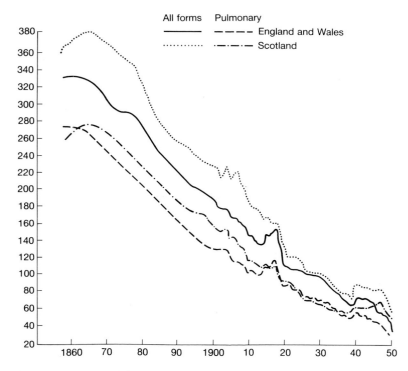

Fɪɢ. ɪ. Standardized death-rates from tuberculosis (all forms and pulmonary) per 100,000 population, England and Wales, and Scotland, 1850–1950.

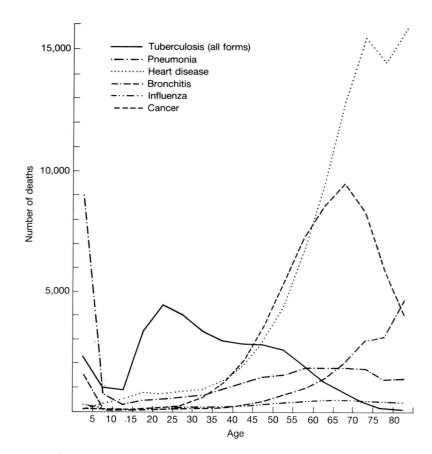

FIG 2. Deaths by ages, from the six chief causes of death, England and Wales, 1930.

Source: NAPT Council Report, 1932.

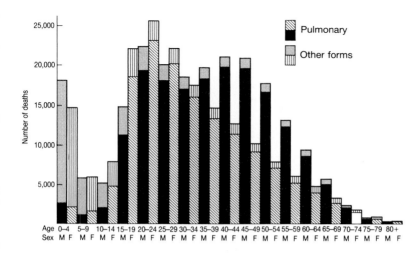

FIG. 3. Tuberculosis deaths by sex and age, England and Wales, 1921–1930.
Source: NAPT Council Report, 1932.

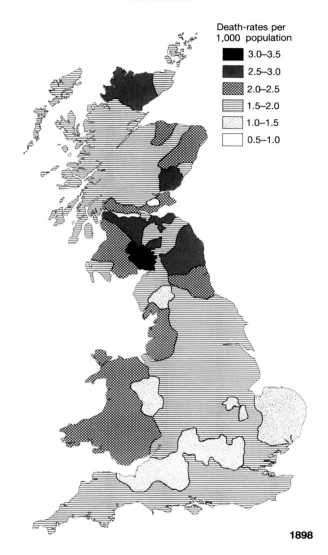

Death-rates per
1,000 population

■ 3.0–3.5

▨ 2.5–3.0

▨ 2.0–2.5

▤ 1.5–2.0

░ 1.0–1.5

□ 0.5–1.0

1898

FIG. 4. Geographical distribution of tuberculosis in 1898 and 1924.
Source: NAPT, *Historical Sketch 1898–1926* (London, 1926).

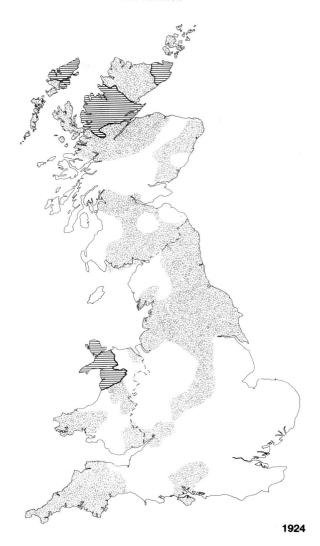

1924

Administrative Counties	Death-rates per 100,000 civil population — Pulmonary Tuberculosis	Other Forms	All Forms
RUTLAND	22	22	44
PETERBOROUGH	44	6	50
DERBY	42	12	54
OXFORD	48	10	58
HERTFORD	49	11	60
WESTMORLAND	48	13	61
BUCKINGHAM	50	13	63
SUSSEX WEST	51	12	63
SUSSEX EAST	53	10	63
ELY ISLE OF	41	22	63
CHESHIRE	55	10	65
SURREY	56	9	65
SUFFOLK EAST	51	14	65
WARWICK	52	13	65
NORFOLK	51	15	66
SOMERSET	53	13	66
WILTSHIRE	56	12	68
YORKS EAST RIDING	52	16	68
HAMPSHIRE	55	14	69
LINCS KESTEVEN	61	9	70
MIDDLESEX	60	11	71
WIGHT ISLE OF	58	13	71
NORTHAMPTON	60	11	71
LANCASHIRE	57	14	71
CAMBRIDGE	59	14	73
GLOUCESTER	62	12	74
YORKS WEST RIDING	57	17	74
YORKS NORTH RIDING	57	17	74
BERKSHIRE	57	17	74
LINCS LINDSEY	58	18	76
SUFFOLK WEST	61	15	76
NOTTINGHAM	61	16	77
KENT	64	13	77
HUNTINGDON	69	9	78
ESSEX	65	14	79
DORSET	62	17	79
SHROPSHIRE	64	15	79
DEVON	66	13	79
LEICESTER	69	15	84
CORNWALL	65	20	85
FLINT	69	16	85
BEDFORD	75	10	85
MONMOUTH	71	15	86
HEREFORD	70	16	86
STAFFORD	70	16	86
WORCESTER	68	19	87
CARMARTHEN	72	17	89
LINCS HOLLAND	67	22	89
DENBIGH	73	19	92
DURHAM	69	26	95
CUMBERLAND	78	20	98
GLAMORGAN	80	19	99
NORTHUMBERLAND	76	24	100
RADNOR	82	19	101
LONDON	90	12	102
PEMBROKE	78	29	107
MONTGOMERY	92	16	108
ANGLESEY	99	21	120
CARDIGAN	111	11	122
BRECON	107	21	128
MERIONETH	116	19	135
CARNARFON	128	28	156

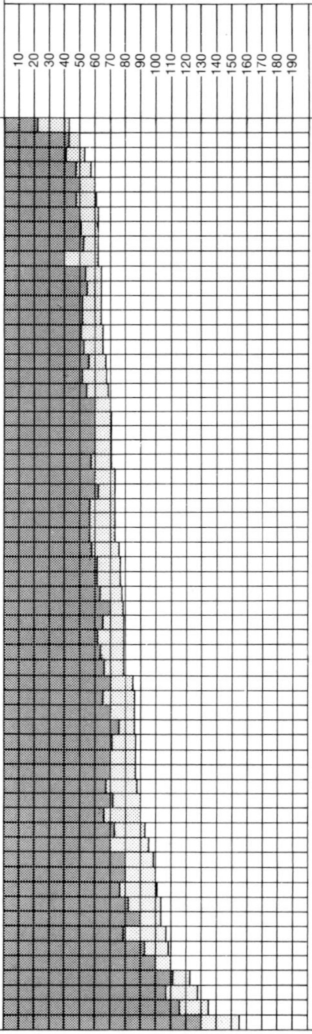

FIG. 5. Death-rates from tuberculosis in administrative counties and county boroughs, England and Wales, 1931.

Source: NAPT Council Report, 1932.

Administrative Boroughs	Death-rates per 100,000 civil population	Pulmonary Tuberculosis	Other Forms	All Forms
BATH		51	9	60
ROCHDALE		48	12	60
CANTERBURY		58	4	62
SOUTHPORT		50	13	63
BOURNEMOUTH		58	7	65
BURTON		52	14	66
DONCASTER		57	9	66
NORWICH		61	9	70
HALIFAX		51	20	71
EASTBOURNE		50	22	72
SMETHWICK		62	11	73
CROYDON		64	10	74
HASTINGS		71	5	76
HUDDERSFIELD		60	17	77
OXFORD		67	12	79
BOLTON		68	12	80
WEST BROMWICH		73	7	80
EAST HAM		70	11	81
SHEFFIELD		68	14	82
BLACKPOOL		73	9	82
BARROW		63	21	84
PRESTON		68	17	85
ROTHERHAM		61	25	86
DERBY		76	10	86
READING		70	17	87
BURY		76	13	89
EXETER		74	16	90
BURNLEY		75	16	91
BARNSLEY		61	32	93
WIGAN		74	19	93
WOLVERHAMPTON		78	15	93
BLACKBURN		75	19	94
NORTHAMPTON		78	16	94
STOCKPORT		84	10	94
BRADFORD		79	15	94
CARLISLE		68	26	94
SOUTHEND		82	13	95
COVENTRY		87	8	95
OLDHAM		77	20	97
WALLASEY		87	11	98
WAKEFIELD		79	19	98
YORK		82	16	98
PORTSMOUTH		83	16	99
SOUTHAMPTON		87	12	99
WEST HAM		86	14	100
BRIGHTON		82	19	101
IPSWICH		82	19	101
WALSALL		93	10	103
BRISTOL		92	12	104
LINCOLN		82	23	105
BIRMINGHAM		92	13	105
DEWSBURY		81	26	107
SWANSEA		92	15	107
PLYMOUTH		86	22	108
LEEDS		92	18	110
WORCESTER		96	14	110
ST HELENS		95	16	111
GLOUCESTER		89	23	112
NOTTINGHAM		93	19	112
WEST HARTLEPOOL		89	24	113
GREAT YARMOUTH		101	14	115
STOKE ON TRENT		98	18	116
DUDLEY		105	12	117
GRIMSBY		94	26	120
BIRKENHEAD		96	25	121
DARLINGTON		107	21	128
MANCHESTER		112	17	129
WARRINGTON		112	18	130
LEICESTER		111	20	131
CARDIFF		106	25	131
LIVERPOOL		116	19	135
NEWPORT		112	24	136
KINGSTON UPON HULL		116	20	136
NEWCASTLE ON TYNE		107	31	138
CHESTER		97	43	140
SUNDERLAND		109	33	142
SALFORD		122	21	143
GATESHEAD		116	32	148
MERTHYR TYDFIL		123	27	150
TYNEMOUTH		121	34	155
BOOTLE		146	15	161
MIDDLESBROUGH		136	27	163
SOUTH SHIELDS		126	46	172

I

A National Problem, 1898–1918

THE founding of the National Assocation for the Prevention of Consumption and Other Forms of Tuberculosis, in 1898, marked the start of a national campaign to eradicate tuberculosis in Britain, which was to gain increasing momentum in the early twentieth century, eventually attracting State involvement. By the end of this period, a comprehensive State-controlled scheme for the prevention and treatment of tuberculosis had been created.

(1) THE NATIONAL ASSOCIATION FOR THE PREVENTION OF TUBERCULOSIS[1]

The NAPT from the start was no insignificant organization. Its founding meeting was attended by leading physicians as well as Lord Salisbury, the Prime Minister, and the Prince of Wales, later King Edward VII. It aimed to attack the problem of tuberculosis in three ways: by educating the public in preventive measures, by campaigning to eliminate tuberculosis from cattle, and by promoting the establishment of institutions for treatment.

The anti-tuberculosis campaign in Britain was part of an international movement. Lord Salisbury pointed out at the inaugural meeting that 'we are very much behind the world in these matters'.[2] France had established a national anti-tuberculosis association in 1891, as had Germany in 1895. In America, the Pennsylvania Society for the Prevention of Tuberculosis had been founded in 1892, and the (American) National Association for the Study and Prevention of Tuberculosis was to be founded in 1904. Other countries also set up associations around this time, for example, Belgium in 1898, Portugal

---

[1] The Association changed its name from the 'National Association for the Prevention of Consumption and Other Forms of Tuberculosis' to the 'National Association for the Prevention of Tuberculosis' in 1919.

[2] An account of the inaugural meeting was given in the jubilee issue of the NAPT Bulletin: *NAPT Bulletin*, 11/5 (1948), 177–81.

and Italy in 1899, Canada in 1900, Denmark and Australia (Victoria and New South Wales) in 1901, Sweden in 1904, Japan in 1908, and Norway and Russia in 1910.[3] International congresses on tuberculosis were held in Paris in 1867, 1888, 1891, 1894, and 1898, in Berlin in 1899, and in Naples in 1900. An international congress was held in London in 1901 organized by the NAPT, at which it was decided to set up an international committee. The International Central Bureau for the Campaign against Tuberculosis was founded in 1902 with its headquarters in Berlin.

Tuberculosis was by no means a new problem in the late nineteenth and early twentieth centuries. Phthisis, or pulmonary tuberculosis, had been described by John Bunyan in 1680 as 'The Captain of all these men of death'.[4] It was estimated from the bills of mortality that 20 per cent of all deaths in London in 1656–60 were caused by phthisis, falling to 12 per cent in 1700, and then rising to 26 per cent in 1800.[5] While a decline in tuberculosis set in around 1850, the disease remained endemic throughout the century. Why then did it suddenly arouse an intensive international campaign in the late nineteenth century?

The most important factor generally held responsible for causing the new anti-tuberculosis movement was the isolation of the causal agent of tuberculosis, the tubercle bacillus, by Robert Koch in 1882, although Britain at least could then be said to be particularly tardy in responding to the discovery. At the founding of the NAPT in 1898, the importance of Koch's discovery was indeed stressed. Sir William Broadbent, personal physician to the Prince of Wales and the first chairman of the NAPT, pointed out that it was now definitely known that consumption was an infectious disease and thus that 'this terrible waste of life . . . is preventable'. The Prince of Wales launched the

[3] F. R. Walters, *Sanatoria for Consumptives in Various Parts of the World (France, Germany, Norway, Russia, Switzerland, the United States, and the British Possessions): A Critical and Detailed Description together with an Exposition of the Open-air or Hygienic Treatment of Phthisis*, 3rd edn. (London, 1905), 20, 71, 124; H. G. Sutherland (ed.), *The Control and Eradication of Tuberculosis: A Series of International Studies* (Edinburgh, 1911), 341, 357, 364.

[4] J. Bunyan, *The Life and Death of Mr Badman* (London, 1680), ed. J. Brown (Cambridge, 1905), 157.

[5] MRC, J. Brownlee, *An Investigation into the Epidemiology of Phthisis in Great Britain and Ireland* (SRS 18; London 1917), 41. Any discussion of the extent of tuberculosis pre-1900 (even post-1900, as will be discussed) is fraught with difficulties: see A. Hardy, 'Diagnosis, Death and Diet: The Case of London 1750–1909', *Journal of Interdisciplinary History* (in press).

national campaign with the rhetorical question: 'If preventable, why not prevented?'[6]

Robert Koch himself had foreseen far-reaching implications in his discovery. Reporting his results to the Physiological Society in Berlin in 1882, he announced that they no longer had to deal with an 'indefinable Something' but with 'a definite parasite whose vital processes were, for the most part, known'.[7] René and Jean Dubos wrote of the impact of the discovery:

What electrified the world was not the scientific splendor of the achievement, but rather the feeling that man had finally come to grips with the greatest killer of the human race. The 'Captain of All the Men of Death' was no longer a vague phantom. The heretofore unseen killer was now visible as a living object; its assailants at last had a target for their blows.[8]

Some time later, Sir Robert Young, physician at the Brompton Hospital for Diseases of the Chest and described as 'the accepted doyen of respiratory disease in Britain',[9] similarly claimed that 'once the cause was known, the problem of prevention and treatment became concrete instead of nebulous. There was no longer any justification for a hopeless, fainéant or resigned attitude to the sufferers from this disease.'[10] Thus a direct causal link was made between the discovery of the tubercle bacillus and the world-wide anti-tuberculosis campaign. According to Dubos, once the cause of tuberculosis was known, preventive measures 'acquired the compelling strength of common sense'.[11]

The isolation of the tubercle bacillus in meat and milk suggested that a preventive campaign should include the control of these sources of infection. Milk in particular was shown to be a common source of infection. The discovery in 1890 that 35 out of Queen Victoria's herd of 40 cows, supposedly of the highest quality, were suffering from tuberculosis indicated the prevalence of tuberculosis in cattle.[12] Starting with Manchester and Glasgow in 1899, local Acts were passed in over one hundred districts in Britain regulating the sale of

[6] *NAPT Bulletin*, 11/5 (1948), 177–8.
[7] R. Koch, 'Die Aetiologie und die Bekämpfung der Tuberkulose', lecture given at the Physiological Society of Berlin, 24 Mar. 1882, *Berliner klinische Wochenschrift*, 19 (1882), 221–30, trans. W. de Rouville, *Medical Classics*, 2 (1938), 853–80.
[8] R. and J. Dubos, *The White Plague: Tuberculosis, Man and Society* (London, 1953), 102.
[9] *British Thoracic Association (The First Fifty Years)* (London, 1978), 72.
[10] *18 NAPT* (1932), 17.   [11] Dubos, *The White Plague*, p. 172.
[12] J. Francis, *Bovine Tuberculosis* (London, 1947), 1 n. 1.

contaminated milk. The Acts permitted local authorities to trace infected milk to its origin and forbid the sale of milk from that cow in their area. However, it was objected to as it involved interference by one local authority in the area of another, and it was pointed out that the same milk could be sold elsewhere. Enforcement of the legislation was moreover variable, and received a setback when Robert Koch announced, at the 1901 Congress on Tuberculosis in London, that the tubercle bacillus of bovine origin was harmless to humans. Action was further postponed until the publication, in 1911, of the Final Report of the Royal Commission on Tuberculosis, which had been set up in 1901 in response to Koch's pronouncement. The Commission concluded that the possibility of the infection of humans from diseased cattle could not be denied and they urged the Government to take action 'to avert or minimise the present danger from the consumption of infected milk'. Yet the outbreak of the First World War led to further delay.[13]

Germ theory also suggested to the NAPT their earliest propaganda effort, an anti-spitting campaign. Expectoration had been condemned as unhygienic prior to the rise of germ theory, but no large campaign had been organized before the NAPT became involved. The NAPT sent 'Do not spit' notices to railway and tramway companies, and by 1901 105,000 leaflets had been issued.[14] They praised highly the campaign in America. Anti-spitting legislation had been passed in New York in 1896, and subsequently extended to other places. The campaign in Britain was never as forceful as that in some parts of the States; for example, in San Francisco, offenders could be fined up to $500 for spitting in public places and plain-clothed policeman rode on public transport to catch offenders.[15] Yet some local authorities in Britain also made spitting punishable by law. Glamorgan County Council was the first to do so in 1902, Liverpool Corporation and some other municipalities followed in 1903, and the LCC introduced a

---

[13] *Final Report of Royal Commission Appointed to Inquire into the Relations of Human and Animal Tuberculosis*, Part II, (Chairman: Sir Michael Foster, replaced by Sir William Power in 1907), Cd. 5761 (1911), 37, 40; Ministry of Health, *A Memorandum on Bovine Tuberculosis in Man with Special Reference to Infection by Milk* (Reports on Public Health and Medical Subjects, 63; London 1931), 23. See also C. Pennington, 'Tuberculosis', in O. Checkland and M. Lamb (eds.), *Health Care as Social History: The Glasgow Case* (Aberdeen, 1982), 89–91; and B. G. Rosenkrantz, 'The Trouble with Bovine Tuberculosis', *Bulletin of the History of Medicine*, 59 (1985), 155–75.

[14] NAPT Council Minutes, 22 Jan. 1900, p. 43; ibid., 15 June 1901, p. 80.

[15] *Jl. NAPT* 2/2 (1902), 51; ibid. 2/3 (1902), 97; ibid. 2/7 (1903), 285; ibid. 2/8 (1903), 338; ibid. 3/3 (1904), 116–17.

by-law in 1903 to make spitting in public places an offence, for which the offenders could be fined up to forty shillings.

The propaganda of the NAPT extended far beyond anti-spitting, however, to encompass health education in general. In 1907, it organized an exhibition which was first shown in Dublin, and then, in 1908, in Whitechapel, London, where it was viewed by over seventy thousand people. The exhibition subsequently went on tour, and was seen in 1909 by over a million people. A caravan for such tours was donated by Sir William Younger, a member of the council of the NAPT, in 1911.

In their exhibition, the NAPT explained the behaviour of consumption, or pulmonary tuberculosis, by analogy with the parable of the sower: the seed was everywhere, it was the soil that was important. The soil was said to be affected by three 'bads': bad food, leading to ill-nutrition, which was 'the great preparation of the ground'; bad air in 'wretched habitations and miserable cabins'; and bad drink, which was alcohol.[16]

This explanation of the behaviour of the disease could have suggested a social reform movement, an attack on living and working conditions and environment in general as harbouring the tubercle bacillus, and an attack on poverty. However, members of the NAPT showed themselves to be very much a product of the middle-class society from which they came, with its fixed assumptions about the poor. Their solution lay in education, just as the solution suggested by Charles Booth to the problem of poverty, following his survey of London from 1889 to 1903 which showed 30 per cent of the population to be living with income less than was required to maintain a level of nutrition adequate for physical efficiency, was to place the poor in labour camps and educate them.[17] Thus, according to Robert Philip, knighted in 1913 for his work related to tuberculosis and a prominent figure throughout the anti-tuberculosis campaign in Britain until his death in 1939,

Individuals and communities must be shown that the disease is maintained through ignorance and folly, and that its removal lies completely in their hands . . . the people must be taught from day to day that tuberculosis comes of their disregard of physiological law for themselves . . . Thereby a higher standard of

[16] NAPT, *Catalogue of Exhibits at the Tuberculosis Exhibition*, Town Hall, Reading, 11–16 Sept 1911, p. 9.
[17] C. Booth, *Life and Labour of the People in London* (London and New York, 1889–1902); A. Fried and R. M. Elman (eds.), *Charles Booth's London* (London, 1969).

national and personal cleanliness will be evolved, in presence of which the tubercle bacillus will be gradually discounted.[18]

The propaganda of the NAPT was often based on scare tactics. Their exhibition of 1907 was later described as a 'cabinet of horrors'.[19] People were to be dragooned into temperate living. Attacking the nineteenth-century image of consumption as romantic or 'poetic', H. de Carle Woodcock, member of the council of the NAPT, wrote in 1912, 'Tubercle is in truth a coarse, common disease, bred in foul breath, in dirt, in squalor. . . . The beautiful and the rich receive it from the unbeautiful poor.' He mentioned two types of non-pulmonary tuberculosis which were particularly disfiguring: 'The scrofula which deforms the already coarsened features of the stunted slum dweller is tubercle. Lupus . . . is a horrible disease which eats away the face; and lupus is due to tubercle.' On the causes of tuberculosis he wrote,

Adolescence is the time of danger, in which the human plant is easily nipped by the frost of ignorance or withered in the hothouse of vice. With more liberty there is more licence. The sedulous cultivation of indoor or outdoor excesses is a broad way leading to destruction. Sexual vice is one horror; the alcoholic habit is another; and the two are seldom found apart from tubercle . . . Legislation has had much to say concerning hours of work and overcrowding of workshops; but it has little to say of physical dirt, and nothing of moral dirt . . . I hope to see the day when tubercle and alcoholism and allied diseases will be under rigorous inquisition . . . Suicides are men who have failed, and are more likely than not to be tuberculous. Tubercle attacks failures. It attacks the depressed, the alcoholic, the lunatic of all degrees.[20]

Such pronouncements might have been counter-productive in the NAPT reform programme, appealing to those who saw tuberculosis as a useful form of natural selection. Eugenics was enjoying widespread support in the early twentieth century. However, among those leading the anti-tuberculosis campaign in Britain, the possibility of hereditary 'diathesis' or an inherited disposition to catch tuberculosis, as expounded by the eugenicist Karl Pearson for example, was played down in favour of personal responsibility through individual lifestyle. Most subscribed to the view of Sheriden Delépine, professor of pathology at the University of Manchester, that it was better, in

[18] *BMJ* 1 (1912), 875.
[19] NAPT Council Minutes, 15 May 1939, p. 1.
[20] H. de Carle Woodcock, *The Doctor and the People* (London, 1912), 184, 202–3.

relation to the anti-tuberculosis campaign, to attach too little than too much importance to the determining influence of predisposition.[21] Nothing was to interfere in the drive to reform the habits of the poor. The anti-tuberculosis campaign was indeed perceived in terms of a religious crusade. In keeping with the NAPT's use of the analogy of the sower, Clive Rivière, physician to the City of London Hospital for Consumption, wrote in 1917, 'Those . . . who obey the dictates of their physical conscience may feel well assured that in them the tubercle bacillus will fall on a stony soil.'[22]

Another feature of the NAPT propaganda was an anti-urban emphasis. Tuberculosis was viewed as a disease of civilization. A series of lantern slides used in their exhibition was captioned:

The anaemic work girls of our towns.
Look at the fisher-lass and see the contrast.
See the pasty-white faces of the city children.
See how different they look after they have been in the country.
The poor fishermen hardly ever contract consumption.
Live as much as possible in the open air.[23]

This was a response to the known prevalence of tuberculosis in the urban slums of Victorian and Edwardian Britain. The NAPT did not attempt to reform urban conditions, but encouraged a retreat back to the countryside as a solution to the problem.

The emphasis on individual responsibility and education rather than on broader social and economic conditions detrimental to health was also evident in the infant and child welfare movements which grew up at this time. This also suggests that too much emphasis should not be placed on the rise of germ theory in bringing about the anti-tuberculosis campaign. It did not take the bacteriological revolution to point to a connection between tuberculosis and the conditions (or habits) of the poor, which was the basis of the preventive work. A more

---

[21] *BJT* 14/2 (1920), 64; K. Pearson, *Department of Applied Mathematics, University College, University of London, Drapers' Company Research Memoirs, Studies in National Deterioration: A First Study of the Statistics of Pulmonary Tuberculosis* (London, 1907), 3, 25. On minimal importance attached to hereditary predisposition, see also C. Rivière, *Tuberculosis and How to Avoid It* (London, 1917), 53; H. H. Thomson, *Consumption, Its Prevention and Home Treatment: A Guide for the Use of Patients* (London, 1910), 12; Woodcock, *The Doctor and the People*, p. 221; *Tubercle*, 1 (1920), 480. An exception to the general view was found in R. D. Powell and P. H-S. Harley (eds.), *On Diseases of the Lungs and Pleurae*, 5th edn. (London, 1911), 510; 6th edn. (1921), 432.
[22] Rivière, *Tuberculosis and How to Avoid It*, p. 127.
[23] NAPT Council Annual Report 1913, p. 101.

important factor in the rise of the anti-tuberculosis campaign appeared to be a heightened concern in the late nineteenth and early twentieth centuries for the physical condition of the people as it affected national efficiency. Britain was facing strong competition as a world power at this time, particularly from Germany and America, and there was a prevalent belief that the cause of Britain's imperial decline lay in the poor quality of its fighters and workers. This concern for national efficiency was intensified by the revelations of the poor physical standards of the recruits in the Boer War of 1899–1902, which led to the setting up of the Inter-departmental Committee on Physical Deterioration in 1903. This Committee drew attention to high tuberculosis rates in urban slums.[24] Tuberculosis did not, however, feature prominently in the report which focused primarily on the health of infants and children, an age group with a relatively low incidence of tuberculosis. Yet, even the tuberculosis prevention programme itself devoted a great deal of attention to children, to prevent the disease from developing at a later stage, as will be further discussed. Tuberculosis cannot be viewed in isolation from the general health movement which arose and flourished in the early twentieth century.

(2) INSTITUTIONS

Another activity in which the NAPT became involved was the promotion of institutions for the treatment of the disease. Underlying this policy was a new confidence in the medical profession and what could be achieved through institutional treatment for tuberculosis.

In the nineteenth century, tuberculosis cases had been generally excluded from voluntary hospitals. Doctors were more interested in acute 'curable' illnesses than chronic 'incurable' diseases among which tuberculosis was included. They wanted to show results in terms of cure and were reluctant to surround themselves with cases which showed the limitations of their professional skills, and which 'blocked' the beds. Thus tuberculosis cases were often relegated to Poor Law institutions. Yet even some of the Poor Law infirmaries which were established in the second half of the nineteenth century strove to emulate voluntary hospitals by concentrating on acute and 'curable'

---

[24] *Report of the Inter-departmental Committee on Physical Deterioration*, Cd. 2175 (1904), 17.

cases, and thus excluded tuberculous patients. Tuberculosis cases were, moreover, even more likely to be excluded from general hospitals once the infectiousness of the disease was recognized.[25] Various kinds of specialized hospitals had appeared in the nineteenth century, including some tuberculosis hospitals. The Royal Seabathing Hospital, Margate, founded in 1791, catered mainly for tuberculosis of the glands, joints, and bones. In London, 4 voluntary hospitals for consumption had been set up by 1860: the Royal Hospital for Diseases of the Chest, founded in 1814 with 80 beds, the Brompton Hospital for Consumption and Diseases of the Chest, 1841, with 321 beds, the City of London Hospital for Diseases of the Chest, 1848, with 164 beds, and the North London Hospital for Consumption and Diseases of the Chest, 1860, with 100 beds. Tuberculosis hospitals were also established outside London in the second half of the nineteenth century, one of the more famous being the Royal National Hospital for Consumption, in Ventnor, Isle of Wight, founded in 1868 with 155 beds. By 1893, there were 17 special hospitals to treat consumption in Britain, with approximately 1,100 beds.[26]

The first of a new type of tuberculosis institution based on 'open-air treatment' was founded by Sir Robert Philip in 1889 in Edinburgh: the Royal Victoria Hospital for Consumption, Craigleith (not residential until 1894). In England, similar institutions were set up in the 1890s, and in Wales the first was founded in 1900. By 1907, there were 96 institutions providing such treatment in England and Wales with 4,081 beds.[27]

Open-air treatment for tuberculosis had preceded the bacteriological revolution in origin and was little influenced by it. Hermann Brehmer, a German physician, popularized the treatment at an institution for tuberculosis which he established at Goebersdorf, Silesia, in 1859. He believed that fresh air and exercise, as a result of their beneficial effect on the heart and lungs, could cure tuberculosis.[28] His institution

---

[25] B. Abel-Smith, *The Hospitals* (London, 1964), 36, 44, 45, 205; R. Gaffney, 'Poor Law Hospitals 1845–1914', in Checkland and Lamb (eds.), *Health Care as Social History*, 44–58; C. Pennington, ibid., 94.

[26] Walters, *Sanatoria for Consumptives*, 2nd edn. (London, 1901), 321–3, 394.

[27] For an outline of the sanatoria established by 1914, including the date of opening, see T. N. Kelynack (ed.), *Tuberculosis Yearbook and Sanatoria Annual*, i, 1913–14 (London, 1914), 191–311.

[28] H. Brehmer, 'Tuberculosis primis in stadiis semper curabilis' (1856), quoted in A. Latham in association with A. W. West, *The Prize Essay on the Erection of the King Edward VII Sanatorium for Consumption* (London, 1903), 5.

became famous and others were modelled on it, including that set up by Peter Dettweiler, a pupil and former patient of Brehmer, at Falkenstein in the Taurus Mountains (near Frankfurt) in 1876, and that founded by Otto Walther at Nordrach-in-Baden, in the Black Forest, in 1888. The direct influence of Walther, in particular, on the British movement can be seen in the names of three sanatoria, Nordrach-upon-Mendip Sanatorium, Somerset (1899), Pendyffryn Hall, Caernarvonshire (1900), commonly known as 'Nordrach-in-Wales', and Nordrach-on-Dee Sanatorium, Banchory, Scotland (1900). T. N. Kelynack, physician to the Mount Vernon Hospital for Consumption and Diseases of the Chest, Middlesex, wrote in 1904 that it was remarkable how many English sanatoria, in their often elaborately illustrated prospectuses, insisted that the 'Nordrach system' was faithfully carried out.[29] Linford Sanatorium, Hampshire (1898), was described as having been built 'as nearly as possible on the lines of Nordrach'. The Vale of Clwyd Sanatorium in north Wales was opened in 1901 'for the treatment of tuberculosis as originally carried out by Dr Otto Walther at Nordrach'. Some physicians and medical superintendents explained that they had travelled to Germany to study Walther's methods. Many of these physicians had suffered from tuberculosis themselves, and they had been treated by Walther. They subsequently set up sanatoria where they would also attempt to maintain their own health.[30]

At the opening of the King Edward VII Sanatorium, Midhurst, Surrey (commonly known as Midhurst Sanatorium) in 1906, it was reported that 'England may now boast that she is on a level with Continental nations, if not ahead of them, in the means which are being taken to cure and stamp out the insidious disease.' It was a visit to sanatoria in south Germany which inspired King Edward VII to endow the sanatorium.[31]

Bold statements appeared in the early twentieth century regarding the curability of tuberculosis by open-air methods. The *Daily Express* reported the opening of Midhurst Sanatorium: 'King Edward Sanator-

[29] T. N. Kelynack, *The Sanatorium Treatment of Consumption* (London, 1904), 13.

[30] S. V. Pearson, *Men, Medicine and Myself* (London, 1946), 32; E. and H. Carling, 'Peppard Common, a Short History', 1938, 3; J. H. Walker, *Open-air Treatment of Consumption, Seven Years' Experience in England* (London, 1899), 4; F. R. Walters, *Domiciliary Treatment of Tuberculosis* (London, 1921), vi; Kelynack (ed.), *Tuberculosis Yearbook 1913–14*, 224, 228.

[31] *Portsmouth Evening Post*, 13 June 1906 (N. D. Bardswell's scrapbook of the opening of Midhurst Sanatorium).

ium/ Not Meant to be a Home for the Dying/ Cures Expected'. The medical superintendent, N. D. Bardswell, said, 'We shall aim to cure our patients', and it was pointed out that 90 per cent of the patients which Bardswell had treated at Mundesley Sanatorium, a working-class sanatorium, from 1901 to 1906, were engaged in active work and were apparently cured.[32]

Jane Walker, who founded the East Anglian Sanatorium in 1901, reported in 1898 that the results of treating 78 cases of tuberculosis by open-air methods from 1892 to 1898 were encouraging, 'even in advanced cases, which a few years ago would have seemed quite beyond the bounds of possibility'.[33] F. R. Walters, who founded Crooksbury Sanatorium in 1900, held that statistics on sanatorium treatment for tuberculosis were 'eminently satisfactory, as they show a very large proportion of apparent recoveries'.[34] Open-air treatment at the Mendip Hills Sanatorium, Somerset, was reported in 1913 to have been 'most successful in saving hundreds of lives since 1899'.[35]

While bacteriology had little influence on the open-air movement, it nevertheless contributed to medical confidence by suggesting a potential curative agent in a bacterial product, 'tuberculin'. Tuberculin was derived from a culture of the tubercle bacillus, proclaimed by Koch in 1890 as a cure for tuberculosis. Experience with tuberculin in Britain was disappointing, however, and it attracted little interest initially. A revival of interest in the treatment in the early twentieth century followed the researches of Sir Almroth Wright, who attributed earlier failures to excessively large doses. Wright treated patients with tuberculin in the Inoculation Department of St Mary's Hospital, where he also treated other infectious diseases by similar methods.[36] By 1912 the use of tuberculin in Britain was increasing, so that the *Lancet* reported a 'general feeling which is setting more strongly in favour of tuberculin treatment', and it was estimated that tuberculin

[32] *Daily Express*, 12 June 1906 (Bardswell's scrapbook).
[33] Walker, *Open-air Treatment*, p. 1.,
[34] Walters, *Sanatoria for Consumptives*, 3rd edn. (London, 1905), p. v; 1st edn. (London, 1899), 48.
[35] Kelynack (ed.), *Tuberculosis Yearbook 1913–14*, p. 250.
[36] 'Report of the Tuberculin Treatment Sub-committee of the Brompton Hospital, 1890', quoted in C. Rivière and E. Morland, *Tuberculin Treatment* (London, 1912), pp. xi, xii–xiii; H. H. Thomson, *Consumption in General Practice*, 2nd edn. (London, 1912), 252. Almroth Wright is known primarily for his work at St Mary's Hospital, London, in the early twentieth century, on immunization against typhoid: V. Z. Cope, *Almroth Wright: Founder of Modern Vaccine Therapy* (London, 1966); see also W. D. Foster, *A History of Medical Bacteriology and Immunology* (London, 1970), 142.

was used routinely in over 200 institutions in Britain.[37] In Germany, the percentage of public tuberculosis institutions using tuberculin increased from 29 per cent in 1905 to 70 per cent in 1910. In 1912, it was recorded that over 80 per cent of patients in certain German sanatoria who had been treated with tuberculin while in the early stage of the disease were cured. All patients at Beelitz Sanatorium, Berlin (accommodating 891 patients), were treated with tuberculin, and in 1910, 86 per cent left partially or totally capable of working.[38] Tuberculin had many enthusiasts in Britain. For example, William Stobie, tuberculosis officer for Oxford, claimed successful results from the use of tuberculin from 1910 to 1915. Sir Robert Philip used tuberculin uninterruptedly, and found it 'a specific remedy of great value'. Sir Clifford Allbutt, Regius Professor of Physic at Cambridge University, believed it probable that with tuberculin as well as sanatorium treatment, the number of cures might be doubled.[39]

Great faith was also placed in the potential achievements of further bacteriological research. Emil Adolf von Behring, professor of bacteriology in Germany who won the Nobel Prize in Medicine and Physiology in 1901 for his work on serum therapy mainly in the treatment of diphtheria, announced in 1905 that he had in view 'a new curative principle' for tuberculosis.[40] The importance of establishing institutions for research was stressed in the early twentieth century. No tuberculosis institution was specifically founded as a research centre in Britain, unlike America where a hospital for tuberculosis was set up on the initiative of Sir William Osler in 1903 as the Henry Phipps Institute, Philadelphia (attached to the University of Pennsylvania from 1910), specifically for research into tuberculosis. Nevertheless, Sir William, then Regius Professor of Medicine at Oxford University, stated at the opening of Midhurst Sanatorium that he hoped that Midhurst would become a centre for the scientific study of the disease. James F. Goodhart, consultant to Midhurst, also held that an important aspect of a sanatorium was that it made possible series of

---

[37] *Lancet*, 1 (1912), 1073; Rivière and Morland, *Tuberculin Treatment*, p. 147.

[38] Rivière and Morland, op. cit., 2nd edn. (1913), 147; see also Thomson, *Consumption in General Practice*, pp. 252, 269; *Astor Committee, Final Report*, ii, Cd. 6654 (1913), 78, 118.

[39] W. C. Wilkinson, *The Tuberculin Dispensary for the Poor* (London, 1923), 66; R. Philip, *GMJ* 79/5 (1913), 330; *Astor Committee, Final Report*, ii. 5.

[40] H. H. Thomson, *Pulmonary Phthisis: Its Diagnosis, Prognosis, and Treatment* (London, 1906), 144.

comparative observations by which a cure might be discovered.[41] The sanatorium movement of early twentieth-century Britain aimed mainly at bringing tuberculosis treatment to working-class patients. A few private, expensive sanatoria were established attempting to attract wealthy patients away from the Continent, where they continued to go, as in the nineteenth century, 'to take the cure', but most of the British sanatoria were charitable institutions for the working and lower middle classes. The NAPT played an important part in this movement. The Pinewood Sanatorium, Wokingham, Berkshire, was established by voluntary funds with NAPT support in 1900. The Knightwick Sanatorium, near Worcester, was founded in 1901 by the Worcestershire branch. Bellefield Sanatorium, Lanark, was opened in 1904 by the Glasgow branch for male patients of the 'artisan and commercial classes'. In 1904 the Blencathra Sanatorium was set up by the Cumberland branch, and in 1910 the Northamptonshire Sanatorium was founded by a local branch. In 1911 the NAPT reported that it had 27 branches in Britain and the colonies, many with their own sanatoria.[42]

Another important voluntary organization was the King Edward VII Welsh National Memorial Association, set up in Wales in 1910, with an initial donation of £150,000 from the wealthy coal-owner, David Davies of Llandinam (Liberal MP for Montgomeryshire, and later Lord Davies). Its aim was 'the prevention and eradication in Wales (including Monmouthshire) of tuberculosis and other diseases, and, in particular the provision of treatment either in sanatoria or other institutions or otherwise of persons suffering from tuberculosis'. Treatment was provided free of charge. By 1915 the Association had 1,586 beds for the treatment of tuberculosis.[43]

The National Association for the Establishment and Maintenance of Sanatoria for Workers Suffering from Tuberculosis was another voluntary organization, founded in 1905. In 1907 it set up Benenden Sanatorium, Kent, which was to be the first of a chain of sanatoria for workers throughout the country. This sanatorium was specifically for

[41] Midhurst Sanatorium Consultant Reports, 9 Oct. 1906, pp. 56–8; ibid., 6 Nov. 1906, p. 66.
[42] NAPT, Catalogue of Exhibits at the Tuberculosis Exhibition, Town Hall, Reading, 11–16 Sept. 1911, p. 1.
[43] PRO MH75/17, Charter of Incorporation, 17 May 1912; see also G. R. Jones, in J. Cule (ed.), *Wales and Medicine* (London, 1975); L. Bryder, 'The King Edward VII Welsh National Memorial Association and its Policy towards Tuberculosis in Wales, 1910–48', *The Welsh History Review*, 13/2 (1986), 194–216.

Post Office employees, who had formed a branch of the Association with 40,000 members. The Association was organized along the lines of a friendly society. Each member paid ½d. a week and was allowed six months' full pay while receiving sanatorium treatment. No provision was made for workers' dependants who contracted tuberculosis.[44]

Midhurst Sanatorium itself was established as a charitable institution. It was intended for patients belonging to a class above the poor who could not afford to go to private sanatoria—officers of the Army and Navy, clergy of all denominations, members of professions and the Civil Service, teachers and governesses, clerks in banks and mercantile houses, and 'the educated classes generally'.[45]

Other sanatoria were founded by private charities. Maitland Cottage Sanatorium, Peppard Common, Berkshire, was founded by Esther Carling in 1899 as the result of a donation for that purpose 'for the treatment of working-class patients', and Westmorland Consumptive Sanatorium and Home was established in 1900 by 'a small band of philanthropists, for working and middle classes'. Kelling Sanatorium for Workers in Norfolk was set up by R. W. Burton-Fanning in 1903, and the Devon and Cornwall Sanatorium for Consumptives was founded in 1903 as a charitable institution. Mount Vernon Hospital, Middlesex, set up in 1904, was described as a 'great philanthropic enterprise'.[46]

There was also some involvement in the sanatorium movement by Boards of Guardians. In 1903, Eastley Sanatorium, Bedfordshire, was built by the Bradford Board of Guardians. In the same year the Daneswood Sanatorium, also in Bedfordshire, was established exclusively for Jews by the Jewish Board of Guardians, and described in 1910 as the best work that had yet been adopted by any public body of its kind in the country.[47] The Liverpool Board of Guardians established Heswell Sanatorium, Cheshire, in 1902. In 1911 the Manchester Board of Guardians acquired property in north Wales and opened a sanatorium there the following year. The Merthyr Tydfil Board of Guardians and the Newport Board of Guardians had also set up sanatoria by 1912.

A few local authorities in England and Wales also became involved. The Lewes Sanatorium was founded by the Lewes Town Council in

[44] A. Latham and C. H. Garland, *The Conquest of Consumption* (London, 1910), 76–7; Kelynack (ed.), *Tuberculosis Yearbook 1913–14*, p. 227; *Jl. NAPT* 3/1 (1904), 88.

[45] Kelynack (ed.), *Tuberculosis Yearbook 1913–14*, p. 264; King Edward VII Hospital, a Brief History, (c. 1978).

[46] Carling, 'Peppard Common', pp. 3–4; Kelynack (ed.), *Tuberculosis Yearbook 1913–14*, pp. 238, 275.

[47] Latham and Garland, *The Conquest of Consumption*, p. 73.

1905 with voluntary aid. By 1906, the Sheffield Corporation had established a sanatorium, and Bristol and Manchester had purchased beds in private sanatoria. The Birmingham Corporation opened a sanatorium, the Municipal Sanatorium, Salterley Grange, near Cheltenham, in 1908, and in 1910 they converted a smallpox hospital into a tuberculosis institution called the City Sanatorium, Yardley Road, Birmingham.[48]

In Scotland, the 1906 Local Government Board (Scotland) Act stated that pulmonary tuberculosis was an infectious disease within the meaning of the Public Health (Scotland) Act of 1897, thereby conferring statutory powers on local authorities to deal with pulmonary tuberculosis along with other infectious diseases. By 1911 local authorities in Scotland were providing 480 beds for the treatment of pulmonary tuberculosis.[49]

Other sanatoria were opened as branches of existing hospitals, generally tuberculosis hospitals. For example, in 1901 the Liverpool Sanatorium, Delamere Forest, Frodsham, was established as a branch of the Liverpool Hospital for Consumption and Diseases of the Chest. The Crossley Sanatorium, Kingwood, Cheshire, was built in 1905 in connection with the Manchester Consumption Hospital. The Brompton Hospital for Diseases of the Chest, London, added open-air wards to the hospital in 1899 and opened a sanatorium at Frimley, Surrey, in 1904 (commonly known as Frimley Sanatorium). Fairlight Sanatorium, Hastings, Sussex, founded in 1908, was managed by the Committee of Management of Margaret Street Hospital for Diseases of the Chest, London.

The expansion of tuberculosis sanatoria in the early twentieth century must be seen in the context of the growth of institutions in general. The decades between 1860 and the First World War saw the proliferation of institutions on a scale rarely known before, which included prisons, asylums, workhouses, and hospitals. There appeared to be a new faith in the medical and social value of institutions; by 1900, as has been noted, they 'had become a universal panacea'.[50] Moreover, they were an attractive object of philanthropy because the donors could see the results of their charity.

[48] LGB, *Bulstrode Report*, Cmd. 3657 (1908), 134, 135; Kelynack (ed.), *Tuberculosis Yearbook 1913–14*, pp. 220, 263, 274, 290.

[49] *6th Annual Report of the Scottish Board of Health 1924*, Cmd. 2416 (1925), 54.

[50] M. A. Crowther, *The Workhouse System 1834–1929: The History of an English Institution* (London, 1981), 57, 58.

Why did tuberculosis institutions in particular attract so much charity? As noted above in reference to the NAPT preventive campaign, tuberculosis was isolated as a disease of special importance because of its tendency to attack young adults, the most productive age group, and in this way was seen to be detrimental to national efficiency. Moreover, the new profession of tuberculosis specialists successfully communicated its own confidence in the curative value of the institutions to a wider public.

Apart from the alleged curative value, another important factor in the establishment of institutions, now that tuberculosis was known to be infectious, was the desire to isolate the source of infection from society as a preventive measure. In his Nobel lecture in 1906, Robert Koch pointed to the decline in leprosy when numbers of the afflicted were isolated, an example which he believed should be followed for tuberculosis.[51] Theodore D. Acland, a physician at the Brompton Hospital and consultant to Midhurst Sanatorium, wrote in 1907, 'As long as the only refuge for a man who is dying of tuberculosis is the Workhouse Infirmary there cannot fail to be much damage done by people refusing to go into the Infirmary and infecting their families by stopping at home.'[52] The final report of the Departmental Committee on Tuberculosis in 1913 recommended the compulsory segregation of infectious cases who could not be adequately segregated in their own homes.[53] H. Hyslop Thomson, a tuberculosis physician, also maintained in 1912 that it was remarkable that the result of segregation on the incidence of leprosy did not suggest the step forward for tuberculosis at an earlier date.[54] However, that the removal of the source of infection was not a priority of the medical profession became evident from the type of case most of the new institutions catered for. They wanted early cases so that they could see results in terms of 'cure', much like the older voluntary hospitals.

Tuberculosis institutions for children with pulmonary as well as non-pulmonary tuberculosis were also promoted in the early twentieth century. The first British sanatorium exclusively for children with all forms of tuberculosis was Stannington Sanatorium, Morpeth, Northumberland, founded in 1907 by the Newcastle Poor Children's Holiday Association and Rescue Agency (an association of Methodist

---

[51] *Lancet*, 1 (1906), 1450.
[52] Paterson Collection IA3 106, letter to M. Paterson, 11 July 1907.
[53] *Astor Committee, Final Report*, ii. 8.
[54] Thomson, *Consumption in General Practice*, p. 176.

origin which had been founded in 1891). In 1908 the famous institution for children with non-pulmonary tuberculosis, the Lord Mayor Treloar Cripples' Hospital, Alton and Hayling Island, was founded as a voluntary institution, with 220 beds by 1919. By 1912 accommodation was being provided in Britain for 300 children with pulmonary tuberculosis and 1,000 with non-pulmonary tuberculosis. The provision for pulmonary cases in particular was considered grossly insufficient at this time.[55]

The effort to provide beds for children with pulmonary tuberculosis is surprising as this form of the disease was relatively rare among children. Yet it was explained that as a result of biopsies and the use of the tuberculin test developed as a diagnostic tool in the early twentieth century, it was becoming clear that the rate of infection with the tubercle bacillus was high among children. Estimates of the percentage of children who actually suffered from tuberculosis varied from 0.3 to 80 per cent, indicating a lack of consensus on what constituted disease rather than just infection, as will be further discussed.[56] However, infection itself was considered important. A new category of 'pre-tuberculous children' was invented, which was interpreted liberally. According to Kelynack, there were almost 40,000 'delicate children predisposed to tuberculosis and other crippling and debilitating ailments' in London in 1908.[57] Again drawing on religious motifs, Sir Robert Philip claimed in the same year that 30 per cent of the school children he had examined showed 'tuberculous stigmata'. In his opinion,

If the conclusion which seems forced on us be correct, that in a majority of instances infection occurs in childhood, we are faced with a problem of totally different complexion and proportion from that which was previously conceived. To solve it we must search for causal conditions in the life of the child.

He pointed out that the incidence of pulmonary tuberculosis showed a steady increase as the child grew and that 'one morbid influence constant throughout the progressive stages of the child's life was the comparative withdrawal from the natural and healthful stimulus of the open air'.[58]

[55] Kelynack (ed.), *Tuberculosis Yearbook 1913–14*, p. 333.
[56] Sutherland and Goss, 'Open-air Schools', in *The Control and Eradication of Tuberculosis*, p. 142.
[57] T. N. Kelynack, in Kelynack (ed.), *Tuberculosis in Infancy and Childhood: Its Pathology, Prevention and Treatment* (London, 1908), 329, 333.
[58] *BMJ* 2 (1909), 258; R. Philip (lecture to International Congress on Tuberculosis, Washington, 1908), *Collected Papers on Tuberculosis* (Oxford, 1937), 70.

The solution was seen to lie in the provision of open-air schools for tuberculous and 'pre-tuberculous' children. These institutions were established under the Elementary Education (Defective and Epileptic Children) Act of 1899, and modelled on that established at Charlottenburg near Berlin in 1904 by a Dr Neufert. The first such school in Britain was opened by the LCC in 1907, at Bostall Wood, Plumstead, Woolwich, London. The following year, schools were set up in Bradford, Halifax, and Norwich, and in 1909 Sheffield established a school where 30 places were reserved for tuberculous children. By 1912, there were about 150 places for tuberculous children in open-air schools established specifically for them and 750 places in general open-air schools in England.[59] Concern about the development of tuberculosis in children was an important influence in the rise of the general open-air school movement of the time.[60] Thus, the anti-tuberculosis movement tuned into the general child-health movement of the early twentieth century, the movement which also led to the setting up of the school medical service in 1907.

Despite the growth of special institutions, many tuberculous patients were still consigned to Poor Law infirmaries. In 1911 over 60 per cent of all beds provided for tuberculous patients were still in such institutions.[61] The President of the Local Government Board, John Burns, claimed in that year that 33 per cent of the total consumptive deaths in London occurred in Poor Law infirmaries.[62] F. S. Toogood, medical superintendent of Lewisham Poor Law Infirmary, estimated in 1908 that about 4,000 cases of consumption were admitted annually to the London infirmaries, with about 2,500 deaths (that is over 50 per cent). During the winter months there was a daily average of nearly 2,500 consumptive cases in the wards.[63] It was estimated on that basis that there were almost 11,000 consumptives admitted to Poor Law

---

[59] *Astor Committee, Final Report*, ii. 112; Sutherland and Goss, in *The Control and Eradication of Tuberculosis*, p. 146.

[60] See also R. Lowe, 'The Early Twentieth Century Open-air Movement: Origins and Implications', N. Parry and D. McNair (eds.), *The Fitness of the Nation: Physical and Health Education in the 19th and 20th Centuries*. History of Education Society Conference Papers, Dec. *1982* (Leicester, 1983), 87; D. A. Turner, 'The Open-air School Movement in Sheffield', *History of Education*, 1 (1972), 58–78; M. Seaborne and R. Lowe, *The English School—Its Architecture and Organisation*, ii, *1870–1970* (London, 1977), 65, 77, 81.

[61] R. Pinker, *English Hospital Statistics 1861–1938* (London, 1966), 62.

[62] *Transactions of NAPT Annual Conference*, London, 19 July 1911, p. 7.

[63] *BJT* 2/3 (1908), 170. See also PRO MH52/99, F. J. H. Coutts, Survey of London Dispensaries, p. 57.

infirmaries in England and Wales each year, and that approximately 10 per cent of the total cost of Poor Law administration was due to tuberculosis.[64] Many of the 21,769 children under the care of Poor Law authorities in workhouses and workhouse infirmaries in England and Wales in 1908 were said to be tuberculous or having 'marked tuberculous tendencies'.[65] It was discovered in 1904 that only 122 out of 695 Boards of Guardians had made any attempt to separate tuberculous patients from other inmates.[66]

(3) DISPENSARIES

As well as an institutional movement for the treatment of tuberculosis, there was also an attempt to reach a wider public through instituting a tuberculosis dispensary movement with staff who would go into the homes of patients. The first tuberculosis dispensary in Britain was set up in 1887 by Sir Robert Philip as the Victoria Dispensary for Consumption and Diseases of the Chest, 13 Bank Street, Edinburgh. Philip had attempted to create a special department for the care of tuberculous patients at a charitable dispensary of which he was in charge, but the managers had not approved of his efforts. He consequently resigned and set up his own dispensary specifically for tuberculous patients. His dispensary was to provide treatment, including tuberculin treatment, but it was to offer more than hospital out-patient departments or general provident dispensaries, for the physicians were also to make house-calls. The main aim of these visits was to influence home conditions and lifestyle, in the patients' interests and that of others living with them:

While caring for the individual in whatever way may be needful, the dispensary regenerates physiologically the dwelling—however humble. It makes the home of the poor man become the nursery of healthy children and cease to be the breeding ground of tubercle-tainted wastrels. Each re-created home is an effective preventorium against tuberculosis.[67]

The entire family was to be examined, a procedure called the 'march past'. Edith McGaw, who founded the first tuberculosis dispensary in

---

[64] Latham and Garland, *The Conquest of Consumption*, pp. 74, 108.
[65] Kelynack, in *Tuberculosis in Infancy and Childhood*, p. 337.
[66] *Jl. NAPT* 3/1 (1904), 83.
[67] *EMJ* 9/4 (1912), 295, 299; *GMJ* 79/5 (1913), 339, *Astor Committee, Final Report*, ii. 110.

England at Paddington, London, in 1909, similarly stressed that tuberculosis was a 'house disease' and that every inhabitant of a home with a case of tuberculosis should come under the dispensary's surveillance.[68]

Apart from the doctor in charge of the dispensary, 'Lady Health Visitors' were employed to carry out much of the visiting. John Burns stressed the value of health visitors in securing separation of infected patients from their families and in teaching them elementary lessons of hygiene.[69] These visitors were clearly descendants of the nineteenth-century 'lady health missioners' whose office had been based on the older Charity Organisation Society belief that the working classes would benefit from direct personal contact with their betters.[70] Women were moreover considered particularly suited to this task; some sanitary authorities had also by this time employed female sanitary inspectors.

In 1910 a Central Fund for the Promotion of the Tuberculosis Dispensary System in London was founded under Lord Glenconner to assist poorer London boroughs to open tuberculosis dispensaries. By 1912 there were 11 dispensaries in London. A dispensary was opened in Glasgow in 1906 by the Glasgow branch of the NAPT, and in Oxford in 1910 by the Oxford branch and Sir William Osler. By 1911, 14 local sanitary authorities in England had set up tuberculosis dispensaries, and 50 other dispensaries were under voluntary management.[71]

Dispensaries had also been established in other countries in the early twentieth century. In 1900 the Emile Roux Anti-tuberculosis Dispensary was set up in France by Leon Charles Albert Calmette, director of the Pasteur Institute in Lille. In Germany, the first 'Charité Clinic' was established in Berlin in 1904, and by 1912 there were approximately 600 tuberculosis dispensaries, established mainly by local anti-tuberculosis associations. By 1915 there were also approximately 450 dispensaries in America.[72]

---

[68] R. S. Walker, 'The Dispensary Idea in London', in J. H. Williams (ed.), *Sir Robert Philip, 1857–1939: Memories of his Friends and Pupils*, (Edinburgh, 1955), 55, 56.

[69] Transactions of NAPT Annual Conference, London, 19 July 1911, pp. 8, 9.

[70] J. Lewis, *The Politics of Motherhood* (London, 1980), 105.

[71] J. K. Fowler, *Problems in Tuberculosis* (London, 1923), 5.

[72] *BMJ* 1 (1904), 1359; D. J. Williamson, in Sutherland (ed.), *The Control and Eradication of Tuberculosis*, pp. 32–9; *Astor Committee, Final Report*, ii. 115; *BJT* 10/2 (1916), 80; see also P. Starr, *The Social Transformation of American Medicine* (New York, 1982), 191–2.

These tuberculosis dispensaries, in Britain and elsewhere, stressed that their functions consisted of diagnosis and health education, not treatment, which was clearly a conscious policy not to alienate GPs by encroaching upon their territory. However, certain dispensaries were set up in Britain for the specific purpose of tuberculin treatment, which as already noted, had many advocates around 1910. The Tuberculin Dispensary League for the Establishment of Tuberculin Dispensaries in the Poorer Parts of London was established in 1909, with the Countess of Mayo as president, and Camac Wilkinson as chairman. The object of the league was to treat the poor gratuitously with tuberculin and to instruct practitioners in the use of tuberculin. A central tuberculin dispensary was set up in London by Wilkinson in 1910, with twelve assistants. Five other tuberculin dispensaries had been established in London by 1914, as well as one in Portsmouth, one in Inverness, and two in Ireland.[73]

Before coming to Britain in 1909, Camac Wilkinson had been a lecturer in pathology and medicine at the University of Sydney, Australia, and honorary physician to the Prince Albert Hospital in Sydney. Wilkinson had attempted to establish a tuberculin dispensary there; his scheme was apparently unanimously adopted by the Municipal Council but then 'stale-mated by some legal difficulty'.[74]

Wilkinson was not well received in Britain. A report in 1911 by Sir Clifford Allbutt, Sir Lauder Brunton, Sir William Osler, and Arthur Latham questioned the reliability of Wilkinson's results by querying the accuracy of his diagnosis, even though, according to Wilkinson, they had not seen him diagnose a single case.[75] They were not, however, alone in their criticism. Wilkinson was unpopular because he was challenging the established rule that dispensaries were not to engage in treatment and so threaten private practice; but worse still, Wilkinson was questioning the value of the tuberculosis institutions themselves. He argued, 'If it can be shown that the simple, direct methods of specific treatment [tuberculin] yielded results even equal to those of sanatorium methods [which his results apparently showed] there is no doubt that sanatoria must give place to tuberculin dispensaries in the

---

[73] Kelynack (ed.), *Tuberculosis Yearbook*, p. 381; W. C. Wilkinson, *The Tuberculin Dispensary for the Poor* (London, 1923), Preface; W. C. Wilkinson, *Tuberculin in the Diagnosis and Treatment of Tuberculosis (Weber-Parkes Prize Essay 1909 with additions)* (London, 1912), 478.
[74] W. C. Wilkinson, *Treatment of Consumption* (London, 1908), 257–61; Wilkinson, *Tuberculin in . . . Tuberculosis*, p. 456.
[75] Quoted in ibid. p. x. See also PRO MH55/148.

solution of the problem as it affects the poor.' He maintained that tuberculin treatment could be given with little cost upon buildings and at one-twentieth of the cost of institutional treatment for each patient. Moreover, it also meant that the patients would not have to give up their jobs to undertake treatment.[76] The MOH for Portsmouth, A. Mearns Fraser, another enthusiastic advocate of tuberculin treatment, pointed out that tuberculin dispensaries could be run for under £600 per annum and therefore many places which could not afford a residential institution would be able to afford a tuberculin dispensary.[77] However, most dispensaries continued to stress their diagnostic and welfare functions, leaving treatment to GPs and tuberculosis institutions.

(4) STATE INTERVENTION

The early twentieth century thus witnessed a growth of sanatoria and dispensaries, mainly by voluntary effort. In 1911, however, the State became involved. Tuberculosis received special attention in the 1911 National Insurance Act. Part 1 of this Act provided free medical treatment by medical practitioners as well as sickness and disability benefits for insured workers. It also provided two additional benefits; a maternity benefit and a 'sanatorium benefit'.

Section 16 of the National Insurance Act (Part 1) provided for free institutional treatment for all insured persons suffering from tuberculosis, and empowered the insurance commissioners to extend such treatment to dependants of the insured. It also provided for the erection of sanatoria and other institutions for the treatment of tuberculosis by local authorities, for which the 1911 Finance Act allocated £1,500,000 to be distributed by the Local Government Board after consultation with insurance commissioners. One shilling and four pence was provided for each insured person for 'sanatorium benefit' per annum, of which 6*d.* was to be used for the remuneration of medical practitioners for home treatment. One penny per person per annum was to be reserved for research, estimated at approximately £57,000 per annum. Legal opinion afterwards decided that the whole research fund need not be expended on tuberculosis work, and this

---

[76] Wilkinson, op. cit., p. 450; see also H. Clark, *The Dispensary Treatment of Pulmonary Tuberculosis* (London, 1915); PRO MH55/148 and MH55/149.
[77] Paterson Collection III F365, Fraser to M. Paterson, 24 Dec. 1910.

fund formed the initial financial basis for the work of the Medical Research Committee (later Council).[78] The sanatorium clauses of the 1911 Act were exceptional; for no other illness was free specialist institutional treatment provided under the Act, and for no other illness were the insurance commissioners authorized to extend treatment to dependants.

Introducing the bill in Parliament, David Lloyd George, Chancellor of the Exchequer, explained that tuberculosis could become a serious drain on the sickness and disability benefit funds which he was proposing to introduce, as a disease to which young adults were susceptible. The disease was known to be a drain on friendly societies—one of the largest friendly societies, the Ancient Order of Foresters, for example, was providing 58 weeks' allowance on average for tuberculosis sufferers, accounting for 25 per cent of expenditure on sick pay. Lloyd George pointed out that one in every three among males aged 14–55 died of tuberculosis in what should be the 'very period of greatest strength and vigour and service', as well as infecting their families in the process. The disease moreover killed 75,000 people per annum in England and Wales and, in his view, if a plague wiped out 75,000 people and then returned to do the same the following year, all the resources of the country would be placed at the disposal of science to crush it.[79]

The tuberculosis clauses of the 1911 Act were clearly inspired by developments in Germany. In 1903 it had been pointed out that the tuberculosis death-rate in Prussia was declining faster than in Britain, and the German insurance schemes and the sanatoria set up under the schemes were largely held responsible for this.[80] Reporting on the International Congress on Tuberculosis held in Berlin in 1905, C. Theodore Williams and H. Timbrell Bulstrode quoted the Privy Councillor, Bielefeldt, who expressed the view that, in Germany, of all the factors concerned in the war against tuberculosis, first place should be accorded to the system of compulsory insurance of the working classes. Resolutions were passed at that Congress to the effect that a system of insurance based on contributions from the employed, the employer, and the State, was desirable, that invalidity should

[78] *Astor Committee, Final Report*, i, Cd. 6641 (1913), 14.
[79] *Hansard*, 5th Series, 1911, xxv (1911), 626. In fact he did not mean that one in three males between those ages died of tuberculosis, but that one in three deaths among males in that age group was caused by tuberculosis.
[80] *Jl. NAPT*, 2/6 (1903), 255, 264; ibid., 2/8 (1903), 336; ibid., 3/3 (1904), 115; ibid., 3/6 (1905), 270.

be included as well as illness in such a scheme, and that the scheme should not be confined to pensions, but should include preventive hygiene and treatment.[81] Thus, discussions in the context of the anti-tuberculosis campaign might have exerted an influence on the 1911 Act in general, and not only on the tuberculosis clauses of that Act. A system of national insurance was also discussed at the 1910 annual conference of the NAPT.

In his report to the Local Government Board on sanatoria, published in 1908, Bulstrode devoted a great deal of attention to the German workmen's insurance system. He pointed out that the invalidity insurance boards in Germany had given special attention to tuberculosis, because, as the organization charged by the State to provide pensions for chronic invalids, they were materially interested in preventing the creation of such invalids. He claimed that their influence in this respect was 'altogether remarkable. It would, in fact, be difficult to overrate it,' and proceeded to explain how the death-rate from pulmonary tuberculosis had been practically stationary in Germany until the 1880s, but that shortly after the introduction of compulsory sick insurance and sanatoria for the insured (the first appeared in 1897), a rapid and continuous decline commenced.[82] Thus, as the *Sheffield Telegraph* pointed out in 1906, the German workmen's insurance boards had recognized that it might be cheaper to incur the cost of curing a man than to have him a permanent invalid on the funds.[83]

Advocacy of State involvement in a curative service for tuberculosis was based on the assumption that the disease could be cured. Lloyd George asserted that the results of treatment in the German sanatoria were 'amazing with a very large number of cures'.[84] Latham and Garland, also impressed by the German State insurance system, urged similar state involvement in Britain:

Statesmen do not appear to have realised either the magnitude of the evil or the amazing advance in our medical knowledge of the subject. They do not realise that the medical profession has acquired such a grasp of the essential facts connected with the disease that the bulk of the scientific work which was necessary to make the eradication of tuberculosis possible, within no distant

[81] *International Congress on Tuberculosis, 1905*, Report of C. Theodore Williams and H. Timbrell Bulstrode, the Delegates of His Majesty's Government, Paris, Cd. 2898 (1906), 27, 28–9.
[82] *Bulstrode Report*, pp. 236, 248, 250, 252, 611, 629–31.
[83] *Sheffield Telegraph*, 14 June 1906 (N. D. Bardswell's scrapbook).
[84] *Hansard*, 5th Series, 1911, xxv (1911), 628.

date, has been accomplished. We know how to prevent and how to cure tuberculosis, and the statesmen must now be made to realise that the eradication of the disease lies in their hands.[85]

Thus Lloyd George pointed out that doctors were confident that they could cure tuberculosis: 'Men who have devoted a great deal of attention to the subject . . . are full of bright hopes that they can stamp it out. But they can only do it if they have the means, and I propose to ask the House to give them.'[86]

Hence the 'sanatorium clauses' of the bill passed through Parliament without difficulty.

In 1912 a Departmental Committee was set up by the Treasury under the chairmanship of Waldorf Astor 'to report at an early date upon the considerations of general policy in respect of the problem of tuberculosis in the United Kingdom, in its preventive, curative and other aspects, which should guide the Government and local bodies in making or aiding provision for the treatment of tuberculosis in sanatoria or other institutions or otherwise'.[87] With a total of twenty members, the committee included prominent tuberculosis specialists, such as N. D. Bardswell, Mearns Fraser, Arthur Latham, Marcus Paterson, Robert Philip, and Jane Walker, as well as Christopher Addison (to become the first Minister of Health in 1919), Arthur Newsholme (Chief MO of the LGB), George Newman (MO of the Board of Education and later Chief MO of the Ministry of Health), and David Davies (chairman of the WNMA). They stressed that one of the most important conditions of any scheme which might be adopted was that it should apply to the whole community and not just the insured, and that the organization of the scheme would best be undertaken by local authorities. First, local authorities were to arrange for residential treatment in their own or private institutions. Second, each one was to establish dispensaries as diagnostic centres and 'clearing houses' (to direct patients to the appropriate form of treatment), to be managed by tuberculosis officers employed by the local authority. Third, the Committee recommended the organization of voluntary 'care committees' to increase the effectiveness of the work of the dispensaries.[88]

[85] Latham and Garland, *The Conquest of Consumption*, pp. 13, 173.

[86] *Hansard*, 5th Series, 1911, xxv (1911), 627.

[87] *Astor Committee, Final Report*, i. 1.

[88] *Astor Committee, Interim Report* (issued to precede the introduction of 'sanatorium

In 1912 the Government agreed to provide local authorities with a sum of money approximately equal to half the estimated cost of treating non-insured persons, including dependants of insured, under any scheme approved by the LGB (known as the 'Hobhouse grant'). The scale of capital grants for dispensaries was settled at £240, not exceeding four-fifths of the cost, and for sanatoria and hospitals, £90 per bed, not exceeding three-fifths of the cost. In a circular issued by the LGB in November 1913, local authorities were urged to establish schemes, and the grants were made statutory by the 1913 Public Health (Prevention and Treatment of Disease) Act, which empowered local authorities to provide free treatment for uninsured tuberculosis patients. In 1915 the LGB issued a circular encouraging the formation of voluntary 'after-care' committees to assist the work of the dispensaries.

Thus a State-financed system for the treatment and prevention of tuberculosis was created. There were fears expressed at the time by the medical profession that the tuberculosis service was an embryonic State Medical Service. It was pointed out in the *BMJ* in 1912 that it was made possible under the 1911 Act to extend all the special benefits granted in relation to tuberculosis to other diseases as the LGB and the Treasury might determine: 'The vista of possibilities is immense. There lies in embryo maintenance or municipalization of hospitals, and indeed the establishment of an extensive State service of doctors. There seems to be no limit.'[89] The *BMJ* pointed to the tendency to push the GP into the background and put the work into the hands of full-time medical officers attached to the dispensaries. The medical officer of health was to be an 'exceedingly important personage in the carrying out of sanatorium benefit', whose purview might be extended to include treatment.[90] In 1913 a GP wrote to the Press bemoaning the fact that with tuberculosis officers being appointed as well as school medical officers, GPs would soon have little left to do.[91] In an attempt to conciliate them, it was constantly stressed that the dispensary staff was not to undertake domiciliary treatment, except in emergencies and for the purpose of consultation. Members of the Welsh branch of the BMA received an assurance from the WNMA, which was to administer the tuberculosis scheme on behalf of local authorities in

benefit' under the 1911 Act on 15 July 1912), Cd. 6164 (1912), 1–22; *Astor Committee, Final Report*, i. 1–17.

[89] *BMJ* 1 (1912), 448.

[90] Ibid., 2 (1912), 392; see also *Hospital Gazette*, 9/4 (1913), 80.

Wales, that officers of the Association would only act as consultants to the GPs, before they agreed to co-operate with the scheme.[92] Yet, with the emphasis of public health moving towards the treatment and supervision of the individual, the demarcation between public health officers and medical practitioners was becoming increasingly blurred; GPs had reason to fear for their territory.

(5) NOTIFICATION

The introduction of compulsory notification of tuberculosis in 1913 further increased the powers of tuberculosis officers and medical officers of health at the expense of GPs, for it required all tuberculosis cases to be notified to medical officers who would then follow up the cases to prevent the further spread of the disease.

Once tuberculosis had been established as an infectious disease, notification became an issue. Compulsory notification of certain other infectious diseases had been introduced by the Infectious Disease Notification Act of 1889 and the Infectious Disease Notification (Extension) Act of 1899, the first enabling local authorities to make notification of certain infectious diseases compulsory in their area, the second requiring it. In London, compulsory notification had been introduced under the Public Health (London) Act of 1891. These Acts had not been introduced without some opposition from GPs who argued that notification interfered with the confidential doctor–patient relationship.[93] Tuberculosis had been excluded from the Acts. It was contended that tuberculosis was different from other infectious diseases in being chronic, so that a short period of isolation would not suffice to prevent its spread, and that if isolation could not be effected then notification served no useful purpose. Notification was thought to jeopardize employment opportunities; as Bulstrode pointed out, 'no human beings . . . are anxious to advertise the fact that they are suffering from a malady which the public are beginning to believe is, as regards infectivity, on a par with small-pox . . .'[94] In reply to this argument, J. (later Sir John) Robertson, then MOH for Sheffield,

[91] S. V. Pearson, *The State Provision of Sanatoriums* (Cambridge, 1913), 34.

[92] PRO MH55/1216, BMA (Welsh Committee), memo of evidence to Clement Davies Inquiry (see Chapter 3, Section 4, After-care), 1937.

[93] A. Hardy, 'Diagnosis, Death and Diet: The Case of London, 1750–1909', *Journal of Interdisciplinary History* (in press).

[94] *Bulstrode Report*, p. 607.

maintained that 'compulsory notification does not mean public notification'.[95] His view that greater knowledge of the distribution of the disease through notification was necessary for research purposes and for adopting effective preventive measures was becoming dominant. At the 1908 International Congress on Tuberculosis, the delegates, 'representing medical science and public health administration', unanimously accepted the principle of compulsory notification of tuberculosis. A resolution was passed at the Congress in favour of compulsory notification as 'an indispensable preliminary to effective and complete preventive measures' against the disease.[96]

Compulsory notification had been introduced in Norway in 1901, in Denmark in 1905, in New York in 1897, and some other parts of the USA by 1906. Scotland introduced voluntary notification in 1903, making it compulsory in some areas in 1906. By 1911 compulsory notification of pulmonary tuberculosis was in force in the areas of Scottish local authorities representing 60 per cent of the population, while other local authorities had adopted systems of voluntary notification.[97] In England, voluntary notification of pulmonary tuberculosis was first introduced in Brighton in January 1899 by Arthur Newsholme (later Chief MO to the LGB), and in Manchester and Sheffield in the same year. By 1903, 27 cities and boroughs, as well as some district councils, had adopted voluntary notification.[98] Sheffield was the first city in England to introduce compulsory notification, which it did in 1903, followed by Bolton in 1905. In 1907 the LGB urged voluntary notification of pulmonary tuberculosis. In 1908 regulations imposed compulsory notification of cases of pulmonary tuberculosis under the care of Poor Law medical officers either at home or in Poor Law institutions. In March 1911 notification was extended, with some exceptions, to hospital cases; in December 1911 to all pulmonary tuberculosis cases; and in December 1912 to all tuberculosis cases, becoming operative from 1 February 1913. In Scotland notification of pulmonary tuberculosis became compulsory in 1912, as did notification of all forms of tuberculosis in 1914.

By the notification regulations, medical practitioners were required to notify medical officers of health within forty-eight hours of first

[95] *Jl. NAPT* 2/4 (1902), 152.
[96] *International Congress on Tuberculosis, 1908*, Report of the British Delegates to the International Congress on Tuberculosis, Washington, Cd. 4508 (1909), 4, 6.
[97] *6th Annual Report of Scottish Board of Health 1924*, Cmd. 2415 (1925), 54.
[98] *Jl. NAPT* 2/6 (1903), 239.

becoming aware that a person was suffering from tuberculosis. School inspectors and medical officers of Poor Law institutions were to submit notifications weekly. The only guidance given in the regulations as to the diagnosis was that it was to have been reached other than solely by a tuberculin test. Article 12 of the regulations stipulated that upon the receipt of a notification, the medical officer, or an officer of the local authority acting under the instructions of the medical officer, should make such inquiries and take such steps as were necessary or desirable for preventing the spread of infection. It was pointed out in article 16 that the medical officer had no power to enforce any enactment which rendered the person, or any other persons, liable to any restriction, prohibition, or disability affecting himself or his employment on the grounds of his suffering from tuberculosis.[99] While the confidentiality of the notifications was stressed by the LGB, the provisions of article 12 meant in effect that notification was not very confidential.

(6) A NATIONAL SCHEME

There were 64 dispensaries in England in 1911; by 1917 there were 371. By 1915, 238 tuberculosis officers had been employed, although in the following three years they were largely replaced by part-time medical officers and their work kept to a minimum.[100] Progress on the building of institutions was also curtailed under war conditions. In August 1914 it was laid down in the Army Orders that men showing any signs of tuberculosis were to be rejected for enlistment. Standards of recruitment were lowered from the end of 1916, and by the end of 1917 men could be accepted who showed signs of past or suspected tuberculosis but who gave a history of two years' good health. The rejections for tuberculosis were numerous even at this stage: 3,874 out of 160,545 men examined in London from January to October 1918 were rejected because of tuberculosis. Arrangements were made in 1915 for all servicemen who contracted tuberculosis on active service to receive free institutional treatment. The number of servicemen recorded as having tuberculosis during the war was low. However, by 1921 as many as 57,985 pensions had been awarded to ex-servicemen

[99] PRO MH55/134, LGB Circular, 20 Dec. 1912.
[100] LGB, *46th Annual Report 1916–17, Supp., Report of Medical Officer*, Cd. 8767 (1917–18), p. xxv.

who claimed to have contracted tuberculosis on active service.[101]

By 1919, English local authorities were providing 97 sanatoria, and using a further 83 isolation hospitals for tuberculous patients. There were in addition 79 voluntary institutions for tuberculosis treatment. While the total number of hospital beds in England doubled between 1891 and 1921, the number of beds for tuberculous patients increased three-fold between 1911 and 1920. The major expansion in numbers of tuberculosis beds between 1911 and 1920 occurred in the public sector. While the proportion of all hospital beds in the public sector was 80 per cent in 1911 and 75 per cent in 1921, 80 per cent of the beds for tuberculous patients in 1911 were in the voluntary sector, but by 1920 this number had fallen to less than 50 per cent.[102]

TABLE 2 *The number of beds for tuberculosis treatment in England (excluding Poor Law institutions)*

Year	Local Authority	Voluntary	Total
1911	1,300	4,200	5,500
1916	6,072	5,821	11,893
1920	8,845	6,936	15,781

Sources: Local Government Board, *45th Annual Report 1915–16* (1916), p. xxi; *On the State of Public Health, First Annual Report of the Chief Medical Officer of the Ministry of Health 1919–20*, Cmd. 978 (1920), 53; *NAPT Handbook of Tuberculosis Schemes in Great Britain and Ireland*, vol. i, *England and Wales*, 2nd edn. (London, 1919), 53, 139. No further breakdown by year during the First World War is given.

In London, the county boroughs managed the dispensaries (the 11 voluntary dispensaries were handed over to the respective boroughs in 1920). The Metropolitan Asylums Board, which already administered London's infectious diseases hospitals, provided and administered tuberculosis institutions. By 1918, the MAB had established two sanatoria, a large children's hospital, and two seaside homes for tuberculous patients. In Wales, the WNMA provided tuberculosis institutions; by 1920 they had 4 sanatoria and 7 hospitals, with 926 beds, and rented a further 262 beds. In Scotland, there were 1,030 beds for the treatment of pulmonary tuberculosis in 1911 (480 under local authorities, and 550 voluntary). By 1920, there were 101

[101] W. G. MacPherson, W. B. Leishman, and S. L. Cummins (eds.), *History of the Great War: Medical Services: Pathology* (London, 1923), 468, 469, 477.
[102] Pinker, *English Hospital Statistics*, p. 48.

sanatoria, hospitals, and other institutions in Scotland, with a total of 3,232 beds for the treatment of pulmonary tuberculosis and a number, not specified, for other forms of tuberculosis.

The first two decades of the twentieth century thus witnessed the emergence of an extensive State-funded organizational network for the treatment of tuberculosis, as well as a heightened effort in preventive work by the NAPT and through the dispensaries. Concern for national efficiency was an important factor in the early twentieth-century anti-tuberculosis movement, arguably more important than the discovery of the tubercle bacillus itself. It did not take the discovery of the causal agent to point to a connection between tuberculosis and the conditions (or habits) of the poor which was the basis of preventive work. Open-air treatment preceded the discovery and was not greatly influenced by it. The importance of the bacteriological revolution, of which the discovery of the tubercle bacillus was a part, lay in its contribution to medical confidence in the early twentieth century.[103] There was in particular a growing confidence in the value of institutional treatment and in medical science in dealing with what was now perceived as a major national problem. The anti-tuberculosis campaign was launched in a positive spirit. Major Greenwood, later professor of epidemiology and vital statistics at the London School of Hygiene and Tropical Medicine, summed up the prevailing mood of the first decade of the twentieth century: 'One faced the problem [of tuberculosis] in a more confident spirit and did not hesitate to anticipate the approaching "conquest of consumption".'[104]

---

[103] The 'bacteriological revolution' occurred in the last 20 years of the 19th century when the causes of the most important bacterial diseases were discovered one by one, including typhoid fever, gonorrhoea, cholera, tuberculosis, diphtheria, tetanus, lobar pneumonia, cerebrospinal meningitis, bubonic plague, undulant fever, and leprosy. Koch's improvements in staining techniques and his development of a method to achieve pure cultivations of bacteria led the way to other methodological advances in bacteriology.

[104] M. Greenwood, 'Epidemiology of Pulmonary Tuberculosis', in *1st CMOH Annual Report 1919–20* (1920), 324.

2

'Pickaxe Cure for Consumptives'

IN 1908, two tuberculosis specialists claimed, 'It may be said without exaggeration that the outlook for the consumptive has, during the past twenty-five years, been completely revolutionized.'[1] The 'revolution' related to the new institutional treatment of tuberculous patients, whereby it was confidently held the disease could be cured. This chapter examines the nature of sanatorium treatment in the early twentieth century which inspired such confidence.

(1) THE LOCATION OF SANATORIA

In the early nineteenth century, consumptives with financial resources were sent off to the south of Europe, to take advantage of the warm climate. By the mid-nineteenth century, fashions had changed, and it was believed that the Alpine heights had a favourable effect on the course of the disease. The Swiss Alps became so popular for those 'taking the cure' by the 1880s that hoteliers tried to hush up the many deaths that occurred and to hurry dying patients elsewhere so as not to damage their health statistics.[2] Robert Louis Stevenson, who had contracted tuberculosis, was persuaded to spend the winter in Davos, Switzerland, in 1880.

British tuberculosis specialists in the early twentieth century held that the advantages of special climates had been greatly exaggerated, that there was no therapeutic advantage in travelling to the Swiss Alps or to the south of Europe.[3] Nevertheless, attention was invariably drawn to local climatic conditions of sanatoria. For example, according

[1] N. D. Bardswell and J. E. Chapman, *Diets in Tuberculosis* (London, 1908), 1.

[2] E. S. Turner, *Taking the Cure* (London, 1967), 208.

[3] Some examples are R. Philip, *BMJ* 2 (1898), 217; C. Allbutt, *British Congress on Tuberculosis, 1901, Transactions* (London, 1902), 3. 176; T. N. Kelynack, *The Sanatorium Treatment of Consumption* (London, 1904), 14; F. R. Walters, *Sanatoria for Consumptives in Various Parts of the World*, 3rd edn. (London 1905), p. viii; R. W. Burton-Fanning, *The Open-air Treatment of Pulmonary Tuberculosis* (London, 1905), 159–60; *Astor Committee, Final Report*, ii. 4.

to the *Tuberculosis Yearbook and Sanatoria Annual 1913–14*, the climate at Merivale Sanatorium, Essex, was well suited for the treatment of tuberculosis, for the atmosphere was dry and bracing, with an abundance of sunshine and very little rain. At Mundesley Sanatorium, Norfolk, the air was 'bracing, dry and very pure with a great deal of sunshine throughout the year'. At Crossley Sanatorium, Cheshire, the climatic conditions were 'specially healthy, dry and invigorating'. Fairlight Sanatorium, Hastings, had 'a maximum of sunshine' and the air was 'invigorating and at the same time sedative'. Although Pendyffryn Hall was situated in Wales, it was said to be outside the rains; mist was rare, and, as a rule, the climate was dry and sunny, and the air pure and invigorating.[4] Midhurst Sanatorium had special meteorological equipment which showed the climate to be mild and equable, as did Eversfield Chest Hospital, St Leonard's-on-Sea, where a meteorological report was included in the annual report: 'We are in the proud position of having no rival with regard to our amount of bright sunshine.'[5]

Special significance was also attached to the presence of pinewoods. Pinewoods could be found at many of the sanatoria, according to the *Tuberculosis Yearbook.*[6] Possibly the founders of the sanatoria believed pinewoods to have a salutary effect, although it was more likely an attempt to emulate Otto Walther's sanatorium situated among the pinewoods of the Black Forest. The *Morning Post* described Midhurst in 1906 as having 'the fragrant and health-giving scent of pinewoods in the air', but there were few scientific writings on the subject.[7]

The British sanatoria also attempted to compete with their Continental counterparts in the beauty of the surroundings. Dartmoor Sanatorium, Devon, sounded more like a holiday resort than a hospital in its advertisement in 1903, situated as it was 'amidst some of the finest mountain and moorland scenery to be found in Britain'.[8] The country around the East Anglian Sanatorium was described by the *Tuberculosis Yearbook* as picturesque, the centre of the 'Constable' district. At Midhurst Sanatorium,

[4] T. N. Kelynack (ed.), *Tuberculosis Yearbook and Sanatoria Annual,* i, *1913–14* (London, 1914), 203, 216, 241, 263, 288.

[5] Ibid., p. 265; Midhurst Sanatorium Annual Report 1908–9, p. 71; Eversfield Chest Hospital Annual Report 1904, p. 18.

[6] Kelynack (ed.), *Tuberculosis Yearbook 1913–14*, pp. 199, 200, 201, 241, 249, 256, 258, 262, 288.

[7] *Morning Post*, 14 June 1906 (N. D. Bardswell's scrapbook).

[8] *BJT* 11/4 (1917), 172.

The ground slopes gently to the south, and is partly clothed with woodland including magnificent pine trees, while the western border consists of open moorland ending in a ravine. The most southerly portion of the property is beautiful park-like ground of considerable extent, and on the upper part of this, backed by a lofty pine grove, at an altitude of 495 feet, the sanatorium has been erected . . . The large tract in front is beautifully sheltered, and has been laid out as terraced gardens, with croquet lawns and flower borders by the well-known landscape gardener, Miss Jekyll.

Pendyffryn Hall was situated at the base of mountains, within sight of the sea. It had over 100 acres of private grounds, comprising parkland, woodland and moorland, and zigzag paths cut through pine and heather almost from the sanatorium entrance to a height of over 1,000 feet.[9]

The rural setting of the sanatoria was part of open-air treatment. However, there were also considerations other than medical which determined the location of sanatoria. Possibly the most important was the public attitude to tuberculosis and institutions for its treatment. Public opposition to having such an institution in the neighbourhood was often pronounced and vocal, as a result of a fear of infection now that tuberculosis was known to be an infectious disease. For example, when the Guardians of South Manchester decided to purchase Plas Ucha, Abergele, Denbighshire, in 1911, to establish a tuberculosis institution for patients from Manchester, local inhabitants became alarmed. They pointed out that Abergele was a seaside resort dependent upon visitors. The Local Government Board granted the Guardians permission to purchase the site in the face of strong local opposition.[10]

In 1913 the WNMA bought a site in the Vale of Clwyd, Plas Llanywyfan, for the North Wales Sanatorium. A neighbour, George B. Behrens, registered a complaint, maintaining that, as the site of the sanatorium reached within 400 yards of his house, it would cause irreparable damage to his property and destroy its value as a residence. He offered to buy the property for the price they had paid, £5,000, as well as donate £500 to the WNMA. A public inquiry was held in 1914 and alternative sites considered. Another site, Fron Bellaf, was objected to by the Llanbedr parishioners who pointed out that in summer almost every house took visitors and that the gathering ground for the public water supply was within 300 yards of the site, which

[9] Kelynack (ed.), *Tuberculosis Yearbook 1913–14*, pp. 253, 264, 288.
[10] *Manchester Guardian*, 2 Jan. 1914, letter to editor (PRO MH96/981).

was in the most populous part of the parish. The parish had a population of 334, and 285 of them had signed a petition against the proposal, 'carried out by one man in a short day's work'. At the inquiry, N. D. Bardswell, medical superintendent of Midhurst Sanatorium, pronounced in favour of the Plas Llanywyfan site on climatic grounds. He maintained that any objection must be based on prejudice or ignorance. He had four children living at Midhurst Sanatorium, and believed there to be no danger of infection. The sanatorium was built at Plas Llanywyfan. In 1930 Behrens sold 271 acres of land to the WNMA.[11]

In 1913, the Departmental Committee on Tuberculosis felt it necessary to point out that a well-conducted sanatorium held no danger for the surrounding community.[12] The Royal College of Physicians also issued a statement in 1914, 'in view of the exaggerated fear of the infectivity of pulmonary tuberculosis entertained by the public', that 'no risk is incurred by living in the immediate neighbourhood of institutions for the treatment of tuberculosis which are properly conducted'.[13] But most sanatoria were situated away from centres of population. Such properties were, moreover, cheaper. The early twentieth century was a period of decline for the British aristocracy, and country estates were often available for sale which were considered suitable for tuberculosis institutions. For example, the WNMA purchased the former residence of 'Madame Patti', Craig-y-Nos, Glamorgan, for a tuberculosis institution, calling it the Adelina Patti Hospital, in 1921. This residence had been built on the lines of a German 'schloss' and subsequently proved very expensive to maintain.[14] The preference from the start was not for a converted mansion but an institution built especially for the purpose.

(2) ARCHITECTURE

One purpose-built institution, Midhurst Sanatorium, possessed 'every up-to-date structural and scientific advantage'.[15] Before deciding on a

[11] PRO MH96/981, North Wales Sanatorium, Public Inquiry, 6 Apr. 1914, pp. 17, 30, 31; *Western Mail*, 18 Dec. 1913 (PRO MH96/981); PRO MH96/981 and 982, North Wales Sanatorium, Purchase of Vron Yw, 1930.

[12] *Astor Committee, Final Report*, i. 4.

[13] LGB, *43rd Annual Report, Supp., Report of Medical Officer*, Cd. 7612 (1914), p. lxii.

[14] *Clement Davies Inquiry*, p. 270.

[15] *Liverpool Post*, 14 June 1906 (Bardswell's scrapbook).

design for Midhurst, an essay competition had been arranged, advertised in twenty-two medical papers in Europe and America, attracting 180 entries. The winning entry was written by Arthur Latham, a physician at the Brompton Hospital, in association with an architect, A. William West. In their essay, they stressed spaciousness, airiness ('the buildings . . . of a sanatorium must . . . be so constructed that the atmosphere within them rivals the outside air in point of purity'), and prevention of dust accumulation.[16] The *Tuberculosis Yearbook* noted an unusual feature at Midhurst Sanatorium which was the step-like façade, which enabled all patients to have a spacious balcony in front of their bedroom, and at the same time did not deprive the room on the floor below of sunshine.[17] The most remarkable feature of the sanatorium, according to *The Times*, was an open-air chapel, an idea conceived by a consultant to the sanatorium, C. Theodore Williams, while visiting Italian mission chapels.[18] Sir Clifford Allbutt, another consultant to Midhurst, reported on the sanatorium in 1906 that 'the freshness and airiness of the building was most striking'. He claimed to have visited most sanatoria, in Britain and abroad, and had seen nothing comparable: 'The air was as pure as outside.' Theodore Williams wrote of the sanatorium in 1906, 'Patients practically live in a thorough draught and seem to enjoy it.'[19]

Frimley Sanatorium was also purpose-built. It contained mainly single-bedded wards, in 'radial pavilions', facing south, south-east, and south-west, specially designed so that no portion of the building was shaded by another. Most institutions, however, did not have the advantage of being specially designed as sanatoria. They were typically converted smallpox hospitals, workhouses, or country mansions. In these cases, 'shelters' or 'chalets' were often added to accommodate the majority of the patients. The shelters were generally arranged so as to maximize sunlight. The King Edward VII Sanatorium, Shropshire, was described by the *Tuberculosis Yearbook* as an aeroplane, the shelters forming the wings and the administration situated in the 'body' of the aeroplane. A special innovative shelter was designed at the Westmorland Consumptive Sanatorium and Home, Meathop. Its features included 'ventilation casements' providing 12-inch airspace underneath,

---

[16] A. Latham and A. W. West, *The Prize Essay on the Erection of the King Edward VII Sanatorium for Consumption* (London, 1903), pp. vii, 26; *Jl. NAPT* 4/2 (1906), 61.

[17] Kelynack (ed.), *Tuberculosis Yearbook 1913–14*, p. 267.

[18] *The Times*, 13 June 1906 (Bardswell's scrapbook); *Jl. NAPT* 4/2 (1906), 73.

[19] Midhurst Sanatorium, Consultant Reports, 6 Sept. 1906, p. 26; ibid. 1 Dec. 1906, p. 102.

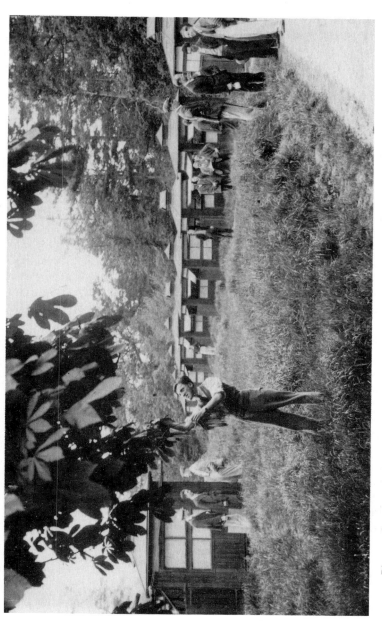

Plate 1. Open-air shelters at a tuberculosis institution (Papworth Village Settlement, founded in 1917 – the shelters were in use there until after the Second World War). *Source*: Papworth Village Settlement Archives.

a 'ventilating pagoda top with louvre ventilators all round, ensuring an upward current of air in the shelter', smooth, enamelled walls, and patent cement floor to reduce the accumulation of germ-breeding dust. Some institutions had revolving shelters to maximize sunlight, for example Pendyffryn Hall, where such shelters had been placed amidst roses and rhododendrons.[20] Shelters were purposely kept simple in construction. It was explained by C. H. Garland and T. D. Lister, who designed the Benenden Sanatorium, that treatment of working-class patients in gorgeous palaces was not only wasteful, but confusing to the patients, for they would come to regard their cure in some way associated with the facilities and luxuries enjoyed in the institution, and return home feeling that it was impossible to keep well. Thus the architecture should be 'of the simplest kind capable of being imitated in all essentials in the average home of the industrial classes'. Education was important in treatment: 'The patient treated in a sanatorium under the natural methods there adopted is taught not only how to live most healthily under his new conditions, but is also taught the whole routine of right living . . .' The likely success of sanatorium treatment (for the working classes) was therefore 'inversely proportional to the magnificence of the buildings and surroundings'.[21] Sir Robert Philip similarly believed that the conditions of the sanatorium should be such as the patients (working-class) could readily realize for themselves after leaving.[22]

In one case education overruled the fresh-air principle. In this instance the sanatorium was situated near a factory, and the coverlets of the patients' beds were often peppered with black smuts in the morning. The theory was advanced that a patient who obtained a cure 'in the smoky atmosphere of his own town' would be less likely to relapse on returning home than the patient who had been sent to the countryside.[23]

Education in 'natural living' also entailed the absence of heating. Marcus Paterson, medical superintendent of Frimley Sanatorium from 1905 to 1912, did not believe heating to be necessary, a conclusion he had apparently reached after experiencing two winters at Frimley

---

[20] Kelynack (ed.), *Tuberculosis Yearbook 1913–14*, pp. 249, 276, 268, 288.
[21] Ibid., p. 227; C. H. Garland and T. D. Lister, *Sanatoria for the People: The State Campaign against Consumption* (London, 1911), 8, 10. See also Garland in *Astor Committee, Final Report*, ii. 51; Garland and Lister, 'A National School for Consumptives', *Lancet*, 1 (1907), 678.
[22] *Astor Committee, Final Report*, ii. 143.   [23] *BMJ* 2 (1911), 170.

without heating as the result of the hot-water heating system freezing and bursting.[24] No heating was originally installed in the South Wales Sanatorium, built in 1913 and opened in 1920, for it was felt that 'both the patients and the disease would be pampered by such methods'.[25] An open-air school for tuberculosis children in Northumberland recorded temperatures inside the schoolroom of 30°F in November 1915.[26] The Brompton Hospital open-air wards were apparently so cold that the physician was known to wear his top coat with the collar turned up on his rounds.[27] Mary Hewins described visiting her sister at the King Edward VII Memorial Chest Hospital, Hertford Hill, Near Warwick (after the First World War). She was told at the gate that she would find her sister at the top of the hill, in a 'cowshed'. She relates, 'It *was* a hut, right at the very top, and all open. They'd each got a little wooden hut, 'bout the size of a garden shed. There was no door, no glass in the windows; the wind and the rain blowed through.'[28]

(3) DIET

One way in which treatment in sanatoria clearly deviated from conditions which could be recreated in the patient's own home following discharge was in the provision of large quantities of food. This resulted from empirical evidence that tuberculosis was a wasting disease, that patients grew progressively thin as the disease advanced. According to Sir James Kingston Fowler and R. J. Godlee in 1898, every patient with tuberculosis should endeavour to increase in weight: 'If he can grow fat he need have little fear that the disease is making progress.'[29] At Frimley Sanatorium, patients were strongly pressured by close medical supervision to eat the food placed in front of them.[30]

In a book on diets in tuberculosis treatment, published in 1908, Bardswell and Chapman reported having tried excessive feeding of

[24] Addison Papers, Box 32: Paterson, evidence before Departmental Committee on Tuberculosis, 28 Feb. 1912, p. 23.
[25] *News Chronicle*, 30 Oct. 1937 (PRO MH96/994).
[26] Northumberland CC Record Office, The Clifton Sanatorium School, Morpeth, NRO 3000/1 School Log Book, p. 37.
[27] S. V. Pearson, *Men, Medicine and Myself* (London, 1946), 16.
[28] A. Hewins, *Mary, After the Queen: Memories of a Working Girl* (Oxford, 1986), 37.
[29] J. K. Fowler and R. J. Godlee, *The Diseases of the Lungs* (London, 1898), 389–90.
[30] M. S. Paterson, *Auto-inoculation in Pulmonary Tuberculosis* (London, 1911), 111.

tuberculous patients at Sheffield Infirmary in 1899. No appreciable improvement in the lung condition had been detected, while the patients' general health, especially the digestive system, had been definitely impaired. They subsequently investigated sanatoria practising 'high-feeding', finding vomiting and nausea to be common among patients, and concluded that overfeeding was 'as unwise a course as can be imagined', for it immeasurably reduced the patients' chances of recovery.[31]

An advertisement for Dartmoor Sanatorium in 1903 stated: 'Patients not made to eat more than they can digest.'[32] Sir Clifford Allbutt was impressed by the 'ingenious clip system' practised at Midhurst by which the amount of each meal consumed by each patient was recorded and compared weekly with the patient's weight. He wrote that at Midhurst there was 'no despotic rule of high feeding, but a diet calculated exactly for each person', and that in any case in which the quantities served were not consumed, 'no stern remonstrance was made but the patient was re-examined, and a fresh estimate made of his needs'.[33]

While overfeeding was generally going out of fashion, diet was still considered an important part of treatment, and progress to recovery was measured partly in terms of weight increases. Fats and milk were considered essential features of the diet of tuberculous patients in the early twentieth century.

(4) GRADUATED LABOUR

Possibly the most important feature of treatment in early twentieth century British sanatoria was the prescription of work. This developed from the walking exercise prescribed as treatment by Brehmer. In Britain, walking exercise alone was not considered suitable, especially for working-class patients. Sir James Kingston Fowler wrote in 1923 that walking exercises were suitable for private sanatoria, but that patients in sanatoria for the 'industrial class', 'cannot be given unlimited freedom of movement for reasons upon which it is not necessary to dwell'.[34]

---

[31] Bardswell and Chapman, *Diets in Tuberculosis*, p. 47.
[32] *BJT* 11/4 (1917), 172.
[33] Midhurst Sanatorium, Consultant Reports, 6 Sept. 1906, p. 24; ibid. 14 July 1907, p. 168.
[34] J. K. Fowler, *Problems in Tuberculosis* (London, 1923), 46.

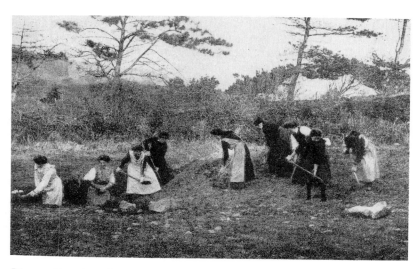

Plate 2. Female patients at a sanatorium doing 'Graduated Labour'. *Source*: *BJT*, 4 (1910), 290. (Bodleian Library, Oxford, Per. 15697 d. 58.)

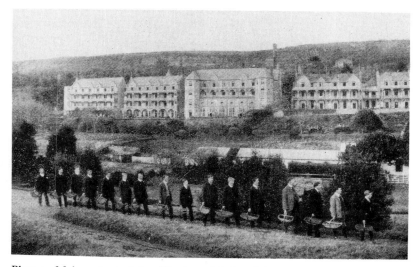

Plate 3. Male patients doing 'Graduated Labour' (the Royal National Hospital, Ventnor, is seen in the background). *Source*: *BJT*, 4 (1910), 289. (Bodleian Library, Oxford, Per. 15697 d. 58.)

Robert Philip described his ideal sanatorium in 1906:

The charge has sometimes been brought against sanatoriums that they tend to produce habits of indolence and idleness. I can conceive of conditions which justify the charge, but it is far from the truth in respect of properly-regulated sanatoriums. While sanatorium life is a life of treatment, it need not, and should not, be for the great proportion of patients an idle existence.

My idea of a sanatorium for the working class is that of a busy hive, where patients, subject to doctor's directions, contribute—some less, some more—by their own regulated efforts to the upkeep and beauty of the place—a kind of working colony.[35]

Many of the early twentieth-century sanatoria introduced work for patients from the time of their opening. But work for patients as part of treatment became associated particularly with Frimley Sanatorium, as its medical superintendent, Marcus Paterson, gave it the status of scientific medicine.

Paterson had introduced work immediately after taking charge of the sanatorium in 1905. He explained that he knew of a navvy with tuberculosis who had worked continuously for forty hours almost without rest a few days before his arrival at Brompton, with no ill effect, showing that patients with relatively advanced disease could still work. He believed that introducing work would do much to meet the objection that members of the working classes were liable to have their energy sapped and acquire lazy habits by sanatorium treatment. It would also make them more resistant to the disease by improving their physical condition, and would enable them, by its effect upon their muscles, to return to their work immediately after discharge. Once they could walk ten miles with no ill effect, the patients at Frimley were given a basket in which to carry mould for spreading on the lawns. After three or four weeks, they were given a spade with which to dig for five minutes and then rest for five minutes, graduating on to larger shovels. Paterson wrote that the patients all expressed the opinion that the work did them good and that the harder they worked the better they felt. Within the first year there were several patients who would over-exert themselves despite all instruction, and use heavier tools than they should have done. In one case, the extent of the disease was increased by over-exertion: 'The necessity of absolute obedience to the Medical Officer's orders was firmly established by such cases.' Hours of recreation were to be regulated just as carefully as hours of work.

[35] BMJ 2 (1906), 1534–5.

Paterson wrote that the results of the new methods of treatment proved beyond reasonable doubt that its principles were sound, although he was unable at the time to give a scientific account of the theory on which they were based. In 1907 A. C. Inman of the Brompton Hospital explained to him Sir Almroth Wright's theory of 'auto-inoculation', and suggested that the reason they were obtaining satisfactory results from the graduated system of labour was that the work caused an inoculation of the patients by their own bacterial products.[36] In this way, graduated labour was given bacteriological explanation. Paterson proceeded to explain his treatment on this basis, using a military analogy:

The aim of the physician is to keep the blood well garrisoned and well armed, swarming with its protective sentinels the anti-bodies so that all invading forces may be overcome at once. [This could be done by injections of tuberculin] . . . or if we allow our patient to exert himself, we make him liberate a certain amount of tuberculin (the poison) or toxin, to overcome which the body immediately re-acts and produces anti-toxin, which at once neutralises or kills the tuberculous poison, and we can bring about this happy result simply by means of exercise or graduated work. Exercise or work, in graduated amounts is therefore, in every sense of the term, scientific treatment.[37]

Paterson explained that when they first started work, many patients were sullen and apathetic, but as a result of the bacterial products influencing their general condition, they were soon transformed into cheerful and lively individuals. Thus the sanatorium, which was 'too often the home of neurotic individuals, mentally and physically deteriorated by long periods of ease and idleness' was transformed into 'a workshop of busy, hopeful men and women'.[38]

The investigations of Sir Almroth Wright and others on the role of the blood in bacterial diseases had therefore, according to Paterson, completely changed their ideas on the diagnosis and treatment of pulmonary tuberculosis. In the past, attention had been focused on the lungs, whereas now it was recognized that tuberculosis was a 'general disease of the blood fluids with a local manifestation in the lung'. The general condition of the patient was more important than the local condition of the lungs. Thus, bacteriology in this instance was used to

---

[36] Paterson, *Auto-inoculation*, pp. 12, 13, 17, 22.
[37] Papworth Archives, M1–20, P. C. Varrier-Jones, 'Tuberculosis and the Working Man: An Appeal to Friendly Societies', 31.
[38] Paterson, *Auto-inoculation*, pp. 59, 218.

justify a holistic rather than mechanistic approach to medicine.[39] At Frimley, all patients received a leaflet on arrival, written by Paterson. The 'Frimley method', described as the accepted form of treatment for pulmonary tuberculosis throughout the world, was explained with its various grades of labour from 1 to 6. The necessity of obedience was stressed:

It will clearly be realised for this careful measurement of work that the doctor, and only the doctor, knows the dividing line between what is useful and what is harmful exertion. Implicit obedience down to the smallest detail of the instructions is therefore essential. Patients have been known, through trivial disregard of their instructions, to have set back their recovery by weeks.[40]

The first stage of treatment was total rest, to control excessive 'auto-inoculation'. The prohibition of visitors was considered essential: 'Visitors will talk, and talking and laughing aggravate a cough and so induce auto-inoculation.' Letters were to be censored to prevent the possibility of a patient being worried by bad news: 'Mental agitation has a deleterious effect, directly or indirectly, by increasing the physical restlessness of the patient and adversely influencing his progress towards recovery.'[41]

Once the patients 'graduated' to the labour stage, the whole day was planned to the minute, from the time they got up at 6.50 a.m. until lights were out at 9.15 p.m. Paterson issued patients with a set of regulations:

[It is] forbidden to walk on the grass, to smoke at other than the times and places specified, to sing, whistle, or make any unnecessary noise, to have anything to eat or drink except at meals without special permission in writing, or to go to other patients' wards.

The men and women are to keep to their own respective parts of the grounds and are not allowed to speak or have any communication with each other.[42]

Walks for men were marked with red stakes, those for women with

[39] On the rise of bacteriology leading to an 'engineering' approach to medicine, see J. Powles, 'On the Limitations of Modern Medicine', *Science, Medicine and Man*, 1 (1973), 15.

[40] PRO MH96/980, WNMA, 'The Treatment of Pulmonary Tuberculosis: Words of Advice and Explanation to Patients Entering a Sanatorium' *c.*1920, 26. (Paterson was medical director of the WNMA from 1916.)

[41] Paterson, *Auto-inoculation*, p. 39.

[42] J. R. Bignall, *Frimley: The Biography of a Sanatorium* (London, 1979), 70; PRO MH96/948, WNMA, 'General Rules and Routine to be Observed by Patients in Residential Institutions', adopted by the Council of the WNMA, 28 Apr. 1916.

green. There were also strict rules on leaving the grounds of the sanatorium. Entering a public house led to instant dismissal. Paterson noted that in the early days of the sanatorium he was regarded as a labour master trying to get so much work out of the patients rather than as a medical man who was endeavouring to cure their disease.[43] A school teacher discharged himself when he was prescribed 'picking up sticks' and threatened to complain to the management committee.[44] However, most patients were persuaded that the strict regime was in their best interests and readily accepted it. The psychological pressure adopted by Paterson is illustrated by the following story: one day Paterson was sitting in his office when he saw a patient who had discharged himself in the act of leaving. He called out to him, 'Oh, by the way, tell your widow to send me a postcard.'[45]

By the end of 1910, 1,674 patients (1,183 men and 491 women) had passed through the graduated labour treatment at Frimley. In 1908 Paterson reported that the patients had dug, manured, and sown over an acre of grass, excavated for the walls of a new reservoir to hold 500,000 gallons of rain water, mixed and laid about 650 tons of concrete, made most of the paths, laid the concrete walk to the dining hall, made a concrete subway 150 yards in length from the engine room to the kitchen, cleared a 20-foot 'fire zone' round the boundary, trenched and sifted about an acre of land, fetched and sifted gravel for the paths, made the terrace and rock garden round the tennis court by the medical officer's house, made a bank round the grounds, and felled and cut into firewood about 100 trees.[6] Bignall rightly commented that, had the system continued, the estate would have been converted into a treeless tract, intersected by trenches and concrete paths, with sunken gardens, concrete-lined subways, and unnecessary new buildings, and believed that by 1910 the pace must have been slackening.[47]

Apart from being used to provide scientific medical justification for the system of labour and for absolute control of the doctor over the

---

[43] Paterson did calculate that by employing patients the amount saved was £10,177 in 6 years: Paterson, *Auto-inoculation*, p. 235.

[44] Bignall, *Frimley*, p. 31. Patients' prescription books are held at the Wellcome Unit for the History of Medicine, Oxford.

[45] P. J. Bishop, 'The History of the Brompton Hospital', *Transactions and Studies of the College of Physicians, Philadelphia, Medicine and History Series* 5, 1/3 (1979), 179.

[46] *Bulstrode Report*, p. 476; R. F. Walters, *Domiciliary Treatment of Tuberculosis* (London, 1921), 252–3.

[47] Bignall, *Frimley*, p. 79.

patient, the theory of 'auto-inoculation' also enhanced Paterson's medical status by involving him in the practice of 'scientific' treatment rather than merely being in charge of a 'home for consumptives'. One of the 'shibboleths' related to tuberculosis that Paterson noted in 1920 was that 'sanatoria are no good', which he attributed to the fact that many members of the medical profession had little experience of sanatorium treatment on modern lines:

It is obvious that the successful treatment of disease needs careful study, yet a great many members of medical staff of the sanatoria of this country have undertaken sanatorium work without special knowledge or training, because they had, unfortunately, contracted tuberculosis in their own practices, and after a period of treatment had turned to such work for the benefit of their own health . . . The truth is that there are many 'homes for tuberculosis' but few sanatoria.[48]

Moreover, the theory of 'auto-inoculation' enabled him to justify, on scientific grounds, increasing the powers of the residential medical officer at the expense of consultants. He wrote, 'It is necessary that the medical superintendent should be given a free hand; no one will do good work if he is being constantly worried by persons who seldom have the inside knowledge and first-hand experience of a competent man on the spot.'[49] Paterson was initially designated resident medical officer with a salary of £200 per annum and worked under the instructions of the Brompton Hospital consultants. In 1906 his designation changed to 'medical superintendent' and his salary rose to £500, rising further to £600 in 1909.[50]

Frimley Sanatorium under Paterson's direction attained a world-wide reputation. At the 1908 International Tuberculosis Congress in Washington, a $1,000 sanatorium prize was divided between Frimley and an American institution, and Paterson won a prize for an essay on sanatorium organization and treatment.[51] Picture postcards were produced for sale, showing men and women patients doing the various grades of work. The lay press reported the activities of the sanatorium enthusiastically. In 1910 the *Morning Leader* reproduced a photograph under the caption 'Pickaxe Cure for Consumptives', and the NAPT collected a series of lantern slides of the Brompton Hospital

[48] M. S. Paterson, *The Shibboleths of Tuberculosis* (London, 1920), 99–100.
[49] Paterson, *Auto-inoculation*, p. 168.
[50] Bignall, *Frimley*, p. 49.
[51] P. J. Bishop, 'The Marcus Paterson Collection', *Tubercle*, 48 (1967), 63.

Sanatorium: 'How patients built a reservoir.'[52] In 1912, H. de Carle Woodcock referred to Frimley as 'a most perfect scheme carried out under the supervision of that most original of innovators, Dr Paterson'.[53] There were many visitors and letters of inquiry. Other sanatorium medical superintendents possibly also saw the advantage of giving work in sanatoria scientific status, of enhancing their own prestige by being involved in scientific treatment, and of obtaining medical justification for the absolute obedience of patients. It was not only tuberculous patients who were thought to benefit from such a regime. In 1910 an American doctor wrote to Paterson that he was hoping to adopt similar treatment for 'certain classes of criminals, dipsomaniacs, drug fiends . . . those exhibiting degenerative symptoms'.[54] Paterson also received a letter in 1910 in response to an article he wrote in *Mother and Home* describing the 'Hard Work Cure for Consumptives', suggesting that his treatment would be ideal for patients with neurasthenia.[55] One commentator did not think the system should be restricted to those already ill, and was building an open-air school in a 'Garden City' where she hoped to 'produce a finer type of physique and a higher degree of mental and moral capacity than is at present known'.[56] Open-air labour was also becoming routine in epileptic colonies established around the turn of the century. The medical superintendent of Langho Epileptic Colony claimed that work was of immense therapeutic value, as measured by less-frequent epileptic fits. Patients who arrived 'dull, surly, and degraded in their habits, . . . after a few months become cheerful and willing workers and careful in their habits'.[57]

Many of the early twentieth-century British sanatoria practised graduated labour. At Kelling Sanatorium for Workers, in Norfolk, all patients worked, even those who were unable to leave the shelters, and their produce was sold for the sanatorium. Some carved wood, others made mats, and others worked in the garden or on the poultry farm.

[52] *Morning Leader*, 23 July 1910 (J. R. Bignall's notebook); NAPT Council Annual Report 1913, p. 99.
[53] H. de Carle Woodcock, *The Doctor and the People* (London, 1912), 224.
[54] Paterson Collection, III, G.372, John C. Gosnell, Seattle, Washington, 1 Sept. 1910.
[55] Paterson Collection, V, B.633, E. B. Tomlin, 12 Nov. 1910.
[56] A. J. Lawrence, *Lancet*, 1 (1907), 836.
[57] The Epileptic Colony, Langho (nr. Blackburn): Annual Report of Medical Superintendent 1909–10 (James Shearer), pp. 9–10 (supplied by J. Barclay, Graduate Student, University of Manchester, Institute of Science and Technology).

Three 'cured' patients were on the permanent staff of the sanatorium as gardener, yardsman, and chauffeur. At Kelling, work was considered to be a therapeutic agent, and idleness 'the worst of curses to the consumptive'.[58]

Other sanatoria which were reported to be practising graduated labour included Benenden Sanatorium, where all the vegetables used in the sanatorium in 1912 were cultivated by the patients under skilled supervision, Westmorland Consumption Sanatorium and Home where patients 'graduated' to quarrying and uprooting trees, and Eldwick Sanatorium for Women and Children, in Bingley, Yorkshire, where patients helped with housework and gardening. Patients at the North Wales Sanatorium accomplished an impressive amount of work on the sanatorium grounds in 1912 and 1913.[59]

Graduated labour was not only practised in working-class sanatoria, but also at those where the patient paid more than a minimum maintenance cost. For example, Pinewood Sanatorium in Bedfordshire, an institution for clerks and others in receipt of a salary or of independent means, who were charged from 2 to 3 guineas per week, had a scheme of graduated labour. Treatment at Crooksbury Sanatorium, in Surrey, a private sanatorium 'for the reception of ladies and gentlemen' at 3 guineas per week, included 'graduated exercise, work and games'.[60]

In his annual report for 1907 as medical superintendent of Midhurst Sanatorium, N.D. Bardswell referred to Paterson's scheme, which he said was initiated after much observation and study, and had proved highly successful in the treatment of pulmonary tuberculosis. He wrote that in consequence of the representation of some members of the consultant staff, similar measures had been adopted at Midhurst. Light work in the gardens and grounds of the sanatorium formed part of regular treatment in place of walking exercise, for both men and women. He stressed that all 'manual exercise' (Bardswell referred to the system as 'manual exercise' rather than 'labour') was carried out under the close supervision of one of the medical officers, and that the patients to whom such work was prescribed were carefully selected – as a rule, not until they could walk from four to six miles a day. The work was to consist chiefly of gardening and poultry farming;

[58] Woodcock, *The Doctor and the People*, pp. 222–3, 224; W. J. Fanning, *Jl. NAPT* 3/8 (1906), 371.

[59] Kelynack (ed.), *Tuberculosis Yearbook 1913–14*, pp. 230, 250, 263, 278, 284, 285; 'Respiratory Tuberculosis in Wales', *CMOH Annual Report 1967* (1968), 187.

[60] Kelynack (ed.), *Tuberculosis Yearbook 1913–14*, pp. 201, 256.

household duties were still left to the domestic staff. An open-air carpenter's shop was erected and fitted by some of the patients, where patients worked under the direction of a county council instructor in carpentry who was himself a patient. Bardswell did not speak of graduated labour in bacteriological terms, but he did believe that such labour had medical value in that it promoted good muscular tone and general well-being, and had a valuable 'moral' effect as it gave patients confidence in their own restored physical powers.[61]

Sir Clifford Allbutt predicted that the proposal to occupy patients at Midhurst Sanatorium in gardening work or farming occupations would prove ineffective except in a very perfunctory way. Many years' experience as visiting Justice of Asylums had led him to conclude that patients who paid from a pound upwards for maintenance (at Midhurst, patients paid up to £5 5s. per week) could not be induced to engage systematically in manual labour. He explained that patients of this class were not used to labour with their hands, it wearied them, and they soon tired of it. It was more practicable at Frimley where the patients were of a class more used to labour. At Midhurst, Allbutt suggested introducing games such as golf.[62]

The provision, or absence, of 'manual exercise' formed the main subject of reports by consultants to Midhurst during the next few years. Theodore Williams regretted in 1906 that the twenty or thirty patients who were employed in gardening at Midhurst did not evince the same zeal and enthusiasm for the work as did the patients at Frimley Sanatorium where inmates of both sexes worked vigorously. Sir James Kingston Fowler was sorry to learn that the attempt to interest the patients at Midhurst in various forms of labour had met so far with little success. He believed that this was in great part due to the adverse influence of the medical men who were under treatment there. He realized that their opinion reflected that generally held on the subject by the medical profession, but pointed out that they had not had the opportunity of observing the remarkable results obtained from the introduction of graduated labour at Frimley Sanatorium. This was,

---

[61] Midhurst Sanatorium Annual Report 1906–7, pp. 7–9; ibid., 1909–10, p. 7. Midhurst had a staff of 75 for 80 patients in 1906 while Frimley had a staff of 28 for 108 patients: J. K. Fowler, Midhurst Sanatorium Consultant Reports, 16 Dec. 1906, pp. 110, 112.

[62] In 1906 charges were reduced from £8 8s. per week to £5 5s.: Midhurst Sanatorium Consultant Reports, 1 Dec. 1906, p. 102; ibid., 9 Jan. 1907, pp. 128–30.

in his opinion, the only real advance made in sanatorium treatment since the method had attracted attention in this country. He recognized that it was impossible to enforce labour by regulation at Midhurst, and that with patients of a higher social position its introduction was difficult, but he hoped that when the medical staff was increased a further attempt would be made. The following year, he reported that he was sorry to hear that the patients who had been employed on the paths had almost given up the work, but was still hopeful that they could be persuaded: 'If a gravel pit can be found on the estate at not too great a distance it would afford an admirable opportunity for carefully graduated labour.'

More favourable reports from the consultants began to appear in 1907. Sir Felix Semon commented on the special feature which 'deserved the warmest of commendations'—that medical officers had succeeded in interesting and regularly occupying patients in gardening, road making, carpentry, and poultry keeping. Sir James Kingston Fowler also noted in 1908, 'I was glad to learn that work out-of-doors was congenial to most of the patients who were fit for it. I never doubted that this would prove to be the case, no matter from what class the patients were drawn.' In 1910, Theodore Williams reported on a visit when he had found a number of patients of both sexes at work in the vegetable garden. Some patients, including several women, were breaking fresh soil with pickaxes, while others were trenching with spades, and others clearing away stones and roots: 'The sun was hot and the nature of the work laborious, but the patients . . . laboured well at their appointed tasks, and seemed quite happy.' Observing the garden work in 1910, Percy Kidd noticed one of the resident medical officers working as hard as anyone.

Sir William Osler urged starting a farm at Midhurst. He believed that its educative value would be great, as farming was eminently suited to a majority of patients after leaving. He regretted that such extra land had still not been purchased in 1912. In his opinion, a grave defect of the sanatorium was the absence of any systematic work for the patients, for 'nothing [was] more injurious to an early consumptive than a period of enforced idleness', regardless of the class.[63]

An advocate of farm colonies specifically for working-class patients, as an extension of sanatorium treatment, was Sir Robert Philip. He

[63] Midhurst Sanatorium Consultant Reports 1906–12. In fact, graduated labour never became successfully established as treatment at Midhurst: Sir Geoffrey Todd, medical superintendent of Midhurst, 1933–79, interview 25 Aug. 1983.

established such a colony, attached to the Royal Victoria Hospital, in 1910 at Springfield, seven miles from Edinburgh. N. D. Bardswell also set up a farm colony for working-class patients at Kinson, Bournemouth, in 1916. Discussing the proposal in 1906, Bardswell referred to the Salvation Army Colony at Hadleigh in Essex for the unemployed, believing that a similar scheme would be very valuable for the tuberculous. Hadleigh was a farm of 3,000 acres purchased by the Salvation Army in 1891, where about five hundred men were trained each year, for an average period of four months. Bardswell pointed out that a consumptive colony would suffer from the additional handicap of having tuberculous labour instead of sound labour, but, by way of compensation, the class of colonists would be better than at Hadleigh, where labour was recruited from the 'submerged tenth'. The colony in his scheme would be 'a finishing school, where men would gain confidence in themselves and their ability to work'.[64]

The reference to the Salvation Army scheme is significant. Close parallels can be detected between the proposed solutions to the problems of unemployment and tuberculosis in the male population in the early twentieth century. As one historian has noted, at that time the creation of farm colonies with a view to restoring workmen permanently to the land was the most widely canvassed solution to the problem of urban unemployment. The Inter-departmental Committee on Physical Deterioration in 1904 recommended labour colonies for reclaiming the 'waste elements of society' and agricultural resettlement for those who had been 'crushed and broken by the wheels of city life'. The Majority and Minority Reports of the Royal Commission on the Poor Laws in 1909 suggested that labour colonies should be used as a means of repressing the 'loafer' and retraining the unemployed. Both the unemployed and the tuberculous were perceived as urban problem groups, and the favoured solution in both cases was to train them in agriculture, with a view to permanent settlement on the land or possibly emigration to the colonies.[65]

Manual labour and labour colonies in the treatment of tuberculous patients gained widespread popularity. Hyslop Thomson claimed in 1912 that manual labour was now recognized as an essential part of

[64] N. D. Bardswell, *The Consumptive Working Man, What Can Sanatoria Do For Him?* (London, 1906), 150–4. The colony only lasted a few years as it was found that the farm work was too heavy for the patients: *BJT* 31/4 Supp. (1937), 89.

[65] J. Harris, *Unemployment and Politics: A Study in English Social Policy 1886–1914* (Oxford, 1972), 141–3; *Report of the Inter-departmental Committee on Physical Deterioration*, pp. 18, 35.

sanatorium treatment.[66] H. de Carle Woodcock wrote in the same year that, at every sanatorium he had visited at home and abroad, cordial agreement had been expressed with the scheme for a labour colony for consumptives.[67]

However, G. (later Sir George) Newman, Chief MO of the Board of Education and later of the Ministry of Health, reported in 1912 that graduated exercises and manual labour formed no part of the treatment in the German sanatoria he had visited. At Hohwald Sanatorium, near Dresden, for example, the patients appeared to spend a large proportion of their time resting. The discipline of the patients did not appear to be strict and on the whole the men looked slack and flabby. Some of the German authorities regarded regulated work as dangerous to the health of patients, others maintained that it required too much supervision, and others that the patients claimed they had come to rest, not to work, and would not co-operate.[68]

Nor were all British sanatoria successful in adopting the scheme. The LGB regretted in 1918 that in many sanatoria insufficient attention was given to the need to provide adequate useful occupation for the patient's mind and body. Without graduated labour, they believed that a prolonged stay in a sanatorium was legitimately open to the charge often made, that it produced deterioration in the character of the patients. They advised: 'Some patients, it is true, refuse to work in a sanatorium saying that they have come there to rest. While avoiding a martinet's attitude, firm but kindly discipline should be enforced, and patients who persistently refuse to carry out the routine work prescribed for them should not be retained.'[69]

Insured patients after 1911 acquired a reputation for complaining. Garland wrote in 1913, 'The mental attitude of the insured workman sometimes shows a tendency to an exaggerated independence. Unless this mental attitude is anticipated, and allowed for, it will be found extremely difficult to apply a scheme of graduated labour.'[70] Servicemen invalided from the Forces with tuberculosis after 1914 also acquired a reputation for complaining as well as for indiscipline. The Ministry of Pensions issued instructions indicating the penalties which

[66] H. H. Thomson, *Consumption in General Practice*, 2nd edn. (London, 1912), 225.
[67] Woodcock, *The Doctor and the People*, p. 224.
[68] *Astor Committee, Final Report*, ii. 118, 120.
[69] LGB, *Annual Report 1917–18, Supp., Report by Medical Officer*, Cd. 9169 (1918), p. lxiii.
[70] *Astor Committee, Final Report*, ii. 51.

could be inflicted on those ex-servicemen who failed to conform to the rules, such as reduction in pensions. Complaints were perhaps an indication that patients were coming to regard treatment as a right and not as charity, an attitude which made manual labour more difficult to enforce, as among paying patients.[71]

(5) EDUCATION

In reply to those who doubted the curability of tuberculosis by sanatorium treatment, it was often pointed out that apart from its curative value, the sanatorium was immensely valuable as an educational institution. Marcus Paterson argued that those who made the claim that sanatoria were no good overlooked the inestimable advantage enjoyed by the sanatorium patients who, having learned the benefits of the hygienic life and returned home, saw that their families adopted a 'rational method of living'.[72] At the opening of Midhurst Sanatorium, Bardswell said, 'Of course all the patients may not be cured when they leave the institution. My aim is to teach them how to cure themselves. They can carry on the treatment even amid the smoke of London itself.'[73] Sir Robert Philip similarly believed the educative value could not be over-estimated: 'The patients learn unconsciously how to treat themselves [by open-air methods] . . . They thus become . . . apostles of the new faith.'[74] In 1904 Kelynack referred to a sanatorium for comparatively poor cases where the visiting physician gave a weekly lecture on the conduct of a healthy life, 'with such results I was assured, that they become enthusiastic missionaries in the cause of hygienic righteousness'. He believed that the chief benefit to the community would prove to be the sanatorium's educational influence on the thought and life of the people, promoting the goal of prevention.[75] S. Vere Pearson, medical superintendent of Mundesley Sanatorium, also claimed that sanatorium treatment had helped to spread 'the gospel of hygiene'.[76] In its 1913 report, the WNMA wrote that the great value of institutional treatment was its educative influence: 'Patients are found to observe the instructions given, and to

---

[71] See also B. Abel-Smith, *The Hospitals* (London, 1964), 248.
[72] Paterson, *Shibboleths*, p. 101.
[73] *Daily Express*, 12 June 1906 (Bardswell's scrapbook).
[74] *BMJ* 2 (1898), 219.
[75] Kelynack, *The Sanatorium Treatment of Consumption*, pp. 16, 27.
[76] S. V. Pearson, *The State Provision of Sanatoriums* (Cambridge, 1913), vi, 3, 55.

a great extent, carry them out on return to their homes. They permeate their families and friends with hygienic standards, and each returned patient becomes in this way a small centre for the improvement of the health standard of the Welsh people.'[77] Each patient treated in a sanatorium would become, according to Drs Wynn and Dixon of Yardley Road Sanatorium, Birmingham, an 'apostle of fresh air and cleanliness . . . [which was] certain to have a wide-reaching influence upon the health of the community. It is also no small thing that for a few weeks the patients should have been subjected to discipline and orderly routine.'[78]

Sir William Osler started a scheme in Oxford whereby poor patients were given one month's sanatorium treatment 'for educative purposes'. Camac Wilkinson commented on the scheme that if a month's instruction in a sanatorium were necessary, they should not confine this valuable instruction to the poor, but should give similar instruction to others who, though not poor, offended quite as often and as grossly against the laws of personal and domestic hygiene. In his opinion, 'All this may be salutary enough, but it hardly touches the serious problem before us of treating consumption, and it is assumed that the poor will be ready to acquiesce in these pleasant excursions to sanatoria for their schooling.'[79]

Wilkinson also queried the source of information that prompted Lloyd George's statement in 1911 that in Germany, 'the results [of sanatorium treatment] are amazing in the number of cures effected'. He referred to the work of Englemann who dealt with the after-histories of many thousands of cases treated in 31 sanatoria in Germany. Four years after discharge from the sanatoria, four-fifths of the patients were either dead or invalids; considerably more than half were dead. Wilkinson argued therefore that sanatoria could have little real effect, when only 30,000 out of the 300,000 tuberculosis sufferers were treated per annum, and of those treated, 15,000 would be dead after four years.[80]

Wilkinson was not alone in doubting the value of sanatoria. It also appeared a serious matter to Halliday Sutherland, formerly medical superintendent of Westmorland Sanatorium, that three tuberculosis

[77] Kelynack (ed.), *Tuberculosis Yearbook 1913–14*, p. 184.
[78] *Astor Committee, Final Report*, ii. 157.
[79] W. C. Wilkinson, *Tuberculin in the Diagnosis and Treatment of Tuberculosis* (London, 1912), 459.
[80] *Morning Post*, 19 May 1911, quoted in Wilkinson, ibid., p. 475.

officers had published 'perfectly accurate figures in the lay press regarding the results of sanatorium treatment' showing that of all the people who received sanatorium treatment during 1914, approximately 80 per cent were dead by 1920.[81] In 1920 Sir George Newman wrote that since 1912 it had seemed to him very serious indeed that three-quarters of the sanatorium cases were dead in five years, in Germany as well as in Britain.[82] In his first annual report as Chief Medical Officer of the Ministry of Health, Newman wrote of the 'disparagement of sanatorium treatment as a costly failure'.[83] The world in general had been talking recently about the failure of sanatorium treatment, according to Clive Rivière in 1920.[84] Sir James Kingston Fowler similarly wrote in 1921, 'It is not uncommon nowadays to read that "sanatorium treatment" has proved a failure and to find a suggestion that the money expended thereon has been wasted and that some sort of conference should be held to decide whether or not the whole system, so far as the State is concerned, should be abandoned.'[85]

---

[81] *8 NAPT 1920*, p. 28.
[82] PRO MH55/164, letter from Newman to R. L. Morant, 4 Nov. 1920.
[83] *1st CMOH Annual Report 1919–20* (1920), 94.
[84] *Tubercle*, 1 (1920), 444.
[85] J. K. Fowler, *Pulmonary Tuberculosis* (London, 1921), 225. See also W. A. Brend, *Health and the State* (London, 1917), 236–44, and *EMJ* 31/3 (1924), 132.

3

The National Tuberculosis Service, 1918–1939

FAR from calling a conference for the dissolution of the national tuberculosis scheme, the immediate post-war climate was favourable to an expansion of the services. A major reason for this was the increase in tuberculosis during the war, checking the decline of the previous fifty years. In particular, after the war, there were estimated to be 58,000 ex-servicemen with tuberculosis attributable to war service.[1] One observer was hopeful that the country's interest in these men would be extended to an interest in the problem as a whole, and that therefore there would be a greater investment in tuberculosis work.[2] Such an interest was in fact manifested in donations from ex-servicemen's funds to the anti-tuberculosis campaign and in an Inter-departmental Committee on Tuberculosis set up in 1919 and presided over by Sir Montague Barlow.

Under the 1921 Public Health (Tuberculosis) Act, local authorities in England and Wales became responsible for tuberculosis prevention and treatment in their respective areas, some 83 county borough councils and 62 county councils (including the LCC). In London, the responsibility was shared between the LCC, the city council, and the 28 metropolitan borough councils. In Scotland, the Public Health (Scotland) Act of 1897 continued to provide the statutory basis of the tuberculosis services, empowering the major local authorities, 31 counties and 24 larger burghs, to administer services. The 1936 Committee on Health Services in Scotland regretted that Scottish local authorities did not have the same powers as were conferred on those of England and Wales by the 1921 Act.[3] The number of people for whom local authorities conducting tuberculosis services throughout

---

[1] W. G. MacPherson, W. B. Leishman, and S. L. Cummins (eds.), *The History of the Great War: Medical Services: Pathology* (London, 1923), 477, stated that there had been approximately 58,000 pensions awarded for tuberculosis contracted in war service by 1921. An earlier estimate (commonly quoted) of the number of ex-servicemen with tuberculosis attributable to war service was 35,000: *Report of Inter-departmental Committee on Tuberculosis*, Chairman: Waldorf Astor; Deputy Chairman who presided, Sir Montague Barlow Cmd. 317 (1919), 5, 7.

[2] *Tubercle*, 1 (1919), 43.

[3] *Public Health* (1941), 158.

Britain were responsible varied greatly, from under 50,000 to over 2,000,000. The cost of the tuberculosis services was borne by local rates supplemented by an Exchequer grant. A specific amount was allocated by the Exchequer for tuberculosis services until the 1929 Local Government Act which replaced a percentage grant for health services by a block grant. In 1921–2, anti-tuberculosis work cost English local authorities £800,000 in rates with an Exchequer grant of £1,100,000. In Scotland anti-tuberculosis services cost approximately £450,000 in 1921–2 in public money (including the Exchequer grant). In Wales, the local authorities came to an agreement with the WNMA, under which the latter operated an anti-tuberculosis service in exchange for an annual grant from local authorities. The cost for 1921 was £180,000, which was reimbursed by the Exchequer on the same basis as in England, apart from interest rates which were reimbursed by a third instead of a half on the grounds that the WNMA could be regarded as half-way between a local authority and a philanthropic society.[4] The proportion of local authority public health expenditure in England taken up by tuberculosis can be seen in Table 3.

TABLE 3 *Local authority public health expenditure in England, 1921–2*

	Local rates %	Exchequer grants %
Tuberculosis	11.0	35.0
Infectious diseases	42.0	Nil
Lunatics (not chargeable to Poor Law)	27.0	0.5
Maternal and child welfare services	12.0	35.0
Mental deficiency	5.0	13.5
Venereal diseases	1.5	10.0
Port sanitary work	1.0	2.0
Blind welfare	0.5	4.0
Total	100	100

Source: Addison Papers, Box 12, 72 (Bodleian Library, Oxford).

The anti-tuberculosis services comprised dispensaries, residential institutions, and after-care committees. This chapter discusses each of these in turn, considering the relative importance which was attached

[4] PRO MH75/1, WNMA deputations to Ministry of Health, 1 Apr. 1924, and MH75/2, 21 Mar. 1928 and 22 Jan. 1929.

to each, as well as local variations. It will be seen that by the end of the period under discussion, the anti-tuberculosis services were coming under criticism as a result of both the emphasis adopted within the individual schemes and the unequal distribution of resources from one area to another.

(1) DISPENSARIES

The administrative head of the tuberculosis service in most areas was the county medical officer or medical officer of health (in Lancashire, Sheffield, and Walsall, there were separate administrative heads). Under the medical officers, tuberculosis officers were appointed by local authorities to take charge of tuberculosis services, based at the dispensaries. Tuberculosis officers were paid at the rate of an assistant medical officer. In Wales, 'tuberculosis physicians' were employed by the WNMA, and performed the same function as the tuberculosis officers in England. In some parts of England no separate tuberculosis officer was appointed; in those places the medical officer undertook the duties of the tuberculosis officer. In 1920, the medical officers of 8 counties and 20 county boroughs were also tuberculosis officers for their areas. In 1931, this was the case for 10 counties and 25 county boroughs (20 and 32 per cent of the total local authorities respectively).[5] In 1932 there were 209 part-time tuberculosis officers in England, who combined tuberculosis duties with other public health work.[6]

A career dealing with tuberculosis, as with other areas of public health, was not prestigious. Many took the job with a view to becoming medical officer, and in this way detracted from the professional status of the tuberculosis specialization itself. It was maintained in 1929 that 'few if any of the 382 [*sic*] approved tuberculosis officers in England began their professional careers with the object of specialising in tuberculosis'.[7] Promotion within the tuberculosis service was to medical superintendence of a tuberculosis institution, but such posts were relatively few in number. Lissant Cox, who became head of the Lancashire tuberculosis service, was told by his friends in 1912 that accepting a post as tuberculosis officer was 'professional suicide'.[8]

[5] *NAPT Handbook of Tuberculosis Schemes in Great Britain and Ireland*, 3rd edn. (London, 1921); ibid., 6th edn. (London, 1931).
[6] *Public Health* (1941), 135.
[7] *Tubercle*, 11 (1929), 136; see also *BMJ* 2 (1949), 153.
[8] Obituary, *BMJ* 2 (1967), 60.

H. de Carle Woodcock described the post of tuberculosis officer in 1921 as a dead-end job, and it was later similarly described by two other tuberculosis specialists, J. Harley Williams and Gregory Kayne.[9] A diploma in tuberculosis was introduced in 1920 at the Welsh National School of Medicine in an attempt to enhance the professional status of the post—the Diploma in Tuberculosis Diseases, TDD (Wales). However, this diploma was neither prestigious, nor required; in 1931 H. D. Chalke, who did not possess the diploma, was chosen as assistant tuberculosis physician for West Monmouthshire, above three candidates with the diploma.[10] Discussing training in tuberculosis in 1950, a leading article in the *BMJ* did not mention the diploma.[11] Training in tuberculosis at the undergraduate level was rare. There were only two professorships in tuberculosis in the country, in Edinburgh (established in 1919 by the Royal Victoria Tuberculosis Trust for Scotland) and at the Welsh National School of Medicine (established in 1920 by David Davies of Llandinam). In 1942, P. D'Arcy Hart of the MRC claimed that there were no departments of tuberculosis worth mentioning in the British Isles.[12]

Co-operation between tuberculosis officers, who were supposedly consultants in tuberculosis, and GPs was poor, as Newman noted in his annual reports as Chief Medical Officer of the Ministry of Health, although he continually expressed confidence that the situation was improving. GPs did not always notify tuberculosis cases to the medical officer and hence to the tuberculosis officer, despite the regulations. The MOH for Leeds threatened in 1928 to prosecute some of the 'worst offenders' among the medical practitioners concerned 'unless they mended their ways'.[13] The MO for Cornwall suspected that many known cases of tuberculosis were not being notified, and carried out an investigation of clinical records, whereby 100 such patients were discovered.[14] In 1944 it was found that in Birmingham there had been for a long time 'an underground war' between certain of the physicians at the voluntary hospitals, headed by a professor, and the tuberculosis service. The physicians had tended to keep patients away from the

[9] TG SMOH Minutes, Special General Meeting, 22 Oct. 1921; J. H. Williams, *Requiem for a Great Killer: The Story of Tuberculosis* (London, 1977), 77; G. G. Kayne, *The Control of Tuberculosis in England, Past and Present* (Oxford, 1937), 146.
[10] PRO MH75/13, F. J. H. Coutts, meeting of Medical Committee of the WNMA, 10 Dec. 1931.
[11] *BMJ* 2 (1950), 1384.   [12] MRC Archives 1615 III, 21 Apr. 1942.
[13] *Tubercle*, 11 (1930), 181.
[14] A. S. Hall, in R. F. G. Heaf (ed.), *Symposium of Tuberculosis* (London, 1959), 94.

service and to send them to private sanatoria. This practice was forced into the open by the tuberculosis allowances scheme introduced in 1943 (see chapter 8, section 1), which was administered by tuberculosis officers who refused to grant the allowances unless the patient had been seen in their department.[15]

Dispensaries were to be the administrative centres of the service. In 1919 there were 398 approved tuberculosis dispensaries in England, increasing to 453 by 1929, and 485 by 1938. Wales had 15 dispensaries and 85 'visiting stations' during this period. Scotland had 22 dispensaries in 1919, increasing to 42 by 1932 (although only 8 of 31 Scottish counties had dispensaries in 1939).[16] The dispensary, as 'a receiving and clearing house and a centre for diagnosis, consultation and observation', followed the model established by Sir Robert Philip in Edinburgh and its functions included home visiting. Tuberculosis officers paid approximately 50,000 visits per annum to patients' homes in England in the 1920s, and tuberculosis nurses or health visitors, approximately 750,000.[17] The setting up of dispensaries, in general, was not an expensive or elaborate enterprise. They were often located in town halls or other public places usurped for the purpose for one or two days a month. For example, in Berkshire such improvised dispensaries were set up at specified times of the month in the Reading Shire Hall, the Maidenhead Town Hall, the Oddfellow's Institute in Newbury, the Church Rooms in Windsor, and the Savings Bank at Faringdon.[18] Most dispensaries were not attached to hospitals. Sometimes locations were shared with the maternal and infant welfare clinics which local authorities were required to set up following the 1918 Maternal and Child Welfare Act. Only in the late 1930s did a few local authorities combine a tuberculosis dispensary with other public health work in a health centre, such as in Bristol and Finsbury, London.

The variation in services provided can be seen from the returns to the Ministry of Health for 1930 relating to the amount of work undertaken. In that year, in Devon there were 662 recorded examinations of contacts of tuberculous patients per hundred tubercu-

---

[15] PRO MH55/1288, Midland Region 9, Birmingham, Tuberculosis, 23 Jan. 1944.
[16] *1st CMOH Annual Report 1919–20* (1920), 52; *10th Annual Report Ministry of Health 1928–9* (1929), 40; *NAPT Handbook*, 10th edn. (London, 1939), 185; *1st Annual Report Scottish Board of Health 1919*, Cmd. 825 (1920), 30; *4th Annual Report Scottish Department of Health 1932*, Cmd. 4338 (1933), 77; *EMJ* 50 (1943), 211.
[17] *9th CMOH Annual Report 1927* (1928), 52.
[18] *NAPT Handbook*, 5th edn. (London, 1927), 4.

losis deaths, in Cornwall 30. In Sheffield in the same year, 496 such examinations were recorded, 10 in Westmorland, 11 in Stockport, 12 in West Yorkshire, 8 in Merthyr and Barrow, and 4 in Bolton. The percentage of X-ray examinations for all new cases and contacts seen in 1927 was 19 in all of England and Wales, 96 in Lancashire, and 9 in Wales.[19]

(2) INSTITUTIONS

The second unit in the tuberculosis schemes consisted of institutions for the treatment of the disease, by far the most expensive element, but also the most attractive to benefactors, as earlier in the century. Institutional accommodation for tuberculous patients expanded during the inter-war period (Table 4) at a time when the expansion of general hospital beds was negligible.[20]

A large proportion of these institutions catered for pulmonary tuberculosis; 85 per cent of the local authority tuberculosis beds in England were for pulmonary cases, although of the beds provided by the WNMA in Wales only 70 per cent were for pulmonary cases.[21] Special arrangements were sometimes made for the treatment of non-pulmonary tuberculosis. For example, bone and joint tuberculosis was usually treated at an orthopaedic hospital, lupus and genito-urinary tuberculosis were often treated in special and general voluntary hospitals, and abdominal and other cases might be treated in a special non-pulmonary block in a tuberculosis institution.

In the expansion of tuberculosis institutions after the First World War, voluntary funds for ex-servicemen played an important part. In 1921 the Joint War Committee of the British Red Cross Society and the Order of St John decided to make grants amounting to nearly £1 million to hospitals and other institutions in England and Wales from their surplus funds; tuberculosis was included in this beneficence.[22] At an international meeting of the Red Cross Society held at Geneva after the war, it was decided to channel some of the resources of the Society

[19] *Medical Officer*, 43 (1930), 135; see also 'Respiratory Tuberculosis in Wales', *CMOH Annual Report 1967* (1968), 190.
[20] R. Pinker, *English Hospital Statistics 1861–1938* (London, 1966), 48.
[21] PRO MH96/1034, WBH, Statistics, England and Wales, 1926 and 1927.
[22] *The Times*, 13 Sept. 1919.

TABLE 4 *Institutional accommodation for tuberculous patients*

(a) England.

Year	Number of Institutions			Number of Beds			Total inc. isolation and general hospitals
	Local Authority	Voluntary	Total	Local Authority	Voluntary	Total	
1921	123	113	236	6,531	7,015	13,546	17,352
1929	166	118	284	12,189	7,684	19,873	22,860
1938	179	108	287	15,609	7,848	23,457	30,614

(b) Wales (WNMA).

Year	Institutions	Beds	
		owned	rented
1921	12	1,128	78
1929	16	1,410	100
1938	18	1,827	182

(c) Scotland.

Year	Institutions	Beds
1921	103	3,558
1929	119	5,114
1938	115	5,500 (approx.)

Sources: (a) *2nd CMOH Annual Report 1920*, Cmd. 1397 (1921), 93; *10th Annual Report Ministry of Health 1938–9* (1939), 234. (b) Glynne R. Jones, 'The King Edward VII Welsh National Memorial Association, 1912–1948' in J. Cule (ed.), *Wales and Medicine* (London, 1975); *NAPT Handbook*, 2nd edn. (1919), 139–40; ibid., 7th edn. (1931), 75; ibid., 10th edn. (1939), 73–4. (c) *3rd Annual Report Scottish Board of Health 1921*, Cmd. 1697 (1922), 20; *1st Annual Report Scottish Department of Health 1929*, Cmd. 3529 (1930), 95; *10th Annual Report Scottish Department of Health 1938*, Cmd. 5969 (1939), 95.

into anti-tuberculosis work.[23] Several tuberculosis institutions in Britain were financed by the Red Cross Society and the Order of St John. Preston Hall, a tuberculosis village settlement in Kent, was founded in 1921 by a Committee for the Industrial Settlement of Wounded Soldiers and Sailors, under the chairmanship of Lord Queensborough. In their appeal for funds they stressed the war service of prospective patients. This institution, accommodating 295 patients, was taken over by the British Legion in 1925.

The terms of reference of the 1919 Inter-departmental Committee on Tuberculosis were 'to consider and report upon immediate practical steps which should be taken for the provision of residential treatment of discharged soldiers and sailors suffering from pulmonary tuberculosis and for their re-introduction into employment, especially on the land'. The Committee pointed out that there was an acute accommodation shortage for tuberculous patients among ex-servicemen as well as the wider public.[24]

In 1919 the Chancellor of the Exchequer appointed a committee chaired by G. H. Murray to consider grants to be allocated to local authorities for tuberculosis institutions. Following an interim report of the committee, grants were settled at £180 per bed, but not exceeding three-fifths of the total cost (they had already increased from £90 per bed with the three-fifths limitation as allowed in 1913, to £160 in October 1918) and voluntary contributions were no longer deducted from the amount eligible for the Exchequer grant as had been the case previously.[25]

Circulars issued by the Ministry of Health in November 1919 and March 1920 encouraged local authorities to establish schemes.[26] The 1921 Public Health (Tuberculosis) Act provided a further inducement for local authorities to establish institutions, for without institutions of their own they had to make arrangements with private institutions for treatment of patients from their locality. In February 1921, however, the Ministry of Health announced that no further schemes would be considered and that schemes which had been approved but not commenced should be postponed. This was part of the Government's retrenchment policy ('the Geddes Axe') in its attempt to deal with the economic depression, which also affected other areas of public

[23] Sub-committee of Oxfordshire Branch of British Red Cross Society County Care Committee Annual Report 1921, p. 6; *Barlow Report*, p. 9.

[24] *Barlow Report*, pp. 1, 5, 6, 7.

[25] PRO MH55/169, Murray Report (1920), 5, 6.

[26] *2nd CMOH Annual Report 1920* (1921), 105.

expenditure. Not until February 1924 did the Government announce a willingness to sanction further grants and loans.[27]

The Barlow Committee also recommended the establishment of tuberculosis colonies and village settlements, and that £250,000 and £1 million should be allocated respectively for such institutions by the Exchequer.[28] The Murray Committee favoured tuberculosis village settlements but believed their development would be on a slow basis.[29] The Ministry of Health set up a committee to consider local authority involvement in the establishment of such village settlements, which was dissolved following the announcement of the economy drive in 1921. A further committee to consider settlements for tuberculous patients was set up under the Labour Government in 1929. However, the only local authorities to attempt to establish a tuberculosis village settlement were Cheshire and Nottinghamshire, both small settlements (Wrenbury Hall and Sherwood Forest) with 26 and 20 'settlers' respectively in 1939.

In 1920 the Ministry of Pensions decided to finance a 'treatment and training scheme' for tuberculous ex-servicemen. For the purpose of the scheme, several of the larger tuberculosis institutions were encouraged to build extensions, the whole cost of which would be borne initially by the Ministry of Pensions, but which after five years could be purchased by the institution at three-fifths of the original cost. Initially the Ministry planned to provide 1,000 places under the scheme, but as the estimated costs were being exceeded, it was reviewed at the end of 1920 and limited to the 410 places already in existence.[30] The scheme was responsible for the development of some training colonies in the 1920s such as Burrow Hill Colony with 80 beds, administered by the NAPT which provided the first 20 beds. This colony was converted into a treatment and training colony for adolescent boys with tuberculosis in 1929.

Under the 1921 Public Health (Tuberculosis) Act, local authorities were only required to provide treatment for those cases which did not come under the purview of the Boards of Guardians, although they were encouraged to treat all cases. Thus, despite the expansion of

[27] PRO MH55/162, Ministry of Health Circular 182, Feb. 1921, Ministry of Health Circular, 1924.

[28] *Barlow Report*, pp. 13–15. For more detailed discussion of the nature of the different types of institutions, see Chapter 6, Section 1.

[29] PRO MH55/169, Murray Report, p. 4.

[30] PRO MH55/165, Ministry of Health Circular 307, 1919; ibid., Conference, 2 Aug. 1922; see also *Tubercle*, 3 (1922), 468.

tuberculosis institutions, in the 1920s many tuberculosis patients were still accommodated in Poor Law infirmaries. In London, for example, a survey revealed that 1,430 tuberculosis patients were accommodated in 25 Poor Law infirmaries.[31] There were 136 tuberculosis patients in Cardiff's Poor Law institution, the 'City Lodge', in 1929, and 220 in 1931.[32] Birmingham dealt with all cases of tuberculosis, including 'Poor Law cases', under its tuberculosis scheme, but it claimed to be the only local authority in England to do so.[33] By contrast, in South Shields all the tuberculosis patients were accommodated in the Poor Law infirmary.[34]

The 1929 Local Government Act, which abolished the Boards of Guardians and delegated their functions to Public Assistance Committees under the control of local authorities, encouraged the appropriation of the former Poor Law institutions for other public health purposes. One thousand tuberculosis beds were added to the tuberculosis services of the local authorities by the appropriation of such institutions. Three Poor Law institutions, as well as accommodation in another 43, were appropriated for tuberculosis treatment. Nevertheless, tuberculous patients continued to be accommodated in Poor Law—now Public Assistance—institutions. The East Sussex MO reported in 1938 that the county tuberculosis scheme was more or less complete with the exception of the treatment and isolation of chronic and advanced cases, for whom the only accommodation available was in Poor Law institutions paid for by the Public Assistance Committee and not the Public Health Committee.[35] In 1934 there were still 5,867 tuberculous patients treated in Public Assistance institutions in England and Wales, and 3,083 in 1938.[36]

While the number of beds for tuberculous patients increased in the 1930s, the number allocated for children with pulmonary tuberculosis declined. In 1929 that number was 1,438 in England (631 local authority and 807 voluntary), but by 1935 it had dropped to 1,274. Even then, the Chief Medical Officer of the Ministry of Health, Sir

[31] PRO MH55/145, LCC, Public Health Committee, Report 528, 2 Nov. 1922, p. 4.
[32] PRO MH96/1041 and 1042, R. Stephenson (Public Assistance Officer) to WNMA, 18 Jan. 1932 and 12 Jan. 1933.
[33] PRO MH52/231, Birmingham City Council, Maternity and Child Welfare and Tuberculosis Services, Investigation Report 1922–5, para. 54.
[34] M. A. Crowther, in P. Thane (ed.), *The Origin of British Social Policy* (London, 1978), 51.
[35] East Sussex County Record Office, 'Tuberculosis, General', 8 (1932–8), 1107, Box 237, Memo by CMO on Tuberculosis, 1938.
[36] *20th CMOH Annual Report 1938* (1939), 136.

Arthur MacNalty, reported that the supply of beds for children with pulmonary tuberculosis exceeded the demand. He explained that this was partly due to the more systematic and routine use of improved methods of diagnosis, including the Mantoux test (a tuberculin test) and X-ray examination (both of which, however, had been available since the early twentieth century). The number of children treated for pulmonary tuberculosis in English tuberculosis institutions dropped from almost 4,000 in 1932 to under 3,000 by 1938, and beds previously reserved for children were being closed or used for some other purpose.[37]

Children treated in tuberculosis institutions in earlier years had often been 'pre-tuberculous', suffering from malnutrition and not tuberculosis at all. There was indeed a policy to treat such potential patients. In 1938 in the West Wales Sanatorium, for example, there were 46 children, of whom 20 were 'definitely tuberculous' and 26 'observation cases'. It was reported that the diagnosis of tuberculosis in children was problematic in the absence of demonstrable disease, and that many were probably suffering from insufficient or incorrect feeding, but nevertheless it was believed that the effect of the sanatorium regime on these children was 'most beneficial'.[38] Similarly in Scotland in the 1920s, treatment was provided for 'tuberculised' children, 'where the diagnosis is by no means certain, but where during a period of observation at the dispensary no improvement in health has been noticeable'.[39]

Some of the tuberculosis institutions accommodated 200 patients or more. Large local authority institutions, which had already been established by 1920, included Hairmyres Sanatorium in Scotland with 250 beds, Yardley Road Sanatorium, Birmingham, with 300 beds, Fazakerley Sanatorium, Liverpool, with 240 beds, Baguley Sanatorium, Manchester, with 322 beds, Killingbeck Sanatorium, Leeds, with 168 beds, and Middleton Sanatorium, Yorkshire West Riding, with 200 beds. By 1931 this list also included Harefield, a Middlesex county sanatorium, with 322 beds, the Cheshire Joint Sanatorium with 240 beds, a Gloucestershire county sanatorium with 250 beds, and a Surrey county sanatorium, Milford, with 300 beds. The number of sanatoria in Scotland with more than 100 beds in 1929 was 19. Scotland in particular had a large number of institutions with

[37] *17th CMOH Annual Report 1935* (1936), 90; ibid., *1938* (1939), 137.
[38] *Welsh Gazette*, 18 Aug. 1938 (PRO MH96/1073).
[39] *9th Annual Report Scottish Board of Health 1927*, Cmd. 3112 (1928), 100.

few beds (44 sanatoria had fewer than 50 beds).[40] In the 1930s the situation changed little in Scotland, while in England some institutions were expanded and others were opened, so that by 1939 there were 28 English local authority institutions each with over 200 beds, as well as 19 voluntary institutions of that size. However, the average number of beds remained much lower, less than one hundred.[41]

Large institutions with modern technical equipment were generally too expensive for individual local authorities to establish. While the 1921 Public Health (Tuberculosis) Act enabled local authorities to form combined schemes, few had done so, largely as a result of local jealousies. The *NAPT Bulletin* maintained in 1945 that the so-called 'National Tuberculosis Scheme' was not one but many schemes since each local authority was virtually independent: 'In England there are some 49 counties and 79 county boroughs, and only five of them have combined together in their war against tuberculosis. The rest go their own way and there is no general staff.'[42] Those 5 local authorities had already combined to form two schemes by 1920: the Staffordshire, Wolverhampton, and Dudley Joint Board for Tuberculosis, and the Warwickshire and Coventry Joint Board. Gloucestershire County and Gloucester County Borough Councils had also formed a joint scheme by 1920, and Berkshire and Buckinghamshire jointly managed a sanatorium, but in other respects remained independent, as did East Riding and the City of York. In Scotland, the Local Government (Scotland) Act, 1929, gave power to two or more local authorities to combine for public health purposes. There were two joint boards for providing tuberculosis services, the Stirling and Clackmannan Joint Sanatorium Board and the South Eastern Counties of Scotland Joint Sanatorium Board. In the 1930s, the Aberdeen town council, and the county councils of Aberdeen and Kincardine combined to form the Aberdeen Regional Scheme of Tuberculosis. Wales was also, as discussed, administered as a joint scheme by the WNMA.

The inequalities of the facilities for the institutional treatment of tuberculosis were evident from the annual returns required by the Ministry of Health. During the year 1924/5, for example, the number of pulmonary tuberculous patients treated per 100 deaths varied from 27.9 in West Hartlepool, to 195 in Leeds. The length of treatment

---

[40] *Public Health* (1941), 159.
[41] Pinker, *Hospital Statistics*, p. 58.
[42] *NAPT Bulletin*, 7/6 (1945), 16. See also PRO MH55/1197, WBH, Brief for Minister of Health, 20 Mar. 1939, p. 50.

varied so that the percentage staying more than three months was 13.4 in Sunderland and 78.2 in Smethwick. The percentage of early cases receiving more than six months' treatment varied from 2.5 per cent in Wallasey to 57.5 per cent in Exeter, and the percentage of advanced cases staying over six months varied from 6.5 per cent in Leeds to 52.9 per cent in Northumberland.[43]

In 1929, the average number of beds per 100 deaths for the 7 authorities of Liverpool, Manchester, Glasgow, Birmingham, Sheffield, Lancashire, and West Riding of Yorkshire was 77, while that for Cardiff, Merthyr, Swansea, and Glamorgan was 42. Sheffield had the most generous supply with 151 beds per 100 deaths. England had an average of 69 beds per 100 deaths in 1929, and Wales 52.[44] Scotland was said in 1931 to have almost twice as many beds per thousand population as England.[45] The JTC drew up a chart showing the variations in 1937 (Table 5).

The variation in the work done in different districts was such that, according to the JTC in 1943, the prognosis of a case of tuberculosis not only depended on the clinical condition of the patient but also on the place of residence:

Mr. X may live on one side of a street which was under the control of an authority which provides every facility for modern treatment and sufficient accommodation to reduce the waiting period of admission to the sanatorium to a matter of a few days whilst Mr. Y, living on the opposite side of the road, may be under the control of another authority which has a small poorly equipped sanatorium so that the unfortunate individual has to wait weeks before he can receive proper care and treatment.[46]

That the prognosis would differ is in fact disputable, as will be discussed later. But what is clear is that resources were not equally allocated under a system of the financial independence of each local authority deriving its income partly from rates. The poorest areas, most in need of the facilities for dealing with a disease generally acknowledged to be associated with poverty, could least afford them.

(3) CHARGES FOR INSTITUTIONAL TREATMENT

The 1921 Public Health (Tuberculosis) Act provided for free institutional treatment for all sufferers from tuberculosis. However,

[43] PRO MH55/130, D. J. Williamson, Returns for 1925, 12 Jan. 1927, pp. 20–2.
[44] PRO MH75/6, WNMA, Proposed Hospital at Sully, 1931, p. 4.
[45] *EMJ* 38 (1931), 152–3. [46] *Tubercle*, 23 (1942), 92.

TABLE 5 *Estimated population, pulmonary tuberculosis deaths, and average number of beds per 100 tuberculosis deaths in different county and county borough areas, England and Wales, 1937*

	Estimated population 1937	Deaths from pulmonary tuberculosis	Average number of beds per 100 deaths
County Boroughs:			
(a) Doncaster, Southport, East-bourne, Blackpool, and Bolton	500,050	253	56
(b) South Shields, Bootle, Middlesbrough, Gateshead, and Tynemouth	509,770	497	33
County Administrative Areas:			
(a) Peterborough, Rutland, Lincolnshire (Holland), Buck-inghamshire, Sussex West, and Southampton	1,242,640	325	74
(b) Cardigan, Caernarfon, Pem-broke, Carmarthen, Merioneth, Anglesey, and Glamorgan	1,230,260	600	52

Source: *Tubercle*, 23 (1942), 35.

the Ministry of Health urged that local authorities should require a contribution from tuberculous patients towards the cost of treatment in those cases in which it could reasonably be demanded, other than ex-servicemen who contracted tuberculosis while on active service.[47]

Collection of contributions from patients was left to the discretion of the local authorities. Practices varied widely. In London, the task of assessment was carried out by local tuberculosis care committees, as recommended by the Ministry of Health. If the patient had an annual income below £160 and dependants, no contribution was demanded. When the income of the patient exceeded £160, the circumstances of the whole family were inquired into, and sometimes a payment required. Small contributions for children, equivalent to the cost of maintenance in a home, were also required.[48]

[47] PRO MH55/136, Circular 257, 3 Nov. 1921, p. 2.
[48] PRO MH96/1030, Ministry of Health Circular 308, 8 May 1922, para. 4; PRO MH55/173, Ministry of Health, 29 May 1926.

Other authorities, including Liverpool, Birmingham, Leicester, and Manchester, adopted no systematic policy of compulsory contributions from patients. The Liverpool Corporation explained that they did not realize that they could claim payments from insured patients, and considered the uninsured generally too poor to pay. The MOH for Birmingham, Sir John Robertson, maintained that it would be unwise to require a payment from patients in Birmingham for they generally came from the working classes, and it would make it more difficult to persuade them to enter the institution and remain for an extended period. The MOH for Manchester, R. Veitch Clark, stated that treatment in Manchester was only provided by the local authority for those cases who could not afford to make their own arrangements, and therefore charges were impracticable. He cited the experience of other contributory schemes, the payment of medical fees for attendance at confinement and the payment towards the supply of milk in the maternal and child welfare schemes, and claimed that the cost of recovering the amount due was often more than the actual sum recovered. He estimated from the London experience that Manchester should recover £1,300, but that the administrative cost would be approximately £600, for they had found that, unlike London, they could not rely on unpaid officials.[49]

Sir Ernest J. Strohmenger, Accountant General to the Ministry of Health, concluded in 1926 that the Ministry's policy of encouraging local authorities to recover charges from patients had been a total failure. The total cost of residential treatment in 1925–6 had amounted to £2,400,000 and total contributions amounted to £30,000. Of this sum, £12,000 had been collected by the LCC, £12,000 by other county councils, and £6,000 by county borough councils. Fourteen county councils and 37 county borough councils had collected no contributions. Even in London the contributions only amounted to 4 per cent of the total costs of the service.

The WNMA did not believe that tuberculous patients should be charged for treatment. In 1928 they resolved that charging any patient for residential treatment 'is quite impractical in Wales and Monmouthshire and is contrary to the principles upon which the fight against tuberculosis was established and has, so far, been conducted'.[50] The

[49] PRO MH55/173, correspondence between the Ministry of Health and the Corporations of Liverpool, Manchester, and Birmingham, 1926–8.
[50] PRO MH96/1036, WNMA, 18 Dec. 1926; PRO MH55/173, WBH, 20 Mar. 1928.

Tuberculosis Group of the Society for Medical Officers of Health and the Metropolitan Sub-group also resolved in 1925 that they were unanimously opposed to the whole principle of assessment for patients' payments.[51]

Sir George Newman disputed Strohmenger's suggestion in 1928 that 2 per cent should be deducted from the expenditure approved for Exchequer grants to encourage local authorities to collect contributions from patients. Providing a remarkably unflattering assessment of the sanatorium, Newman claimed that, although it provided the best known treatment for tuberculosis, it was not an attractive or popular institution: 'Everyone who has any margin of financial resource, or who can by any screwing and saving, keeps outside, if he can.' He pointed out that attempts to impose compulsory recovery of expenses in other fields of public health such as fevers, venereal diseases, and the school medical service provision of meals, had failed. Moreover, he added, tuberculosis was a disease which created poverty; it was not a short and foreseen episode like maternity for which there was indeed maternity benefit, but 'a long, drawn-out and blighting disability of the gravest kind'.

The only exception, according to Newman, was in the case of children. Just as charging a penny for school meals in the late nineteenth century had been seen as fostering a sense of parental responsibility, so Newman argued that requiring a contribution from parents for treatment of children would increase their self-respect and also be in the child's own interest. This he argued despite his own recognition of the failure of charges for school meals. He maintained that if no charges were made, the family had more to spend while the child was away and therefore might regard the child as a financial encumbrance on return.[52] A. B. Maclachlan of the Ministry of Health held a similarly cynical attitude to family ties; he argued that unless a charge were made, parents might be disposed to place obstacles in the way of receiving their child back again and to make life somewhat unpleasant for the child concerned.[53]

Sir John Robertson replied to this argument that in Birmingham during the sixteen years they had been treating tuberculosis, they had

[51] TG SMOH Minutes, 23 May 1925; Metrop. Sub-group Minutes, 20 Feb. 1925.
[52] PRO MH55/173, Strohmenger, 3 Jan. 1928; Newman, 21 Jan. 1928. On charges for school meals, see B. B. Gilbert, *The Evolution of National Insurance in Great Britain: The Origins of the Welfare State* (London, 1966), 307.
[53] PRO MH55/173, Birmingham Town Clerk to Robertson, 23 July 1926, and Strohmenger to Manchester Town Clerk, 16 June 1927.

known no case where there had been any desire on the part of the parents to keep their children in the institution. On the contrary he wrote that no week had passed but that they had to urge the parents to permit their children to stay in the sanatorium for a period sufficiently long for the cure of the patient.[54] The high premature discharge rate among children in tuberculosis institutions, discovered in an investigation in 1922, supports that view.[55]

Cambridgeshire County Council experienced difficulties in collecting contributions from patients in the 1920s. They demanded a contribution from insured patients of half their sickness or disablement benefit. However, patients could not always keep up weekly payments, as they received their benefits in a lump sum on leaving the institution, and yet, owing to their insecure future, were reluctant to commit themselves to paying on leaving. Moreover, as insured persons, they felt that free treatment was their due (as it had been before 1921), and in the institutions they often met patients sent by other local authorities, who were not required to pay. It was also pointed out, when the question of payments was being discussed in 1935, that demanding payments led to friction between patients and tuberculosis officers and added to the difficulties experienced by patients when they were suddenly confronted with the fact that they were suffering from a disease which would alter the whole course of their lives. In view of the small amount collected anyway, 2.5 per cent of the total costs in 1933, it was decided in 1935 to abandon compulsory payments.[56]

In Salford, contributions were collected from tuberculous patients until 1929. They had found that the 'Gilbertian' situation had arisen whereby the Corporation was assessing the patients and a voluntary charitable body was paying the contributions.[57] The LCC also abandoned compulsory payments in 1929, only accepting voluntary contributions from those who wanted to make a payment and could afford it, and the contributions were paid into the county fund.[58]

The Isle of Wight CC continued to require payments until 1942 when it wrote to the Ministry of Health asking for the official view in

    [54] PRO MH55/173, 24 July 1926.
    [55] *Tubercle*, 3 (1922), 443; see also M. S. Rice, *Working-class Wives* (London, 1939), 15, n. 1.
    [56] Cambridgeshire CC Public Health Tuberculosis Sub-committee, Minutes, 13 July 1935.
    [57] PRO MH55/173, Newman, 21 Jan. 1928; ibid., Ministry of Health to Salford Town Clerk, 5 Feb. 1929.
    [58] PRO MH55/1129, LCC Scheme for the Treatment of Tuberculosis in London 1936, LCC 3194, (London, 1936).

the light of the small amount collected and the small number of patients able to make contributions. The Ministry replied that it had formed the view that recovery of expenses from tuberculous patients was not desirable, and believed that the number of local authorities who demanded payment from tuberculous patients at that time was relatively few.[59]

(4) AFTER-CARE

In 1920, Newman reported that voluntary after-care committees had been established in many districts, as recommended by the LGB in 1915. However, he added that while some had done valuable work, in most cases their endeavours had not been sufficient to cope with the needs as a result of a lack of funds. Yet, rather than recommend subsidies for the work of the committees, he advised: 'Apart from material assistance, after-care committees can encourage ex-patients to make the best of existing conditions.'[60] The financial problems associated with this long drawn-out illness, often involving the loss of earnings, were considerable. Unless the patient were an ex-serviceman, under the 1911 National Insurance Act an insured worker who contracted tuberculosis would receive 10s. per week for the first 13 weeks of sickness (subsequently extended to 26 weeks), and 5s. disability benefit thereafter. By 1922 these benefits were 15s. and 7s. 6d. respectively, and by 1942 they were still no higher than 18s. and 10s. 6d.[61] These benefits were well below Seebohm Rowntree's stringent 'human needs minimum'. The only other recourse, and the only recourse for the uninsured, was private charity or the dreaded Poor Law (or 'Public Assistance' after 1929).

The 1921 Public Health (Tuberculosis) Act empowered local authorities in England and Wales to provide after-care for tuberculous patients. They were permitted to provide office facilities for after-care

---

[59] PRO MH55/1288, Isle of Wight CC, TO to Ministry of Health, 7 Nov. 1942, and reply (Deputy Senior MO), 11 Nov. 1942.

[60] *2nd CMOH Annual Report 1920* (1921), 101.

[61] By contrast, ex-servicemen with tuberculosis aggravated by military service received 37s. 6d per week plus allowances of 9s. 2d. for wife, 7s. 1d. for first child, and 5s. 5d. for each other child: MRC, *Report of Committee on Tuberculosis in War-time* (SRS 246; London, 1942), 20. For dependent wives there was no assistance available, financial or otherwise (as is also discussed in Chapter 7), making it difficult for them to accept institutional treatment.

committees; and £2 per thousand population per annum for the relief of patients could be included in the expenditure approved for an Exchequer grant. This arrangement continued until the 1929 Local Government Act replaced the percentage grant to local authorities for health services with a block grant. Local authorities were still empowered to provide after-care, which was later incorporated into the 1936 Public Health Act.

After-care work in tuberculosis was based on the principles of the old Charity Organisation Society, which had pioneered 'case-work' in Britain. Under the COS system, social workers inquired carefully into the backgrounds of their clients and those who were found worthy were given help, such as cash and tools to carry on a trade or assistance in finding a job, and were regularly visited until they could 'stand on their own feet'. Those whose 'condition is due to improvidence or thriftlessness and there is no hope of being able to make them independent in the future' were left to destitution or the Poor Law. Leaders of the COS argued that many charities were encouraging the 'demoralization' of the poor by handing out benefits in cash and kind too readily and with no attempt to ensure long-term improvement in the client's condition.[62] Likewise, tuberculosis after-care committees were told to inquire carefully into the finances of the whole family, and those who would have been poor had tuberculosis not intervened, or who could not be made financially independent again, were to be left to the Poor Law. In 1923, F. J. H. Coutts, Senior MO in the Ministry of Health, in charge of supervising anti-tuberculosis work, outlined the role of the tuberculosis after-care committees:

The tendency of some Care Committees, in the past, has been to consider that their main function was to provide material assistance, usually in the form of financial help, and the labours of such Committees have had little success . . . their true function is not attained if they merely transform themselves into a kind of additional Public Assistance Committee . . . Care Committees should . . . constantly keep before them the importance of avoiding as far as possible anything that will undermine the patient's self-reliance, and find ways of giving assistance whilst safe-guarding the patient's self-respect and independence. The aim should be to help the patient to help himself rather than to allow him to be dependent upon others.

It is important that a patient should be taught that, although his disease has left him with a, perhaps permanently, damaged life requiring constant care, self-denial and watchfulness on his part, it is still his duty to seize every

62 On COS, see P. Thane, *Foundations of the Welfare State* (London, 1982), 22.

opportunity of becoming a useful and self-supporting member of the community. It follows, therefore, that a Care Committee should restrict the actual giving of financial assistance as much as possible.[63]

In the opinion of S. D. Rowlands, TO for Gateshead, financial assistance should not be given, as it tended to stop the initiative of the individual patient.[64] Nevertheless, just as many who subscribed to COS principles found it difficult to abandon to destitution or the Poor Law those who were in desperate and immediate need, so many of the tuberculosis after-care committees in the event performed the function of a charitable organization helping those in the most desperate need. For example, the tuberculosis after-care committee for the Borough of Hastings reported in 1925 that quite a number of 'advanced and helpless cases' were on their books: 'They are cheered by our visits, their last days rendered more comfortable by little extras, and in several instances it has been possible to provide . . . nursing requisites, which were not easily available from any other source.' Typical help given by the committee for such cases was one pint of milk and one egg per day, and half a pound of butter and one tin of Ovaltine per week.[65]

As with dispensary and institutional provision, there was great variation in after-care work performed from one area to another. The *NAPT Handbook* recorded that 68 out of 122 English local authorities had made no after-care arrangements in 1919, and neither had 53 out of 125 authorities by 1939. More county boroughs than counties had made arrangements. While Somerset, Shropshire, and Surrey had 26, 25, and 19 after-care committees respectively in their counties, in some other areas of England the work was done by the local tuberculosis officer, public health committee, the Insurance Committee, the Council of Social Service, the Guild of Help, or the Hospitals' Committee. After-care work in Wales (as will be further discussed) was negligible. Only 46 of the 110 after-care committees affiliated to the NAPT in 1942 received grants from local authorities.[66] The importance attached to after-care work by local authorities in general therefore must be assumed to have been minimal. Much depended on the initiative of the local medical officer of health, tuberculosis officer,

[63] *9 NAPT 1923*, pp. 275–7.   [64] *18 NAPT 1932*, p. 122.
[65] East Sussex County Record Office, HH58/7, Borough of Hastings Tuberculosis Care Committee Annual Report 1924–5 (1925), 5; Borough of Hastings Tuberculosis Care Committee Minute Books, 1930s.
[66] *Tubercle*, 23 (1942), 86.

public health committee, or voluntary after-care committee. The TO of Wallasey, for example, set up a malnutrition clinic for children in 1923 (attached to the tuberculosis dispensary) which he believed was an important preventive agent.[67]

As noted in the Political and Economic Planning Report on Health Services in Britain in 1936, after-care work had not been developed in Scotland.[68] By 1938, out of the 55 tuberculosis schemes in the counties and burghs of Scotland, only 9 had after-care committees. Some of those were synonymous with the pubic health committee which, in the view of the *EMJ*, meant that they were not after-care committees in the real sense of the term.[69]

Some local authorities had special rehousing schemes for families with tuberculous patients. Sheffield, Middlesbrough, and Leeds were pioneers in this area. The Sheffield Corporation introduced a re-housing scheme in 1928. The rent charged was carefully proportioned on a sliding scale to the income and size of the family and was subsidized by the Public Health Committee. By 1933, 171 families had been rehoused, at a cost of £700 per annum. Middlesbrough introduced a similar scheme in 1931. By 1935, 61 families with a tuberculous patient had been accommodated on a Corporation housing estate; £300 per annum was allowed by the Corporation for this purpose, rising to £500 in 1934. Leeds also started a scheme in 1929 whereby 10 per cent of the council houses built (almost 400 by 1942) were 'sunshine' houses, in which the windows could be completely opened on one side, for families with a tuberculous patient. By 1936, 241 families had been rehoused, with subsidized rent. Glasgow introduced a similar scheme for rehousing tuberculous patients in 1929, and by 1949 new houses had been allotted to 1,849 families with a tuberculous patient. By 1939, rent differentiation schemes existed in 110 local authorities, some of which gave special preference to tuberculous patients.[70]

Various employment schemes operated for tuberculous patients as well, financed by local authorities, modelled on a scheme in New York,

[67] *Medical Officer*, 42 (1929), 217; *Tubercle*, 12 (1930), 31.

[68] Political and Economic Planning, *Report on Health Services in Britain* (London, 1936), 288.

[69] *EMJ* 50 (1943), 216.

[70] Details on rehousing schemes are found in PRO MH96/1030, 1934, and 1935; *16th CMOH Annual Report 1934* (1935), 80; *Tubercle*, 20 (1939), 281, and ibid., 23 (1942), 153. For Glasgow, see B. R. Clarke, *Causes and Prevention of Tuberculosis* (Edinburgh and London, 1952), 148.

Altro Workshop, which had been set up by a Committee for the Care of Jewish Tuberculous in 1915. The best known scheme in Britain was the 'Factory-in-the-Fields' set up voluntarily in Leeds by an ex-sanatorium patient for ex-servicemen with tuberculosis. The factory, where firewood was chopped and firelighters and brushes produced, employed approximately 100 men with tuberculosis in 1925. In 1927, following closure of the factory owing to financial problems, the Corporation of Leeds purchased it for £10,000, and reorganized the work. Forty men were now employed, at a cost to the Corporation of around £2,000 per annum.[71] The LCC also financed a scheme known as 'Spero Workshops'. In Hull, the Public Health Committee started a scheme in 1924 which provided work for 6 tuberculous men as official attendants at the various motor parks in the city; by 1938, approximately 45 men had been employed there. Five ex-patients were regularly employed in Sheffield Corporation hospitals as gardeners, porters, or carpark attendants. A few other small schemes existed, but all the schemes together, including those financed voluntarily, did not employ more than 300 ex-sanatorium patients in 1939, although possibly more were employed in the sanatoria themselves.[72]

Some areas had more comprehensive anti-tuberculosis schemes than others. The scheme in Edinburgh was described in 1937 as 'world famous'. It was still based on the model established by Sir Robert Philip in 1887, and included institutional treatment and after-care.[73] The Edinburgh scheme was not, however, typical of schemes in Scotland. In England, the Lancashire tuberculosis service was widely praised as a model scheme. This scheme co-ordinated institutional treatment with after-care and home treatment. The Lancashire CC gave a grant to voluntary after-care committees amounting to a third (a half after 1929) of their costs, and in areas with no after-care committee the Council commissioned the dispensary staff to be responsible for after-care in their area. The Central TO for Lancashire, Lissant Cox, boasted that the whole of Lancashire was covered by a 'complete and comprehensive scheme', and that the tuberculosis work was 'well organised with a close combination of the hospital, dispensary and domiciliary sides of the work, which enables the problem of prevention and treatment to be seen as a whole'.[74]

[71] *Tubercle,* 23 (1942), 7.
[72] Ibid.; *24 NAPT 1938,* p. 10; *NAPT Bulletin,* 9/5 (1946), 149.
[73] *EMJ* 44 (1937), 288.
[74] Lancashire CC, Annual Report of Central Tuberculosis Officer 1927, 87; J. D.

The organization of the tuberculosis service in London was based on a three-cornered arrangement by the LCC, the MAB, and the metropolitan borough councils, until 1930 when the MAB was abolished and its functions taken over by the LCC. From 1920 the 28 metropolitan borough councils and the city council administered the dispensaries, the MAB managed the tuberculosis institutions, and the LCC was the official overseer of the tuberculosis service. Lissant Cox was critical of the bureaucracy of the scheme in London. He pointed out that if institutional treatment were decided upon by the tuberculosis officer at the dispensary, the recommendation had to go to a different authority, the LCC, and when patients were sent to an institution they came under yet another authority, the MAB. Thus, 'the dispensary or public health side of tuberculosis in London is divorced from the institutional side'. Nor did the abolition of the MAB alter the situation, according to Cox, as there was still little co-ordination between the dispensaries and the institutions.[75]

Nevertheless, a great deal of after-care work was carried out in London. One unusual scheme developed in London was the removal of babies at birth from tuberculous mothers; if they were still infectious after twelve months the mothers were encouraged to foster out the children to relatives or make other arrangements. There was also a scheme which started in 1925 for the boarding out of children of a tuberculous parent; a grant of £3,000 per annum in 1930, rising to £15,000 per annum by 1939, was paid by the LCC to the Invalid Children's Aid Association for that purpose. Approximately 200 were boarded out per annum. Voluntary after-care committees existed in the majority of the metropolitan boroughs. The after-care committee attached to Paddington dispensary was particularly active, with an open-air school and a Sea and Sun Club to arrange holidays for tuberculous children and mothers. After-care committees in 12 boroughs ran handicraft classes for ex-sanatorium patients. The LCC paid a grant of £500 per annum to the Spero Workshop for tuberculous ex-sanatorium patients and provided a market for the wood bundled in the factories. Spero had been started in 1923 by the Central Fund for the Industrial Welfare of Tuberculous Persons which previously, under a different title, had been responsible for the

Marshall and M. E. McClintock (eds.), *The History of Lancashire County Council 1889–1974* (London, 1977), 31, 295; see also *17 NAPT 1931*, pp. 161–2, and *21 NAPT 1935*, p. 30.

[75] *14 NAPT 1928*, p. 133; *20 NAPT 1934*, p. 47.

voluntary tuberculosis dispensaries in London. The LCC also employed 12 tuberculous ex-patients and 5 boys each year from the NAPT Burrow Hill Colony in its Parks Department. As already noted, London pioneered open-air schools for delicate or 'pre-tuberculous' children. By 1939 there were 15 open-air schools in London for 2,000 children (6 of which, accommodating 500 pupils, were reserved exclusively for confirmed tuberculosis cases). Open-air classes were also held in the London parks, attended by over 6,000 children. Thus, even if the institutional side of the scheme was separate from the dispensary, after-care, and preventive aspects, the tuberculosis service in London was active in all areas.[76]

This was not the case in Wales, where anti-tuberculosis services came under the charge of the WNMA. The WNMA did not consider after-care to lie within its purview; it perceived its function as providing an institutional service. On the other hand, local authorities felt that, as they were paying large sums of money to the WNMA for anti-tuberculosis services, all aspects of the campaign should be adequately covered.

In 1937, when the WNMA was drafting its budget for the next five years, with annual expenditure estimated to exceed £380,850 by 1941–2, the Welsh local authorities staged a protest. Alderman Waterhouse of Flintshire CC pointed out that the expenditure upon services operated by the Association swallowed up to 50 per cent of the gross expenditure on health services in the county of Flint: 'Having regard to the fact that tuberculosis is responsible for only 7 per cent of the deaths in Wales it seems to us that this expenditure is all out of proportion.' Lloyd Williams of Denbighshire CC calculated that the expenditure of the Association would mean five-eighths of the county's total expenditure on public health and asked: 'Was it strictly fair that the 93 per cent of the deaths from the other causes, which they would wish to see reduced, should have only 50 per cent of the public health expenditure?' A Monmouthshire councillor pointed out that during the previous year his Council had paid a 6.5 pence rate to the Association, and only spent 3.8 pence on maternity and child welfare. The high cost of tuberculosis services was held responsible for the small amount available for maternal and mental services.[77]

[76] *17 NAPT 1931*, p. 150; *20 NAPT 1934*, p. 37; *24 NAPT 1938*, pp. 8, 28; *NAPT Handbook*, 10th edn. (London, 1939), 22; G. Gibbon and R. W. Bell, *History of the London County Council 1889–1939* (London, 1939), 306.

[77] *Western Mail*, 30 Jan. and 17 Mar. 1937 (PRO MH75/26).

The WNMA had included provision for after-care in this budget for the first time, allocating £10,000 per annum for this purpose, calculated from Lancashire's experience. However, after-care accounted for only a small part of the increased budget which also included provision for a new hospital in Swansea and a new research department. The dispute over finances led to the setting up of the Committee of Inquiry into Anti-tuberculosis Service in Wales and Monmouthshire in 1937, chaired by Clement Davies, Liberal MP for Montgomeryshire and later leader of the Liberal Party. The main question to be decided by the committee was whether preventive and after-care work should be undertaken by the WNMA or local authorities.[78]

The Committee concluded that preventive and after-care work, because such work touched on every aspect of public health, was rightly the responsibility of local authorities. It strongly reprimanded the local authorities and the Welsh Board of Health for neglecting preventive work—housing, sanitation, and after-care of ex-sanatorium patients. The rural areas were seen as the main culprits, in contrast to the 'public-spiritedness' of some of the depressed industrial areas of south Wales. The WNMA was praised for conducting an efficient institutional service. Yet, in focusing blame on local authorities and the Welsh Board of Health, the Committee of Inquiry did not question whether the WNMA, however efficiently it provided a hospital service, was in the best public interest of Wales.[79] Lissant Cox maintained in 1941 (a viewpoint which was repeated by MacNalty two years later) that 'the very excellence of the Memorial Association scheme on the diagnosis and treatment side seems to have been an excuse for neglect on the preventive side'.[80] Local authorities found themselves paying for an increasingly expensive curative service as well as for research. In England local authorities did not become so involved in tuberculosis research, but left it largely to the MRC paid for by a direct Exchequer grant and not by local rates. Following the Inquiry, local authorities in Wales were required to introduce preventive measures independently, involving an even greater expenditure on tuberculosis. By 1942, 10 of the 17 local authorities in Wales had established an after-care scheme

[78] PRO MH75/26, WNMA deputation, 27 Apr. 1937.

[79] See L. Bryder, 'The King Edward VII Welsh National Memorial Association and its Policy towards Tuberculosis in Wales, 1910–48', *The Welsh History Review*, 13/2 (1986), 194–216.

[80] *Public Health*, (1941), 138, 162; A. S. MacNalty, *The Reform of the Public Health Services* (Oxford, 1943), 68.

for tuberculous patients, while others were formulating schemes for doing so. At the same time the expenditure of the WNMA increased to £360,000, an increase which was agreed to by the local authorities almost unanimously. The heightened concern for tuberculosis in Wales resulting from the publicity given to the Inquiry probably accounted for this subsequent acquiescence. Two councillors described the increases from £235,000 to £360,000 in five years (an increase of 53 per cent) as alarming, and believed that, as a result of these high charges to the Association which dealt mainly with treatment, there was a danger of crippling other public health services. Yet, another commentator expressed surprise that there should be any objections so soon after the publication of the Anti-Tuberculosis Inquiry.[81]

During the inter-war period, tuberculosis became an integral part of the public health services of the local authorities. By the late 1930s there were two respects in which the service was coming under criticism. First, the system whereby initiative depended on individual authorities and on the financial capacity of local ratepayers was criticized as inefficient and causing an uneven distribution of resources. As in other areas, such as general hospitals, there were demands for greater central control and co-ordination. F. Temple Clive, medical superintendent of Benenden, for example, pointed out in 1940 the 'amazing discrepancies which exist in the facilities available to tuberculosis patients in different parts of the country'. He asked, 'Should not the whole problem of tuberculosis be dealt with on a national basis, not subject to the vicissitudes, financial or otherwise, of Local Authorities?'[82] Thus there were demands for a national health service. Second, there was some criticism of the direction of resource allocation within the individual schemes. The major emphasis of the service was on institutional treatment, which had also attracted voluntary contributions after the war. Little status and finance accrued to dispensaries and their administrators. Even Lancashire, held up as a model because the public health and institutional sides of the service were co-ordinated, spent 70 per cent of its tuberculosis funds on institutional treatment (the percentage in Scotland was 85).[83] The scheme in Wales was criticized on this score. In 1939 the Committee

[81] PRO MH75/31, WBH, Hughes to Rowland, Conference with local authorities, 10 Mar. 1939; ibid., 28 Mar. 1939, pp. 10–12.

[82] *Lancet*, 1 (1940), 291.

[83] *24 NAPT 1938*, p. 60; *10th Annual Report Scottish Board of Health 1928*, Cmd. 3304 (1929), 201.

of Inquiry into Anti-Tuberculosis Service in Wales and Monmouthshire pointed out that 'Early attention to the sociological problems
arising from the occurrence of tuberculosis in a household is often as
urgent in the interests of the patient and of the family as the medical
treatment of the individual sufferer.'[84] MacNalty also maintained in
that year that 'A striking feature of the modern outlook on
tuberculosis is the public recognition of its social and economic
setting. Tuberculosis is no longer solely a disease of medical
significance and relegated entirely to the physician and the surgeon.'[85]
Thus there were demands for greater social security for tuberculous
patients. Two important aspects of the post-Second World War
welfare state, the national health service and social security, were
therefore being advocated in the inter-war period in the context of
tuberculosis. In the following chapters the nature of epidemiological
studies and the preventive and curative measures adopted in the inter-
war period will be discussed. These led to the demand for a better
social security system and at the same time, paradoxically, for an
increasing investment in, and greater access to, the existing (curative)
services.

[84] *Clement Davies Report* (London, 1939), 102.
[85] A. S. MacNalty, preface to P. D'Arcy Hart and G. P. Wright, *Tuberculosis and Social Conditions* (London, 1939), p. v.

4

Causal Factors in Tuberculosis

THE causal connection between tuberculosis and such factors as housing, sanitation, nutrition, race, and certain modes of behaviour was widely studied and discussed in the inter-war period. This chapter considers the reasons for a heightened interest in this issue at that time, the problems inherent in the available data, the results of major studies, and the viewpoints of dominant authorities in the field. A very clear division emerged between those who believed in individual responsibility for contracting the disease and those who considered environment the dominant factor. The discourse penetrated far beyond the academic arena to the political world, charged as it was with social and political implications.

(1) EPIDEMIOLOGICAL RESEARCH

Research into all aspects of tuberculosis—epidemiology, aetiology, bacteriology, and methods of prevention and cure—expanded in the inter-war period following the establishment of the 'National Tuberculosis Service'. The Departmental Committee on Tuberculosis had recommended in 1913 that 'concurrently with the measures for prevention, detection and treatment, provision should be made for increasing by way of research the existing knowledge of the disease and of methods for its prevention, detection and cure'.[1] Major Greenwood, later president of the Royal Statistical Society and professor of epidemiology and vital statistics at the London School of Hygiene and Tropical Medicine, equated knowledge with the power to control. He looked forward in 1919 to a time, within the next decade, when more statistical information would be available so that 'much which is now speculative or hypothetical will be put to the proof and our knowledge of the epidemiology of phthisis and power to control the disease thereby extended'.[2]

[1] Astor Committee, Final Report, i. 13.
[2] M. Greenwood, 'The Epidemiology of Pulmonary Tuberculosis', in 1st CMOH Annual Report 1919–20 (1920), 348.

The importance attached to research led to the establishment of the Medical Research Committee, financed by the 'sanatorium benefit' funds created under the 1911 National Insurance and Finance Acts (until 1920 when it became the Medical Research Council receiving a direct Exchequer grant). The central institute of the MRC, for which one-third of the funds was allocated, included a department of statistics, as well as departments of bacteriology, pharmacology, and applied physiology. Epidemiology was to be studied by the statistics department under John Brownlee, formerly medical superintendent of Rushill Hospital, Glasgow, and a disciple of the statistician, Karl Pearson. The department began with a study of tuberculosis in the boot and shoe industry on which a report was published in 1915. It was also reported to be considering tuberculosis in the printing trade.[3] However, the work of the department was interrupted by the First World War when it became involved in compiling army medical statistics. Following the war, Brownlee continued to direct the statistics department until his death in 1927, and Major Greenwood was appointed chairman of the statistical committee in 1920, which after 1927 was transferred to the London School of Hygiene and Tropical Medicine where Greenwood had been appointed professor.

The initial investment by the MRC in statistical research seemed surprising to Landsborough Thomson, writing its history.[4] It can in fact only be explained in the context of the early importance attached to tuberculosis in the research programme of the Medical Research Committee, an emphasis which was not subsequently sustained. After 1918, no further major epidemiological studies into tuberculosis were initiated by the MRC until 1947, apart from one in association with the Industrial Fatigue Board in 1929 on the printing trade.[5] This neglect occurred despite the fact that the Registrar-General continued to record excessive tuberculosis incidence in certain industries including the boot and shoe industry. The shift of interest of the MRC was clearly related to the research interests of its administrators, specifi-

[3] MRC, *First Report of the Special Investigation Committee upon the Incidence of Phthisis in Relation to Occupations: The Boot and Shoe Industry* (SRS 1; London, 1915); *MRC 1st Annual Report 1914–15*, Cd. 8101 (1914–16), 25.

[4] A. L. Thomson, *Half a Century of Medical Research, i, Origins and Policy of the Medical Research Council (UK)* (London, 1973), 114.

[5] MRC and Industrial Fatigue Research Board, A. B. Hill, *An Investigation in the Sickness Experience of Printers (with Special Reference to the Incidence of Tuberculosis)*, 54 (London, 1929); A. M. Stewart and J. P. Hughes, *BMJ* 1 (1949), 926; ibid., 1 (1951), 899.

cally its secretary, Sir Walter Fletcher. The MRC did not play a major role in tuberculosis research, despite its initial association with 'sanatorium benefit'.[6]

It was pointed out in 1948 that it was curious that of all the generous bequests for research into serious diseases, few were concerned with tuberculosis, a disease which accounted for more deaths between 15 and 24 years of age in Britain than any other condition.[7] One bequest was the Dorothy Cross Research Fellowship, established in 1929, to be administered by the MRC and valued up to £800 per annum. Dorothy Cross, who died of tuberculosis in 1927, left £40,000 to her mother who decided to devote the whole of it as a memorial to her daughter and son (who had also died of tuberculosis) for research into tuberculosis. An indication that tuberculosis research was not perhaps a priority of the MRC was that the Second Secretary, Landsborough Thomson, attempted in 1935 to have the fellowship extended to include other branches of medical study. It was only the obstinacy of Mrs Cross that prevented this.[8] Another endowment for research into tuberculosis was the Cecil Prosser Research Scholarship, valued at £200 per annum, established in 1925 at the Welsh National School of Medicine. The largest endowment for tuberculosis research was that bequeathed by J. M. G. Prophit, a Calcutta merchant who had died in 1924 and left £120,000 for medical research to be divided equally between tuberculosis and cancer, which, on the death of his sister, the surviving beneficiary, became available in 1931.[9] In general, tuberculosis did not attract as much beneficence for research purposes as did cancer. G. D. H. and M. I. Cole pointed out in 1937 that the financial provision for research into the causes and treatment of cancer had been lavish in comparison with the provision made for research into most other diseases, which they attributed to the fact that cancer was a disease hardly less prevalent among the rich than among the poor.[10]

Much of the research into tuberculosis in the inter-war period was carried out and financed by organizations and individuals directly

---

[6] L. Bryder, 'Tuberculosis and the Medical Research Council, 1911–1939', *SSHM Bulletin 37* (1985), 68–71.

[7] *NAPT Bulletin*, 11/4 (1948), 140.

[8] *Daily Chronicle*, 29 Aug. 1929 (MRC, 1615, i); MRC, 1615, iii, Thomson to Treasury Solicitor, 4 Feb. 1935.

[9] For the results of the survey see M. Daniels, F. Ridehalgh, U. H. Springett, and I. M. Hall, *Tuberculosis in Young Adults, Report on the Prophit Tuberculosis Survey 1935–1944*, Royal College of Physicians (London, 1948).

[10] G. D. H. and M. I. Cole, *The Condition of Britain* (London, 1937), 105.

concerned with the prevention and treatment of the disease. The WNMA had an active research department, and financed a few epidemiological studies such as those by H. D. Chalke, J. Glyn Cox, and R. C. Hutchinson. The NAPT financed one major survey on tuberculosis in Tyneside in 1933, which cost £2,500.[11]

In the USA, the National Tuberculosis Association sponsored much research, with a large source of finance from its annual seal sales amounting to £2 million sterling by 1929. The first major investigation conducted by the NTA, but sponsored by the Metropolitan Life Insurance Company who contributed $200,000 to the work, was the Framingham Community and Health Demonstration, carried out from 1916 to 1923, under which approximately a third (5,000) of the population of Framingham, 'a typical American industrial community', was examined for tuberculosis. The anti-tuberculosis campaign in the USA was subsequently described as 'solidly based on scientific research'.[12] The NTA appointed a committee on medical research in 1921, and the research plan adopted was, according to R. H. Shryock, unusually comprehensive in scope. During the next twenty years the NTA distributed about $650,000 in various research grants, 'a scale of support which was unusual among societies dealing with a single disease'.[13]

The British counterpart, the NAPT, had fewer resources at its disposal, although it did have some—appeal campaigns from 1926 to 1929 raised over £110,000 for the work of the Association, and seal sales which commenced in 1933 had raised more than £50,000 by 1939.[14] These campaigns were conducted by 'idle ladies' of the upper classes in the nineteenth-century tradition, and included a dinner at the Mansion House in London which raised over £17,000, as well as balls, dances, and bridge parties in various parts of the country. Ivy Titchfield (the Marchioness of Titchfield, later the Duchess of Titchfield, and chairman of the NAPT from 1938) was prominent in

[11] F. C. S. Bradbury, *Causal Factors in Tuberculosis* (London, 1933); Chalke Report; PRO MH55/1192, WNMA, J. G. Cox, Report of an Investigation into the Incidence of Tuberculosis in the County of Anglesey and the Urban District of Barry (Cardiff, 1937); R. C. Hutchinson, 'Tuberculosis in a Welsh Parish', *Tubercle*, 2 (1921), 345–9.

[12] M. M. Torchia, 'Tuberculosis among American Negroes: Medical Research on a Racial Disease, 1850–1950', *Journal of the History of Medicine and Allied Sciences*, 32 (1977), 256.

[13] R. H. Shryock, *American Medical Research, Past and Present* (New York, 1947), 111, 112.

[14] NAPT Council Annual Report 1928, p. 1; ibid., 1938, p. 15.

organizing the campaigns, her 'energy and charm' being held largely responsible for their success.[15] According to P. D'Arcy Hart, the NAPT was a 'society for ladies and gentlemen'.[16] Tuberculosis specialists did not regard the NAPT as a professional organization, dissociating themselves from it by setting up their own association, the Tuberculosis Society. Founded in 1911, the Society had 200 members by 1919. Withdrawing from the NAPT meant, however, that it did not have the resources of NAPT at its disposal. Nor was there close contact between the NAPT and the MRC.[17] The NAPT itself, unlike the American Association, was primarily concerned with the education of the public in the means of prevention rather than with research.

The more professional body, the Tuberculosis Society, amalgamated in 1928 with the Society of Medical Superintendents of Tuberculosis Institutions (founded in 1919), to form the Tuberculosis Association. Research by the TA, according to its History, was conducted on a 'financial shoestring'.[18] A Tuberculosis Group of the Society for Medical Officers of Health was also formed in 1920 (one of the first SMOH Groups which were formed from 1919) and had 180 members by 1930. Its primary aim was 'to promote study and discussion of subjects relating to the prevention and treatment of tuberculosis and to safeguard the interests of all members of the medical profession specially interested in the control of the disease'. While one of the aims of the TG SMOH was 'to collect and co-ordinate statistics', its main attention was focused on ensuring that salaries of tuberculosis officers did not fall below the minimum laid down by the Ministry of Health.[19] Sub-groups of the TG SMOH were also founded in 1920, including a Metropolitan Sub-group with similar aims to the central Group. Other organizations founded at this time included the North Western Tuberculosis Society (initially the Lancashire and Westmorland Tuberculosis Society), and the North of England Tuberculosis Society.

An attempt was made to pool the resources of the various groups for

[15] NAPT Council Minutes, 26 July 1926, p. 119; ibid., 24 Jan. 1927, p. 135.

[16] P. D'Arcy Hart, interview, 20 May 1983. Indeed Philip said in 1933 that the NAPT was not a doctors' association and they wanted 'laymen' to have 'more than an equivalent voice in discussions': *19 NAPT 1933*, p. 47.

[17] MRC 205/1.

[18] *British Thoracic Association (The First Fifty Years)* (London, 1978), 74.

[19] SMOH C14/I, Minutes of Special General Meeting, TG SMOH, Constitution, 22 Oct. 1921; the setting up of a Salaries Committee was reported at a previous meeting, 14 Jan. 1921.

research purposes in 1924 when the Joint Tuberculosis Council was founded under the chairmanship of T. Peyton, county TO for Cheshire. The JTC aimed to co-ordinate the work of various organizations interested in the study and treatment of tuberculosis, to promote study and research, and act as an advisory body to Government departments, local authorities, and others. In 1938 membership included six representatives from the TA, three from the TG SMOH, two from each of the NWTS, the NETS, the WNMA, the NAPT, and the BMA, one from the council of the SMOH, one from the (newly formed) Society of Thoracic Surgeons of Great Britain and Ireland, one each from the Ministry of Health and Ministry of Pensions, as well as ten other members of the medical profession, whom the Council decided to co-opt. The majority of the members had local authority (or WNMA) appointments. A research committee was set up by the Council in 1924 under the chairmanship of Roodhouse Gloyne, pathologist at the City of London Hospital for Diseases of the Chest and editor of the *Tubercle*. The Council did not succeed in channelling the resources of the NAPT into research. The JTC became in effect a subsidiary of the TA, or at least the TA saw it that way judging from the amount of space in the aforementioned official History of the TA devoted to the JTC before it was eventually amalgamated with the TA in 1966. Although it was financed by a subscription from its members and a grant from the MRC, the JTC was constantly faced with the problem of inadequate staff and facilities for having its reports edited and published 'in a proper fashion'.[20] In the late 1930s some attempt was made to amalgamate the various societies. The NAPT was said to be the most resistant to the idea, specifically the chairman, Sir Robert Philip.[21]

While research was not co-ordinated or financed as well as in the USA, the various organizations were responsible for stimulating discussion and research which could be reported in the journals devoted to tuberculosis subjects, specifically the *British Journal of Tuberculosis* and the *Tubercle*, founded in 1907 and 1919 respectively. The publication of scientific papers was a part of the process by which tuberculosis officers sought acceptance in the scientific medical community as specialists, as well as being a result of their increasing specialization. ·

[20] PRO MH55/1120, JTC memo, 6 July 1936, pp. 1–2.
[21] PRO MH55/1124, Jameson to MacNalty, 28 July 1937.

(2) DATA ON WHICH RESEARCH WAS BASED

The existence of the dispensaries themselves further facilitated research. For no other disease was there such a large body of statistics available. The tuberculosis dispensary was described in 1925 as 'an out-patient department, stocked with drugs which are mostly placebos, or an annexe of an office for the compilation of statistics'.[22] Paddington dispensary, for example, was reported to be engaged in an 'interesting inquiry': 'By means of statistical cards we are tabulating details concerning the environment in which every patient who has passed through our hands has lived or still lives.'[23] Lissant Cox reported on the Lancashire scheme: 'Special mention may be made of the arrangement whereby a tuberculosis health visitor writes out a report on the environmental conditions of every new case of tuberculosis.'[24] Notification records, although sometimes initially kept separately by the medical officer of health, were generally held at the dispensaries.

Data from notification records did not, however, form a reliable basis for research. Notification was not administered very thoroughly at first, but the disorganization caused by the First World War was held responsible. The Ministry of Health issued regulations in 1921 stressing the importance of keeping the notification records up to date. In 1924 further regulations were issued when Newman discovered that 'in some areas, the tuberculosis notification register was either non-existent or had not been revised and kept up to date, so that the Medical Officer of Health was unaware as to the number of notified cases of tuberculosis in his area'.[25] A third set of regulations was issued in 1930. However, a committee set up in 1945 by the JTC to discuss the notification of tuberculosis, reported: 'Revision of the registers in some districts is rarely done and thus statistics based on existing registers may be highly misleading.'[26]

Evidence suggested that even those who did attempt to keep the records up to date did not have accurate data at their disposal. M. Greenwood and A. E. Tebb wrote in their report for the Medical Research Committee in 1919,

---

[22] *The Lancet*, 1 (1921), 258; G. S. Woodhead, C. Allbutt, and P. C. Varrier-Jones, *Papworth: Administrative and Economic Problems in Tuberculosis* (Cambridge, 1925), 62.
[23] *19 NAPT 1933*, p. 123.
[24] PRO MH55/1202, Anti-tuberculosis Committee for Wales, memo of evidence, April 1938, p. 6.
[25] *6th CMOH Annual Report 1924* (1925), 91.   [26] PRO MH55/1142.

We have spent much time in collating the returns made to various Medical Officers of Health and published in their annual reports during the past few years and find ourselves in complete accord with the opinion frequently expressed by the Medical Officers, viz. that the number of notified cases do not at present give any real idea of the distribution of the disease, and that the rates are not even useful indices of comparison between district and district.[27]

The incompleteness of tuberculosis notifications is suggested by the fact that many cases of the disease had reached a late stage before being notified. For example, of the 1,239 deaths from tuberculosis in Liverpool in 1923, 22 per cent were not notified until after death, 13 per cent within one month of death, and 34 per cent within twelve months of death. Some districts had even less complete records. Kenneth Fraser, CMO for Cumberland, reported in 1935 that 'as in previous years, almost exactly half of the tuberculosis cases were not notified before death or not until within three months of death'. Scotland had a similar experience; in 1921–3, 45 per cent of the deaths from pulmonary tuberculosis were unnotified or notified within three months of death. In 1928, in England and Wales, death preceded notification in 4,593 cases. Nor was there much improvement over time; in 1950, 2,704 cases were notified after death. In Scotland in 1941, 28 per cent were notified after death or within one month of death.[28]

There is evidence to suggest that some cases escaped notification even after death. Sir Robert Philip said in 1918:

. . . mortality statistics as published by the Registrar-General include only deaths certified by the patients' doctor as having occurred from tuberculosis. It is common knowledge that many deaths occur from tuberculosis which are not thus certified, either because the disease has not been recognised or because it has been described euphemistically. What the patient died of and what he is said to have died of are not always one and the same thing. Many deaths are labelled as from pneumonia, bronchitis, measles, whooping-cough, or influenza, which are really referable to tuberculosis.[29]

[27] MRC, M.Greenwood and A. E. Tebb, *An Inquiry into the Prevalence and Aetiology of Tuberculosis among Industrial Workers, with Special Reference to Female Munition Workers* (SRS 22; London, 1918), 12.

[28] *Journal of State Medicine*, 35/6 (1927), 334; *Tubercle*, 13 (1932), 202, and ibid., 17 (1936), 564; A. S. Hall, in F. R. G. Heaf (ed.), *Symposium of Tuberculosis* (London, 1957), 93; *EMJ* 50 (1943), 213.

[29] R. Philip, 'Present Day Outlook on Tuberculosis', Inaugural address at the institution of the Chair of Tuberculosis in the University of Edinburgh, *EMJ* 20/5 (1918), 293–4.

These two problems, the failure to diagnose the disease and the failure to acknowledge it, persisted in the following three decades.

Diagnostic problems were discussed by the notification committees, formed by the JTC in 1929 and again in 1945 to consider the under-reporting of the disease.[30] It was generally recognized that tuberculosis infection was ubiquitous, that virtually the whole population passed through the phase of primary infection. Disagreement arose concerning the point at which the infection became a disease and therefore should be notified. It was pointed out that there was no evidence that the grosser primary manifestations were more liable to lead to progressive tuberculosis than the minimal reactions which passed undetected. Early symptoms of the disease were moreover far from clear-cut, and were often confused with those of other illnesses. The 1945 committee pointed out that the relations between tuberculosis and such conditions as ischio-rectal abscess, erythema nodosum, phlyctenular conjunctivitis or sarcoidosis were unclear; these conditions might be manifestations of active tuberculosis and if so, they came within the scope of the notification order, but in reality they were rarely notified. The diagnosis of tuberculosis in children was considered particularly problematic.[31]

The widespread use of X-rays by the 1930s did not necessarily make diagnosis more accurate. As Heaf pointed out, X-rays required interpretation and a misreading could lead to active tuberculosis being incorrectly diagnosed. The introduction of mass miniature radiography during the Second World War created a new problem of cases which were borderline between infection and disease. In some countries, such as Denmark, X-ray evidence alone was not considered adequate to prove the existence of the disease; bacteriological confirmation was also required before notification.[32]

It was suggested in 1929 that two grades of notification should be introduced: 'Beyond all doubt' and 'probably tuberculous'. J. Williamson of the Ministry of Health objected that this would lead to confusion and the proposal was rejected, but the suggestion gives some indication of the extent of the problem. A 'long and heated' debate took place at one of the notification committee meetings in 1929 as to whether GPs should be required to notify cases with suspicious symptoms, provided those symptoms could not be accounted for by

---

[30] PRO MH55/157 and MH55/1142, JTC, Reports of Meetings of Notification Committee, 1929 and 1945.
[31] *EMJ* 46 (1939), 565.   [32] Heaf (ed.), *Symposium of Tuberculosis*, p. 9.

evidence of some other (non-tuberculous) condition, or whether they should be required to have some corroborative evidence of tuberculosis before notifying a case. The committee decided to specify when notification should be carried out. However, F. J. H. Coutts objected that GPs might resent this as implying that they were not competent of forming an opinion as to whether a given case was one of tuberculosis or not, and in the event no specifications were laid down. 'Provisional intimation' was again suggested by the committee in 1945, although a BMA representative at the meeting objected that this would create a precedent in the generally accepted principle of notification which would be 'undesirable and inappropriate'.[33]

There is also evidence to suggest, as previously mentioned, that GPs consciously neglected to notify tuberculosis cases. The reason for this failure may have been carelessness or inefficiency. A. Stephen Hall, chest consultant for Buckinghamshire CC, suggested that notification was regarded as an 'administrative nuisance of trifling importance compared to their life-saving work with the patient'.[34] A councillor from Stepney blamed the inefficiency of panel doctors.[35] C. H. C. Toussaint, TO for Bermondsey, considered overwork of panel doctors in industrial areas an important factor.[36]

However, it was much more likely to be a conscious choice on the part of the GP not to notify. The decision may have resulted from a reluctance to lose the patient to the tuberculosis dispensary, or to another doctor who offered a diagnosis more acceptable to the patient, or it may simply have resulted from a sense of compassion for the patient. Heaf admitted in 1939 that 'It is not uncommon for a patient with definite early symptoms of tuberculosis to escape notification because the physician wishes to avoid the effect of such an action on the general life and future of the individual.'[37] The diagnosis of tuberculosis was thought to be particularly damaging to children. Jane Walker referred to the stigma that often followed such a diagnosis and believed that they should be more guarded against making it.[38] N. Tattersall, Chief Clinical TO for the City of Leeds (appointed Principal MO of the WNMA in 1943), discovered cases of tuberculous children sent to Knaresborough Emergency Hospital for treatment

[33] PRO MH55/157 and PRO MH55/1142.
[34] Heaf (ed.), *Symposium of Tuberculosis*, p. 93.
[35] *15 NAPT 1929*, p. 34.
[36] TG SMOH Metrop. Sub-group Minutes, 16 Dec. 1938.
[37] *Tubercle*, 20 (1939), 350.   [38] Ibid., 1 (1920), 252.

in 1941 who had not been notified. He was told that notification was objected to because of the handicap to the individual in later years, especially with respect to life assurance.[39] A report by the British Paediatric Association in 1943 pointed out that doctors often hesitated to notify because they realized that the majority of children diagnosed in the early stage of infection recovered completely, but that once notified the stigma remained and could lead to unnecessary invalidism.[40]

While it is possible that doctors delayed such a verdict as long as possible because of undesirable consequences for the patient, it could not damage the patient in the final stages of the disease or at death. Yet there are indications of a reluctance to notify even at this late stage, as Stephen Hall wrote, 'out of consideration for the prejudices of the relatives . . . feeling that after all the poor man was dead and that there was no need to perpetuate trouble'.[41] Sir John Robertson pointed out in 1927: 'Long ago it was said that we doctors and statisticians juggled with the figures relating to tuberculosis by attributing deaths to bronchitis and pneumonia which ought to have been attributed to tuberculosis in order to spare the feelings of the relatives of the patient. To a very limited . . . extent this is true . . .'[42]

The JTC notification committee maintained that many of the objections to notification by patients arose from lack of discretion in the visiting of persons in their homes and at their places of employment, and the neglect to treat information about the tuberculous person as confidential. The notification regulations of 1912 had stressed the confidentiality of notification, but at the same time had imposed upon local authorities the responsibility of following up the notified case to prevent the further spread of the disease. It was pointed out by the committee that it was not sufficiently known that if the notifying doctor desired that no public health officer should visit the home of the patient, the wish was generally respected. By so deciding, however, the GP must be assumed to have taken over the responsibility for seeing that everything possible was being done to limit the spread of the infection and to deal with the cause of the patient's breakdown.[43] Even when the notification was received after

[39] PRO MH55/1142, N. Tattersall, 3 Dec. 1941.
[40] *Archives of Disease in Childhood*, 18/95 (1943), 158.
[41] Heaf (ed.), *Symposium of Tuberculosis*, p. 67.   [42] *13 NAPT 1927*, p. 12.
[43] PRO MH55/157, Unrevised Report of JTC Notification Committee, Jan. 1929, D. J. Williamson (11 Nov. 1929).

death, the home in which the patient had lived was to be investigated and disinfected.[44] It was pointed out in *Public Health* that strictly speaking, only the medical officer of health, or through that officer the sanitary inspector, had the right of entry into the homes of notified cases, but in practice the tuberculosis officer and tuberculosis health visitor were rarely challenged when they visited.[45] Sometimes even the after-care committee became involved—the after-care committee for Hastings borough reported in 1926 that 'As soon as a fresh case is notified, investigation is made to find out if help is required . . .'[46]

The JTC committee wrote of the wide variation among doctors:

In practice some extremists do not notify at all, or only such patients as are about to die. Some will notify only when the sputum is found to contain tubercle bacilli; others when it seems likely that notification will in some way assist the patient; others when notification seems likely to assist prevention. Others, again, will notify cases with a few physical signs alone, and some do not yet realise that non-pulmonary cases are notifiable.[47]

The responsibility for failure to notify did not always lie with the GP. The Minister of Health in 1934, Sir Edward Hilton Young, referred to the frequent delay on the part of the patient in seeking medical advice.[48] The reasons suggested by various tuberculosis officers for this delay included 'the fear and dread with which the disease is held by the lay person', a sense of fatalism, the social stigma attached to the disease, the prospect of supervision and threatened invasion of his or her home by the authorities, and finally and possibly most important of all, the fear of losing his or her job as a result of being discovered to be tuberculous and the financial consequences for the patient and family which this entailed.[49] The reluctance of many families at this time to agree to post-mortem examinations also made difficult the confirmation of the diagnosis after death.

Thus there is much evidence to suggest that the records on which epidemiological studies in the inter-war period depended were in fact unreliable, particularly morbidity statistics but also mortality statistics. However, it is still likely that the data, albeit unreliable, give an

---

[44] *16th CMOH Annual Report 1934* (1935), 76.   [45] *Public Health* (1941), 133.
[46] East Sussex Record Office, HH58/7, Hastings Borough Care Committee Annual Report 1925–6.
[47] PRO MH55/157, unrevised Report of JTC Notification Committee, Jan. 1929.
[48] *15th Annual Report Ministry of Health 1933–4*, Cmd. 6446 (1934), 69.
[49] See for example *Tubercle*, 11 (1930), 540. For a further discussion of the stigma attached to the disease, see Chapter 7, Section 2.

impression of general trends. Indications are that, if anything, the disease was often more prevalent than the figures suggested. The reluctance to be stigmatized as tuberculous might have prevented the notification of upper-class families and there is evidence to suggest under-reporting here—Dr Prest, medical superintendent of Ayrshire Sanatorium in Scotland, said in 1927, 'Of course, among the upper classes, who can go off to Switzerland and say nothing about it, that is a very good thing; . . . but it is necessary, unfortunately, at the present time, before any working person can be treated in a sanatorium, for them to be notified.'[50] Yet working-class families in fact had much more practical reasons for not seeking medical advice and for avoiding notification: loss of employment which might make the difference between poverty and the Poor Law for the patient and his or her family. Moreover, a sense of fatalism which was said to prevent patients from seeking attention was apparently most prevalent in Wales, an area where the rates were already higher than the national average.[51]

Thus, the data give an indication of the prevalence of tuberculosis although they cannot be taken as definitive. It seems clear from the statistics that there was a general decline commencing around the mid-nineteenth century, which continued in the twentieth century. However, it seems equally clear from the statistics that there were some exceptions to the general trend of decline, which also attracted attention at the time. First, there was an increase in tuberculosis death-rates during the First World War, particularly among young women. Second, in the post-war period , rates continued to be high in areas of depression and unemployment, reflected once again above all in young female death-rates. Finally, rates remained high in certain industries, such as the slate industry, where the presence of silica predisposed to tuberculosis.

(3) EPIDEMIOLOGICAL RESEARCH: THE FIRST WORLD WAR

Between 1913 and 1918 the respiratory tuberculosis death-rates increased by approximately 25 per cent in England and Wales, and 35 per cent among women aged 20–5. The 1918 influenza epidemic might have contributed to these increased rates, although by 1917 the

---

[50] *13 NAPT 1927*, p. 31.
[51] *Clement Davies Report*, p. 14.

percentage increases over 1913 were already 17 for the whole population and 22 for females aged 20–5.[52] In Scotland the increase was not so marked but was still in evidence, with a 9 per cent increase among all female deaths from pulmonary tuberculosis from 1914 to 1918. In his history of civilian health during the First World War, J. M. Winter has postulated two reasons for the rise in tuberculosis death-rates during the war: first the transfer of large populations to urban centres of war production and their concentration in munition factories, and second, the deterioration in housing conditions and the postponement of necessary demolition and sanitary work by local authorities. He claimed that virtually all observers accepted that the rise in tuberculosis death-rates was 'a negative and largely unavoidable consequence of the concentration of large numbers of factory workers working under considerable stress and living in inadequate housing'. He quoted 'one observer' who stated that 'tuberculosis deaths were a direct outcome of "overcrowding, overwork and overstrain" but not of poor nutrition'.[53]

Housing and working conditions were undoubtedly important factors in the rise of tuberculosis death-rates during the First World War. However, modern epidemiologists would not dismiss malnutrition as a possible predisposing cause of tuberculosis in the way Winter does or claims contemporaries to have done. Indeed, it is not true to say that contemporary observers denied any role played by nutrition. Major Greenwood, E. L. Collis (Mansel Talbot Professor of Preventive Medicine [later Emeritus Professor], University of Wales), T. H. C. Stevenson (the Registrar-General), and Sir George Newman were among those who, immediately after the war, stressed the importance of malnutrition in causing the rise in respiratory tuberculosis during the war. Newman wrote in his annual report for 1921, 'The close association of poverty or lack of nutrition with a tendency to higher tuberculosis death-rates is increasingly evident.'[54] According to Collis, the evidence drawn from the First World War was conclusive that nutrition was a factor ruling mortality from the disease in early adult life. He explained that tuberculosis death-rates increased dramatically with the tightening of the blockade and restriction on food consump-

[52] *CMOH Report 1939–45* (1947), 59.

[53] J. M. Winter, *The Great War and the British People* (London, 1986); for a critique, see L. Bryder, 'The First World War: Healthy or Hungry?', *History Workshop Journal*, 24 (1987), 141–57.

[54] *3rd CMOH Annual Report 1921* (1922), 62–3.

tion in Germany; and that in Denmark, rates increased when food consumption was restricted owing to the export of essential food stuffs and fell when such exports were stopped in 1917. Collis cited the dramatic decline in tuberculosis death-rates in Britain immediately after the war (9 per cent below the 1913 rate by 1920) as evidence of the greater importance of nutrition over housing conditions, pointing out that the fall occurred while overcrowding was prevalent as a result of inadequate housing, and when nutrition had improved (at least in the first few years following the war, before the onset of the depression). He believed that the fall, as in the fifty years before the war, was coincident with a rise in real wages.[55]

The rise in the death-rate among young women was believed by some to be associated with their employment in the munition industries, although, as Greenwood pointed out, there was no statistical evidence available to support this. F. J. H. Coutts attributed the rise to the overstrain associated with industrial conditions as well as to their state of nutrition. However, the death-rate also increased in the age group 5–14, and industrial employment could not explain this rise. Stevenson suggested that these children may have suffered from a change in diet, such as deprivation of fats. A study of tuberculosis death-rates and female employment in the 28 London boroughs in 1911–13 showed a negative correlation between the index of employment for women and the tuberculosis rates. Greenwood thought that this probably reflected the overriding influence of better nutrition compensating for the ill effects of industrial environment, explaining, 'the parlous state of unemployed or casually employed widows with dependants is notorious'.[56]

L. Cobbett, lecturer in pathology at Cambridge University, writing on tuberculosis in 1930, claimed that diet was 'of the utmost importance' in transforming latent tuberculosis cases into active cases during the First World War. He cited the experience of mental asylums. These suffered from severe food restrictions during the First World War, and also experienced a dramatic increase in tuberculosis death-rates; Cobbett believed the two factors to be related.[57]

[55] *14 NAPT 1928*, pp. 78–9; *Journal of State Medicine*, 23/3 (1925), 122; *Western Mail*, 2 July 1927 (PRO MH96/1111).

[56] Greenwood, in *1st CMOH Annual Report 1919–20* (1920), 334, 341; *14 NAPT 1928*, p. 62; *48th LGB Annual Report 1918–19, Supplement, Report of Medical Officer*, Cmd. 462 (1919), 105.

[57] Cobbett, *Journal of Hygiene*, 30 (1930), 79–103. On severe wartime rationing in mental hospitals, see MRC 2169/1, note for Jameson.

Greenwood also isolated the case of mental asylums, with their 'epidemic' of tuberculosis during the war (16.5 deaths per 1,000 residents in 1910–14, 31.9 in 1915–19, and 13.7 in 1920–4) as an 'unintentional illustration of the fact that a principal determinant of mortality is nutrition'.[58]

To support further his argument of the greater importance of overcrowding and stress related to industrial employment over nutrition, Winter pointed out that tuberculosis rates also rose in the first two years of the Second World War, when nutrition was satisfactory owing to effective wartime rationing. In fact, the rise did not approach the magnitude of that of the First World War (see Chapter 8, Section 1). Moreover, after the first two years, the rates for England and Wales fell below the pre-war level at a time when the housing problem (which Winter had considered so important in causing the rise in the First World War), exacerbated by the bombing, had by no means been solved. At the end of the Second World War, there was an estimated immediate need for half a million more houses. The major difference between the two world wars (apart from the 1918 influenza epidemic) was clearly related to nutritional levels, with rationing operating much more successfully in the Second World War.

(4) EPIDEMIOLOGICAL STUDIES: ECONOMIC DEPRESSION AND UNEMPLOYMENT

Nutrition appeared to have played an important part in causing the rise in tuberculosis death-rates during the First World War, or at least this was the dominant view among contemporary observers. The importance of the state of nutrition as a predisposing factor in tuberculosis continued to be stressed after the war. In 1924 Newman noted that there had been an increase in mortality from pulmonary tuberculosis in 1923 in certain areas and maintained that 'the conditions associated with lack of employment seemed to be the probable explanation'. He quoted the 1923 annual reports of the tuberculosis officers for Sunderland and Newcastle-upon-Tyne who attributed the increased tuberculosis death-rates in their areas to undernourishment and general distress resulting from unemploy-

[58] M. Greenwood, *Epidemics and Crowd-Diseases: An Introduction to the Study of Epidemiology* (London, 1935), 342.

ment.[59] In his report for 1926, Newman pointed out that the rate of decline of tuberculosis varied in different districts, that in Middlesbrough the high mortality was attributed to the amount of unemployment and the resultant underfeeding during the last four years, and that also in Wolverhampton, industrial depression was suggested as the cause for the steady rise since 1922 in the death-rates from tuberculosis.[60]

Not all medical commentators considered unemployment an adverse factor influencing rates of tuberculosis. In response to the 1926 report of the tuberculosis officer for Lancashire, the medical correspondent for the *Manchester Guardian* remarked,

Dr Cox's assumption that unemployment is an 'adverse factor' is not borne out by his own results, or by those in other affected areas either as regards tuberculosis or other forms of sickness. Deplorable as its effects are, unemployment is not nowadays allowed to involve absolute destitution, and enforced leisure, by removing people from the still unhealthy conditions of many forms of labour, by lessening the consumption of alcohol, even in some cases by restricting the diet, and increasing opportunities for obtaining fresh air, appears to result in a lowering of the death-rate from many of the principal diseases which affect the community.[61]

By 1930 a change of emphasis in the annual reports of the Chief Medical Officer can be detected. He no longer quoted medical officers of health or tuberculosis officers attributing the tuberculosis death-rates in their areas to malnutrition and unemployment. In his 1930 report, Newman pointed out that the distribution of mortality varied widely from area to area and that there were differences among the sexes. But, he wrote, the reasons were at present obscure. The only suggestion he made was that the stress of life had materially increased since the latter part of the nineteenth century.[62] No reference was made to nutrition. In 1932 he remarked upon the importance of nutrition, pointing to the responsibility of the parent in this respect.[63]

The change of emphasis is no doubt related to the mounting attack on the Government by social investigators and nutritionists who were arguing that the Government's social policies were causing widespread

[59] *6th CMOH Annual Report 1924* (1925), 93, 94.
[60] *8th CMOH Annual Report 1926* (1927), 123.
[61] *Manchester Guardian*, 30 Oct. 1926 (PRO MH96/1120).
[62] *12th CMOH Annual Report 1930* (1931), 86.
[63] *13th CMOH Annual Report 1932* (1933), 113.

malnutrition.[64] Given Newman's commitment to the view that 'though specially sought for, of evidence of widespread malnutrition there is none', and that there was 'no available evidence of any general increase in physical impairment, in sickness or in mortality, as a result of the economic depression or unemployment', it is hardly surprising that the causes of the high tuberculosis rates in depressed areas were sought elsewhere.[65]

Some medical officers of health continued to attribute the high tuberculosis rates to poverty and malnutrition. In 1932 the County MO for Durham, K. Falconer, wrote, 'One is forced to the conclusion that want and impoverishment, following in the train of long-continued unemployment and low wages, are amongst the chief exhaustive factors of such an unduly high phthisis rate.'[66] In 1933 the County MO for Oxfordshire, H. C. Jennings, conducted an investigation into some factors affecting the incidence of tuberculosis in the county of Oxfordshire. He examined records of every case notified from 1913 to 1932 inclusive and plotted purchasing power with tuberculosis incidence, and concluded, 'When the purchasing power of the community is high the incidence of and death rate from pulmonary tuberculosis both tend to be low and vice versa.'[67] Ralph M. F. Picken, Mansel Talbot Professor of Preventive Medicine, Welsh National School of Medicine, and formerly MOH for Cardiff, said at the 1933 NAPT Conference, 'Poverty has long been recognised as a prime factor in the causation of tuberculosis, principally through its effect upon nutrition.'[68]

In 1933 Newman referred to the problem of the rise of mortality in

[64] For a discussion of nutritional studies and infant mortality during the inter-war period and the political implications, see J. Lewis, *The Politics of Motherhood* (London, 1980), 175–90; J. Macnicol, *The Movement for Family Allowances, 1918–45: A Study in Social Policy Development* (London, 1980), 43–74; C. Webster, 'Healthy or Hungry Thirties?', *History Workshop Journal*, 13 (1982), 110–29 and 'Health, Welfare and Unemployment during the Depression', *Past and Present*, 109 (1985), 204–30; C. Petty, 'The MRC's Inter-war Dietary Surveys', in J. Austoker and L. Bryder, *A History of the Medical Research Council, 1913–50* (forthcoming); M. Mitchell, 'The Effects of Unemployment on the Social Condition of Women and Children in the 1930s', *History Workshop Journal*, 19 (1985), 105–27.

[65] *13th CMOH Annual Report 1932* (1933), 16, 34, 39–40; *14th CMOH Annual Report 1933* (1934), 219–21.

[66] Quoted in R. Titmuss, *Poverty and Population: A Factual Study of Contemporary Social Waste* (London, 1938), 173.

[67] *Oxford Times*, 26 Oct. 1934 (Churchill Hospital, Oxford); *Oxfordshire CC Annual Report on the County Health Services 1933* (1934), Part 2, p. 23.

[68] *19 NAPT 1933*, p. 42.

the industrial areas of south Wales, Merthyr Tydfil and Rhondda Urban Valley, in the age group 15–25 and 25–35. In Merthyr Tydfil County Borough, the young adult (15–25 years) mortality rate from pulmonary tuberculosis had risen for males from 131 per 100,000 population in 1921–5 to 197 in 1930–2, and for females from 185 to 268 in the same period (the rate for all of England and Wales in 1933 in this age group was 79 for males and 107 for females). By way of explanation, Newman wrote,

Many social and geographical features of coal mining districts favour tuberculosis; such as the loss of sunlight in the deep and narrow valleys in which the villages are situated, the tendency to crowd into small rooms and halls, some lack of playfields and facilities for open-air recreation, sometimes an unsuitable dietary and the tendency to conceal the presence of tuberculosis. In the case of young women economic depression has accentuated another factor—their migration to domestic service, a migration often followed by their breakdown and return home when the disease is found to have already reached an advanced stage.[69]

C. E. McNally, honorary treasurer of a Committee against Malnutrition set up in 1931, responded to Newman's analysis:

Now the geographical social conditions [in south Wales] have presumably not changed over the last few years. There is no evidence that the valleys are deeper and narrower today than formerly, and migration to service does not account for the increase in male mortality . . . We have already drawn attention to the fact that Sir George Newman, in his Report on the Effects of Unemployment on Health, has omitted to mention the increase in tuberculosis in the distressed areas. Now, in this section, he fails to diagnose the cause of this increase.[70]

J. E. Tomley, member of the council of the WNMA and secretary of the Montgomeryshire Insurance Committee, carried out a study of the 'special areas' of Wales in 1935. He pointed out that the decline in the death-rate from pulmonary tuberculosis from 1921–3 to 1931–3 was 22.7 per cent for England and Wales, 12 per cent for Wales, 2 per cent for Glamorgan and 2.3 per cent for Merthyr Tydfil, while Monmouthshire and Brecknockshire showed an increase of 0.6 and 2.5 per cent respectively over this period. He wrote that in the days of prosperity in the south Wales coalfields, mortality from pulmonary tuberculosis in

[69] *14th CMOH Annual Report 1933* (1934), 123.
[70] C. E. McNally, *Public Ill Health* (London, 1935), 168–9. See also W. S. Gilmour, *Journal of State Medicine*, 43 (1935), 567.

Glamorgan tended to be low. In his opinion, there seemed little doubt that the distressed economic conditions were in large measure responsible for this unfavourable position, with the reduced income through the depression in the coal industry causing many families to live under conditions bordering on starvation.[71]

In an unpublished report by the Ministry of Health of an inquiry conducted in 1936 into the effects of continued unemployment on health in certain areas in south Wales, it was pointed out in regard to tuberculosis that the population in the areas of economic distress had not shared in the decline in the tuberculosis death-rate at ages 15–35 which had been general in England. While in 1921–5 the death-rate from pulmonary tuberculosis for males aged 15–35 was lower in Glamorgan and Monmouthshire than in England and Wales, the rates in 1933–4 were much higher in these two coal-mining counties, although no explanation was offered in the report.[72]

The official denial of a relationship between malnutrition and tuberculosis continued with Sir Arthur MacNalty as Chief Medical Officer of the Ministry of Health. In his first report in 1935 he wrote,

Attention is drawn from time to time to the considerable variations in mortality from tuberculosis in different parts of England and Wales. The subject has received much study over many years, but it is difficult to elucidate by reason of the fact that a high or low rate of mortality in an area is never the result of one factor but of a considerable number of factors synchronising . . .

The relative shares of influence of poor nutrition, overcrowding and other factors which affect persons of both sexes and at all ages are . . . difficult to determine.[73]

MacNalty wrote in the preface to the report published in 1939 by P. D'Arcy Hart and Payling Wright on tuberculosis and social conditions which correlated the high tuberculosis rates among young females with low incomes: 'It is gratifying to note that during recent years there has been a decline in the incidence and mortality of respiratory tuberculosis in young adults.' He pointed out that the close association between poverty and tuberculosis had been recognized for

[71] PRO MH55/1121, J. E. Chapman, Notes on High Rates of Tuberculosis Mortality in Certain Counties of Wales, 1935. PRO MH55/1197, Statistics show death-rates to be comparatively low among coal-miners (apart from anthracite coal where the presence of silicosis was important); see also MRC, P. D'Arcy Hart and E. A. Aslett, *Chronic Pulmonary Disease in South Wales Coalminers*, (SRS. 243, Part 1; 1942), 155.

[72] PRO MH55/1197, WBH, 20 Mar. 1939, pp. 19, 21.

[73] *17th CMOH Annual Report 1935* (1936), 82.

many years, with tuberculosis leading to poverty, and poverty favouring tuberculosis. On the causes of tuberculosis he did not commit himself to any single explanation: 'There is a complex interaction of a considerable number of factors, and the respective shares taken by the various individual factors in the production of tuberculosis are difficult to assess.' He concluded by pointing out that he took no official responsibility for the conclusions and views expressed in the report, although he described it as an important contribution to the statistical study of the disease.[74]

The NAPT found itself drawn into the debate following a paper presented at the 1929 Annual Conference by H. A. Mess, director of a Bureau of Social Research for Tyneside set up in 1925 to research into the industrial depression in Tyneside. In his book on Tyneside, Mess had drawn attention to the mortality figures from pulmonary tuberculosis for the area (see Table 6). Moreover, he pointed out that the present tuberculosis death-rate in Jarrow was as high as it had been thirty years previously.[75] In his paper at the conference, he pointed to overcrowding and poor and irregular diet as the two most important factors in causing tuberculosis in the area. That overcrowding was not the most important factor was suggested to him by the fact that two areas in the survey, Blaydon and Newburn, had very bad housing but quite good tuberculosis figures. Mess also pointed out that the pit villages and mining towns of the county of Durham had usually remarkably low tuberculosis death-rates in spite of abominable housing. He considered that the factor of ship-building, with its 'violent fluctuations and extreme irregularity of incomes' was most important, and concluded,

It is at least suggestive that the worst tuberculosis figures on Tyneside are found in the towns with a great deal of casual labour. And it is possible that a partial explanation of the relative immunity of the coal-mining population is to be found in the fact that, until recently, coal-mining was an occupation which, whatever other disadvantages it may have had, did give fairly steady employment.[76]

The NAPT council appointed F. C. S. Bradbury, a tuberculosis officer in Lancashire (who was to succeed Cox as Central TO for

---

[74] P. D'Arcy Hart and G. P. Wright, *Tuberculosis and Social Conditions in England with Special Reference to Young Adults, a Statistical Study* (London, 1939), vi.
[75] H. A. Mess, *Industrial Tyneside* (London, 1928), 114.
[76] *15 NAPT 1929*, p. 15.

TABLE 6 *Comparative death-rates from pulmonary tuberculosis 1921–5*

Area	No./1,000
England and Wales	0.858
Industrial Tyneside	1.188
Jarrow	1.719
Blaydon	0.881

Source: H. A. Mess, *Industrial Tyneside* (London, 1928), 110.

Lancashire CC in 1946), to conduct a survey from a 'more strictly medical standpoint'.[77]

Bradbury investigated 2,963 families and 1,033 tuberculous persons in the two towns of Blaydon and Jarrow in Durham, and considered the following factors statistically—poverty, occupation of tenements and flats, Irish nationality, undernourishment, bad ventilation of homes, insanitation of houses, number of children in the family. He concluded:

It is apparent that the association of tuberculosis with poverty is of greater importance than with any of the other conditions studied. The principal means by which poverty is found to cause tuberculosis are the overcrowding and undernourishment which are the chief distinguishing features between poor and not poor families in the area studied.

Bradbury considered the relationship between tuberculosis and undernourishment to be statistically more significant than that between tuberculosis and overcrowding, and that poverty caused tuberculosis rather than tuberculosis causing poverty. He pointed out that no attempt had been made to trace the association between the incidence of tuberculosis in the two areas and the prevailing types of employment—mining in Blaydon and ship-building in Jarrow. He noted, however, that in Blaydon, while tuberculosis was rather less common in the families of miners than others, unemployment was also less common in the miners' families.[78]

The Tyneside Inquiry Committee of the NAPT, chaired by F. J. H. Coutts, chose to single out a different point for comment in the foreword of the study: 'Attention may be directed to one interesting point which helps to account for the disproportionately high mortality

[77] NAPT Council Annual Report 1930, 11.
[78] F. C. S. Bradbury, *Causal Factors in Tuberculosis* (London, 1932), 34, 39, 53, 96, 98.

from tuberculosis in Jarrow, viz. the racial factor. Dr Bradbury's figures appear to show that the high proportion in Jarrow of persons of Irish origin is directly correlated with the high incidence of tuberculosis.'[79] This was the factor which received wide notice in the Press at the time. According to Ellen Wilkinson (known as 'Red Ellen', Labour MP for Jarrow, 1935–47), 'The local Press leapt joyously at this useful excuse.' Wilkinson described the vicious cycle of low wages, lower allowances, and malnutrition passing on to one or other of the deficiency diseases, and concluded, 'There is no mystery about the high tuberculosis rate of Jarrow.'[80]

In 1935 Major Greenwood considered the tuberculosis rates in various districts in London:

Passing from the most to the least prosperous group, although general mortality (standardized) increases no more than 29.9 per cent, mortality from tuberculosis increases by more than 60 per cent. This relation, striking as it is, falls far short of that observed in Paris by Hersch, who was able to express the mortality from tuberculosis in the various administrative divisions of Paris almost as a mathematical function of a measure of poverty. Still, even the English data suffice to bring out the essential potency of this economic factor . . .[81]

In 1921 the Registrar-General calculated mortality rates from pulmonary tuberculosis in five social class groups, pointing out that the mortality for Class I, aged 20–5, was little more than one-third of the average of all social classes for that age group.[82]

In the discussion of the causes of the high tuberculosis rates in depressed areas or among the lower socio-economic groups, the 'blaming the victim' explanation was often invoked. For example, Sir John Robertson explained the differences in tuberculosis death-rates between poorer- and better-class districts in Birmingham in terms of the 'ignorance and carelessness of the inhabitants' and believed it to be wonderful that more young people did not contract tuberculosis, 'for

---

[79] Ibid., Foreword.

[80] E. Wilkinson, *The Town that was Murdered: The Life-history of Jarrow* (London, 1939), 222, 244.

[81] Greenwood, *Epidemics and Crowd-Diseases*, p. 358. M. L. Hersch, Professor of Statistics, University of Geneva, calculated in 1920 that the rate for the poorest district in Paris was six times as great as that for the richest: *Revue d'économie politique*, 3 and 4 (1920), quote in T. H. C. Stevenson, *Journal of the Royal Statistical Society*, 84 (1921), 96–7.

[82] *The Registrar-General's Decennial Supplement, England and Wales, 1921, Part 2, Occupational Mortality, Fertility and Infant Mortality* (1927), p. xviii.

so large a number are living unhealthy lives in one direction or another'.[83]

High tuberculosis rates provided an excellent opportunity to censure the behaviour of young people, who were it seems particularly vulnerable to the excitement and stress of modern urban life. L. E. (later Sir Leonard) Hill pointed out that the death-rates in country areas were on average 35 per cent lower than in the cities for males and 30–3 per cent for females, and explained, 'In the last decades, the rush and excitement of modern city life has increased . . .'[84] R. C. Wingfield, medical superintendent of Frimley Sanatorium from 1920 to 1945, believed that 'in spite of generations of endurance of the artificialities of civilisation, man is still an animal, designed and ordained to live his life in the open air, and disease is part of the penalty that he has had to pay for disregarding this law'.[85] F. R. G. Heaf (later professor of tuberculosis at the Welsh National School of Medicine), who had examined in detail the lives of 120 young adults suffering from pulmonary tuberculosis, also blamed the 'speed' of modern life: 'The youth of today does not lead the peaceful life that he did twenty or thirty years ago,' as did Sir Robert Philip, who spoke of the 'devitalizing influence of restlessness, irregular hours, and the thoughtless misuse of leisure time' of modern youth.[86] James Watt, medical superintendent of King George V Sanatorium, Godalming, came to a similar conclusion after inquiring into the histories of 100 young adult male patients at the sanatorium.[87] S. Vere Pearson, medical superintendent of Mundesley Sanatorium from 1905 to 1949 and chairman of the JTC from 1937 to 1940, maintained that the influences which often excited tuberculosis were chiefly concerned with city life. The three most important factors in his opinion were the increase in the amount of travelling that was entailed in getting to and from work, the lack of facilities for recreation in the open air, and the sense of irritation and anxiety which was so frequently associated with

[83] *13 NAPT 1927*, p. 16; *14 NAPT 1928*, p. 144.

[84] MRC, L. E. Hill, *The Science of Ventilation and Open-air Treatment*, (SRS 52, Part 2; 1920), 183, 185. The Registrar-General later pointed out that diagnostic facilities were often better in urban than rural areas, and thus differences might be accentuated: *Registrar-General's Statistical Review of England and Wales for the Year 1950* (NS 30; London, 1952), Tables, Part 1: Medical, 120.

[85] R. C. Wingfield, *Modern Methods in the Diagnosis and Treatment of Pulmonary Tuberculosis* (London, 1924), 64.

[86] *18 NAPT 1932*, p. 84; *22 NAPT 1936*, p. 15.

[87] *18 NAPT 1932*, p. 74.

vocations followed and circumstances encountered in big cities.[88] These theories did little to account for the high tuberculosis rates found in certain rural areas of Wales and the Highlands and Islands of Scotland.[89] Modern life was considered particularly damaging to young women of all classes. It appeared to Bardswell to be more than coincidence that the increase in tuberculosis rates among young women should have been first noticed in 1901 and become more marked since (see Table 7)—a period which had seen the emancipation of women, and a profound change in their social habits following their entry into competitive wage-earning. He had inquired into the life-histories of many young female tuberculous patients. He noted the varying degrees of fatigue over a long period consequent upon the nature or conditions of employment. He also observed the want of rest and late hours to bed, around 11 p.m., most commonly the result of recreation, such as the 'pictures' or dancing at the end of a long day's work, but not infrequently due to evening- and night-work, reading for examinations, night-classes or helping in the home. Neglected colds and unsatisfactory meals—often a poor breakfast owing to late getting up and a cheap but inadequate lunch—were also found to be common. All these were considered contributory factors to their breakdown.[90] Jane Walker, medical superintendent of East Anglian Sanatorium from 1900 to 1938, stated in her presidential address to the TA in 1932 that many of the occupations held by women involved more arduous exertion than had been customary for them to undergo, and that few causes were more powerful to determine the outbreak of pulmonary tuberculosis than physical over-exertion.[91] Maurice Davidson, physician to the Brompton Hospital, similarly believed that the effect of hard physical labour in the case of factory girls was definitely of some importance in the aetiology of tuberculosis. He had also often noted the 'sudden . . . outward manifestation of active pulmonary tuberculosis following the occurrence of some unusual expenditure of mental energy, brain work, severe emotional stimulus, grief, shock, and so forth . . .' and believed that 'psychological energy plays no small part in the lives of young

[88] Empire Conference on the Care and After-care of the Tuberculous, *BJT* 31/3 (1937), 150; *The Times*, 4 May 1937 (PRO MH96/1030); S. V. Pearson, *Men, Medicine, and Myself* (London, 1946), 188.

[89] *6th Annual Report Scottish Board of Health*, Cmd. 2416 (1925), 57; *7th Annual Report*, Cmd. 2674 (1926), 61; *9th Annual Report*, Cmd. 3112 (1928), 96. See also M. Flinn (ed.), *Scottish Population History* (Cambridge, 1977), 414, and above Fig. 4, pp. 10, 11.

[90] *18 NAPT 1932*, p. 68.   [91] *Tubercle*, 14 (1932), 136.

TABLE 7 *Death-rates from pulmonary tuberculosis per 100,000 population in England and Wales, 1851–1929, and percentage decline*

Age group	(a) 1851–60	(b) 1901	(c) 1929	% decline	
				(a) to (b)	(b) to (c)
Males					
10–15	76	19	11	75	42
15–20	240	80	63	67	21
20–25	405	167	107	59	36
25–35	403	215	119	47	45
35–45	402	289	149	28	48
45–55	384	313	173	19	45
55–65	335	252	136	25	46
65–75	239	159	89	33	44
75+	93	60	33	35	45
Females					
10–15	129	40	23	69	42
15–20	352	100	100	72	0
20–25	430	129	134	70	+4
25–35	458	164	109	64	33
35–45	419	186	77	56	59
45–55	313	149	60	52	60
55–65	239	112	48	53	57
65–75	164	83	40	50	52
75+	72	31	20	57	35

Source: Ministry of Health, A. S. MacNalty, *A Report on Tuberculosis*, Reports on Public Health and Medical Subjects, 64 (HMSO, 1932), 8.

women of today, not only in their working hours, but more especially perhaps in their off-time'.[92] The histories of 44 young women who had died of tuberculosis in Bristol in one year were analysed by the TO for Bristol, Campbell Faill, who 'tentatively suggested that "summer time" encouraged young people to be actively engaged in games etc., until late at night', thus lowering their resistance.[93] In 1934 MacNalty referred to the widely held view that the change in the pattern of mortality from pulmonary tuberculosis among young women was related to the changes in their lifestyles which had occurred since

[92] *Tubercle*, 17 (1936), 539, 540.
[93] Ibid., 19 (1938), 376.

1900—'associated as these changes are with a more strenuous life generally'.[94]

However, these views had been reached without considering a comparable control group who had not contracted tuberculosis. One investigation of tuberculosis and social habits of young women in London showed no significant difference in behaviour between the tuberculosis cases and the control group.[95] Bardswell himself admitted that there was a group of patients, 'by no means a small one', whose lives were well ordered, and whose conditions at work and at home left little or nothing to be desired. The explanation he offered was that these patients had proved unequal to cope with their circumstances owing to some inherent lack of resistance (although tuberculosis specialists in general did not dwell on the possible role of heredity in tuberculosis in this period).[96]

Querying the 'strain theory' in tuberculosis causation, A. (later Sir Austin) Bradford Hill of the Royal Statistical Society (later Emeritus Professor of Medical Statistics, London School of Hygiene and Tropical Medicine) asked whether the 'increasing strain and speed of modern life' varied so much that it could account for a decline of 31 per cent in the death-rate of young females in Bradford between 1911–13 and 1929–31, and a rise of 27 per cent in Manchester, a decline of 20 per cent in Derby and a rise of 30 per cent in Birmingham, a rise of 35 per cent in Lambeth and a decline of 12 per cent in Stepney. He also questioned the part played by increasing employment of women as the proportion of women in employment did not change from 1911 to 1931 and only increased very slightly in the age group 14–25. The percentage of young females in employment in fact only changed from 58.4 in 1871 to 56.3 in 1901, to 62 in 1911, 62.2 in 1921, and 65.1 in 1931 (for all ages, the rates were 32.5 per cent in 1911 to 34 per cent in 1931), that is, not a significant change. Hill also pointed out that the distribution between the various sectors—clerical, domestic, and factory—had not altered significantly. The proportion in personal service changed only from 39 per cent to 35 per cent between 1911 and 1931, in clerical work from 2 to 10 per cent in the same period, and in textile work from 13 to 10 per cent.

[94] Ministry of Health, A. S. MacNalty, *A Report on Tuberculosis*, Reports on Public Health and Medical Subjects 64 (1932), 10. See also H. M. Vernon, *Health in Relation to Occupation* (London, 1939), 137.

[95] F. J. Bentley, *Journal of State Medicine*, 42/5 (1934), 256; *The Practitioner*, 85/807, (1935), 314.

[96] *18 NAPT 1932*, p. 68. On heredity see also Chapter 7, Section 2.

Percy Stocks calculated the death-rates from tuberculosis of women in those jobs and found that the rates were lower than for all females in the social class from which they were likely to have come (class III). Hill also pointed out that county boroughs with a higher proportion of females in paid employment had lower pulmonary tuberculosis death-rates.[97] To this it could be added that the rates of female employment in Wales remained relatively low, yet tuberculosis rates were excessive —while the pulmonary tuberculosis mortality rate for females aged 15–25 in England and Wales was 98 per 100,000 population in 1934, that for Glamorgan for 1933–4 was 195, for Monmouthshire, 186, and for Merthyr Tydfil, 311.[98] The experience of other countries is also revealing. Two American tuberculosis specialists described the 'slight increase' in the tuberculosis death-rate for young women aged 15–24 in twentieth-century Britain, which, they wrote, had been ascribed to the increased employment of young women in industry and the migration of relatively susceptible girls from the country districts seeking work in the towns. They commented, 'The steadily increasing industrial employment of women in this country [America] has not as yet been reflected in a higher tuberculosis mortality in women, even at the ages of highest susceptibility'.[99]

Subsequent studies of epidemiology of tuberculosis over the past century based on 'the cohort model' have shown that the patterns of decline were relatively constant among all age groups calculated by cohorts and that the check in the decline among young females in the early twentieth century was not therefore to be regarded as an anomaly.[100] V. H. Springett, Adviser in Chest Diseases to the Ministry of Health, who made a special study of the epidemiology of tuberculosis, wrote in 1952 that the decline over the past century was on a fundamental age/sex pattern—high in infancy and higher at that age for males than females, low for both sexes in childhood, rising at puberty, with an earlier rise among females than males, and reaching a maximum in adult life, with a fall in later life, greater among females.

[97] A. B. Hill, *Journal of the Royal Statistical Society*, 99/2 (1936), 264, 266, 268–9, 281, 285; J. Lewis, *Women in England 1870–1950* (Sussex, 1984), Tables 4 and 5, p. 147, Table 10, p. 156.
[98] PRO MH55/1197, WBH, Brief for Minister of Health, 20 Mar. 1939.
[99] H. D. Chadwick and A. S. Pope, *The Modern Attack on Tuberculosis* (New York, 1942), 17.
[100] V. H. Springett, *The Lancet*, 1 (1952), 521–5, 575–80; J. J. Collins, 'The Contribution of Medical Measures to the Decline of Mortality from Respiratory Tuberculosis: An Age-Period-Cohort Model', *Demography*, 19/3 (1982), 409–27.

He believed that the death-rates were determined by the rates of infection which usually occurred in young adults; some of those infected would die immediately, others surviving for many years with sometimes long periods of good health. The decline in tuberculosis death-rates was believed to be associated 'with a general improvement in living conditions in the widest sense', an improvement which he pointed out was first checked in the early twentieth century.[101] The high rates among young women in depressed areas may have been related to a greater susceptibility of that group under adverse economic and social conditions to contract the disease, or it may be that they bore the brunt of the poor conditions particularly severely, for example, receiving a smaller share of the family's food.

MacNalty also pointed to the building of 4 million houses between 1918 and 1938 as an important factor in the declining tuberculosis rates.[102] However, others pointed out that families most likely to contract the disease and those already with a tuberculous patient were the least likely to afford the higher rents involved in the new dwellings. Some local authorities gave tuberculous patients and their families priority in council houses, as has been noted, but according to the Kent MO in 1938, this was of limited use (unless the rents were very heavily subsidized, which they were in a few cases), for it led to a decline in the amount of income expendable on food.[103] M'Gonigle and Kirby did not include tuberculosis among the diseases which increased following the transferral of slum dwellers to a housing estate with consequent reduced expenditure on food, but from his experience R. M. F. Picken thought such an increase was a likely corollary.[104]

(5) EPIDEMIOLOGICAL RESEARCH: EMPLOYMENT AND
PERSONAL HABITS

The nature of work and working conditions were also undoubtedly important factors in the epidemiology of tuberculosis. Certain industries persisted in registering excessive tuberculosis rates. As already noted, the MRC carried out a study of tuberculosis in the boot

[101] *The Lancet*, 1 (1952), 579.
[102] *20th CMOH Annual Report 1938* (1939), 133.
[103] 'Papworth Sims-Woodhead Memorial Laboratory Research Bulletin 1940', p. 25.
[104] *19 NAPT 1933*, p. 42; G. C. M. M'Gonigle and J. Kirby, *Poverty and Public Health* (London, 1936).

and shoe trade in 1915. They held that the excessive tuberculosis rates in the industry resulted from the failure to attract robust workers (the nature of the work not being very physically demanding), and from the lack of ventilation. No other studies were carried out in this industry before 1947, despite the fact that the Registrar-General continued to record high rates.

Industries with particularly high tuberculosis rates were those with pneumoconiosis risk which predisposed workers to tuberculosis (see Table 8). Tuberculosis itself was not a scheduled disease under the Workmen's Compensation Act. At least in one instance, the weight of scientific medical evidence was used to delay the extension of workers' compensation, that is in the north Wales slate industry. In retrospect, pneumoconiosis is thought to have been responsible for the high tuberculosis rates which prevailed in the area.[105] However, this was far from accepted in 1927 when T. W. Wade (Principal MO of the

TABLE 8 *Death-rates from tuberculosis among males in certain industries which had more than twice the tuberculosis death-rates for all occupied and retired males (taken as 1,000), England, 1921–3*

Occupation	Deaths
Tin and copper miners	8,394
Metal-grinders	4,117
Slate masons and slate-workers	3,341
Potters' mill workers, slip-makers, potters	2,625
Barmen	2,613
File-cutters	2,407
Drafters and brush-makers	2,314
Costermongers, hawkers, and street sellers	2,234
Earthenware, china, etc., kiln and oven men	2,167
Brass foundry, furnacemen, and labourers	2,118
Stevedores	2,113
Cutlers	2,075
Masons, stone-cutters, and dressers	2,050
Metal glazers, polishers, buffers, and moppers	2,024

Source: M. Greenwood, *Epidemics and Crowd Diseases: An Introduction to the Study of Epidemiology* (London, 1935), 358.

[105] J. R. Glover, *et al.*, 'Effects of exposure to slate dust in North Wales', *British Journal of Industrial Medicine*, 37 (1980), 152–60.

Welsh Board of Health) was sent into the region to investigate. Wade himself concluded that the inhalation of slate dust was an important factor in predisposing the workers to tuberculosis, and that contrary to popular belief, the tuberculosis of the slate workers was not less infective than other cases. Not only did the employers and the doctors working in the area reject his conclusion; he was not supported by subsequent investigations, those by C. H. Sutherland and S. Bryson of the Ministry of Mines in 1930, and by H. D. Chalke, assistant tuberculosis physician for Monmouthshire, appointed to carry out the survey by the WNMA in 1933. Chalke's report did, however, result in the setting up of a tuberculosis visiting station with X-ray apparatus in the area, and in 1937 the tuberculosis physician reported that a year's work had led him to the conclusion that slate dust was an important predisposing cause of tuberculosis locally. In 1939 slate miners were included under the Workmen's Compensation (Silicosis) Act, as were other slate workers in 1946.[106]

Reasons advanced by medical practitioners in north Wales for the high tuberculosis rates included a racial disposition to contract the disease, and the local tendency to intermarry exacerbating such a predisposition. Generally, however, the subjects most dwelt upon by the local medical commentators were the personal habits and customs of the people, including an over-addiction to tea, overeating on Sundays, an unsuitable rather than insufficient diet owing to house-wives' ignorance of food values, the tendency of young slate workers to stint themselves in order to spend more on clothing for Sundays to equal or better their peers, the habit of crowding houses with furniture, and the tendency to congregate in crowded ill-ventilated chapels and to neglect outdoor exercise. Also considered relevant were 'the national characteristics of the Welsh, for example, the intense conservatism of their social habits, the closeness and tenacity of their family relationships, and their fatalistic outlook . . .'.[107] R. C. Hutchinson, medical superintendent of Baguley Sanatorium, Man-chester, wrote his MD thesis on tuberculosis in a parish in Carmarthen, in which he pointed out that the unhygienic mode of life found in this parish was partly a result of poverty, but to a much greater

---

[106] See L. Bryder, 'Silicosis, Tuberculosis, and the North Wales Slate Industry', in P. Weindling (ed.), *The Social History of Industrial Health* (London, 1985), 108–26.

[107] *The Times*, 5 May 1937 (PRO MH96/1030); PRO MH55/1191, WNMA, memo for Clement Davies Inquiry, Nov. 1937, p. 22; Chalke Report, 1933, pp. 18, 43, 82, 85; *Clement Davies Report* (London, 1939), 36.

extent a result of bad tradition, which he believed made the tuberculosis problem all the more difficult to solve.[108] One personal habit, which was also a middle-class habit, was not subject to censure or implicated as predisposing to tuberculosis, and that was smoking. At the 1933 NAPT conference, the belief that the cocktail habit and excessive smoking were responsible for a great deal of tuberculosis was described as 'humbug' by Bardswell.[109] Nor did Dubos agree with the idea that smoking predisposed to tuberculosis. He described how, in the nineteenth century, every vice or form of unconventional behaviour had been regarded as a cause of consumption. He quoted one nineteenth-century physician who believed that his patient's phthisis had been caused by 'inordinate use of tobacco', and added that the waltz had also been considered a cause.[110] Smoking was permitted in sanatoria for male patients in the inter-war period, and one patient had even formed the impression that tobacco was an enemy of the tubercle bacillus.[111] At Eversfield Hospital, it was specified that male patients were permitted to smoke, but that smoking was only advisable after meals and when sitting down.[112] A pamphlet issued to patients leaving a sanatorium advised against smoking, pointing out that smoking immediately before meals interfered with the taste and spoiled natural appetite.[113] Not until 1960 did the JTC publish a report on 'Smoking in relationship to tuberculosis and chest diseases', and in 1962 the TA (now the BTA) resolved at its AGM that smoking should be banned at all future meetings.[114]

The consumption of alcohol was thought to predispose to tuberculosis, although only in excessive quantities. MacNalty pointed out in 1932 that the increasing sobriety and temperance of the British people must be a contributory factor of some importance in the decline of

---

[108] *Tubercle*, 2 (1921), 345–9.
[109] Reported in *Western Mail*, 15th July 1933 (PRO MH96/1056).
[110] R. and J. Dubos, *The White Plague: Tuberculosis, Men and Society* (London, 1953), 197.
[111] A. Dick, *A Walking Miracle* (London, 1942), 30. See also *Tubercle*, 1 (1920), 188: tobacco smoke was said by the editor of the *American Review of Tuberculosis* to be 'mildly stimulating and tending to repair [the infected lung]'. It should be noted, however, that a commentary on *A Walking Miracle* stated that 'A man with or without tuberculosis who smokes 2oz. of dark flake a day in hospital is clearly an ass (or his physician is)': *Lancet*, 2 (1942), 292.
[112] Eversfield Hospital Annual Report 1916, p. 34; ibid. 1926, p. 29.
[113] PRO MH96/986, WNMA, Advice to Patients who Leave a Sanatorium Fit for Work, 26.
[114] *British Thoracic Association*, p. 66; *Tubercle*, 48 (1967), 219–26.

tuberculosis.[115] Chalke did not find alcohol to be an important factor in the high tuberculosis rates in north Wales, for alcohol consumption was low among the inhabitants.[116] James Watt believed 'over-exertion of any kind, physical, mental, or sexual', to be a factor of greater significance than the consumption of alcohol in predisposing to tuberculosis.[117]

Barmen experienced an incidence of tuberculosis well above the national average (see Table 8), which was thought to be related to their easy access to alcohol and tendency to over-indulge.[118] However, another factor which may have been important in this context was the persistent habit of spitting in public houses. Chalke found spitting to be prevalent in Wales in the 1930s, and one commentator held that if spitting could be eradicated then tuberculosis would be wiped out.[119]

The twentieth century witnessed a general decline in tuberculosis mortality rates in England and Wales. However, national figures can be deceiving as they obscure regional and occupational variations. The districts with high tuberculosis rates, and rates which were not falling as rapidly as the national rates, coincided with those areas most heavily affected by unemployment and economic depression. Observers on the spot, such as Bradbury and local medical officers of health and tuberculosis officers, often commented on the adverse influence of economic conditions. Those subscribing to the 'general strain of modern life' theory were often, with some exceptions, medical superintendents, remote from the realities of working-class life. Imbued with the dominant ideology of self-help, their focus of attention was on individual responsibility and reformation of the personal habits of the poor, and it was they who dictated much of the preventive work carried out in this period.

[115] Ministry of Health, A. S. MacNalty, *A Report on Tuberculosis* 64 (1932), 28–9.
[116] Chalke Report, p. 17.
[117] *18 NAPT 1932*, p. 74.
[118] *Journal of State Medicine*, 33 (1925), 101; *14 NAPT 1928*, pp. 81–2; *BMJ* 2(1949), 230.
[119] PRO MH75/15, Chalke Report, unrevised, 1931, pp. 33, 61, 87; John Guy in C. W. Hutt and H. H. Thomson (eds.), *Principles and Practice of Preventive Medicine*, i (London, 1935), 368.

5

Fighting Infection

METHODS of preventing the spread of tuberculosis which were advocated and attempted with various degrees of commitment and success included the isolation of tuberculous patients, preventing people with tuberculosis from working in food trades, the control of milk supplies, vaccination, education, the provision of open-air schools, and the boarding out of susceptible children. It will be argued in this chapter that policies involving compulsion and interference in personal liberties were shied away from in favour of policies involving persuasion. The latter approach was not only cheaper but also suited the dominant ideology of those leading the campaign, specifically their belief in self-responsibility for contracting the disease.

(1) COMPULSORY ISOLATION

Compulsory isolation as a preventive measure was recommended by the Departmental Committee on Tuberculosis in 1913, particularly in those instances where the patient's surroundings were such as to increase the risk of other people being infected.[1] The first report of the Medical Research Committee in 1915 included among its recommendations the power to suspend from employment individuals suffering from pulmonary tuberculosis in an infectious state.[2] Various tuberculosis specialists recommended compulsory isolation as a preventive measure, including Sir James Kingston Fowler and Marcus Paterson.[3] Paterson wondered why the same powers of enforcing isolation of the insane did not also apply to the tuberculous, the latter in his opinion being just as dangerous (to themselves as well as to the

[1] *Astor Committee, Final Report*, i. 8.
[2] MRC, *First Report of the Special Investigation Committee upon the Incidence of Phthisis in Relation to Occupations: The Boot and Shoe Industry* (SRS 1; 1915), Appendix 3, p. 29.
[3] J. K. Fowler, *Problems in Tuberculosis* (London, 1923), 47; M. S. Paterson, *The Shibboleths of Tuberculosis* (London, 1920), 201.

community) as the former. Before 1925, local Acts had given several local authorities the power to isolate compulsorily infectious cases of tuberculosis, starting with St Helen's (Lancashire) in 1911, and Liverpool, Bradford, and East Ham in 1913. Eight other local authorities followed in the next two years, and Swansea in 1920. The Local Legislation Committee of 1925 recommended that the power become more general, and it was included in the 1925 Public Health Act which also extended the powers of local authorities (other than the LCC) in other matters relating to public health. By section 62 of the Act, local authorities could secure, with the consent of a court of summary jurisdiction, the removal to hospital of a person suffering from pulmonary tuberculosis in an infectious state and without accommodation adequate to prevent the spread of infection (in other words, compulsory isolation applied only to the poor). Local authorities were not allowed to use notification records to gain the information because of the confidentiality of the records, but were reliant on some other source. The local authority could be called upon to contribute to the maintenance of dependants. This was later incorporated into section 172(5) of the Public Health Act of 1936.

The injustice of the situation in which those who willingly went to hospital did not receive assistance for their dependants whereas those who went forcibly did, was referred to by the WNMA in 1942.[4] However, the Ministry of Health replied that the anomaly was theoretical as the powers of compulsory removal were seldom invoked. Only one instance was reported in England in 1928, one in 1929, three in 1930, three in 1931, and no instances were reported in Wales.[5] MacNalty maintained in 1932 that the majority of infectious persons suffering from tuberculosis were only too glad to avail themselves of the medical care and skilled nursing which they obtained in a hospital. In a minority of cases when the patient or the patient's family had at first opposed the removal to hospital, knowledge of the powers of compulsory removal had been sufficient to ensure eventual compliance.[6] The required payment of maintenance for dependants possibly deterred local authorities from more regular use of the powers.

The handling of foodstuffs, particularly milk, by sufferers from

---

[4] PRO MH96/1031, WNMA, General Purposes Committee, 27 Mar. 1942, p. 3; Clement Davies, *Hansard*, 5th Series, 1941–2, 381 (1942), 80.

[5] PRO MH96/1031, WNMA, 27 Mar. 1942, p. 6; PRO MH55/133, Ministry of Health memo, 6 Feb. 1934.

[6] Ministry of Health, A. S. MacNalty, *A Report on Tuberculosis* 64 (1932), 56.

tuberculosis was considered an important channel for the spread of infection. By 1925 the Ministry of Health had received numerous complaints from local authorities who had discovered through notification records several cases of active pulmonary tuberculosis in people engaged in the milk trade, but had been unable to do anything about it because of article 16 of the 1912 tuberculosis regulations as to the confidentiality of notifications. F. J. H. Coutts pointed out that the total extent of contamination of milk supplies by tubercle from human sources was probably insignificant compared to the extent of contamination by bovine infection. Nevertheless, the Ministry of Health decided that, as milk was the most readily contaminated of all foods, in this case a departure from the principles of article 16 was justified. Regulations were thus issued in 1925 empowering local authorities to prevent persons with infectious tuberculosis from working in the milk trade. For the purpose of applying those regulations, a local authority could use information obtained from notification records. It was specified that they might be required to pay compensation for damages suffered by the application of the regulations.[7]

These regulations were used sparingly, in two cases in 1928 (one of which received compensation for loss of employment), one case in 1929, four in 1930 (three of which were paid compensation), and two in 1931. Medical officers of health also cited instances in which the affected person was persuaded to leave the job voluntarily. Coutts suggested that the amount of compensation payable was a deterrent to their more frequent use by local authorities.[8]

Infection was also possible through the handling of other foodstuffs, although this means of infection was not considered extensive enough to warrant general legislation. However, beginning with Torquay in 1923, 33 local authorities had passed local Acts by 1934 which enabled them to apply the restrictions in the milk trade to other food trades. Compensation was also payable, but local authorities were not permitted to use the notification records to discover the cases. The Ministry of Health found no evidence of these powers being used.[9]

---

[7] PRO MH55/133, The Public Health (Prevention of Tuberculosis) Regulations, 1925.
[8] PRO MH55/133, Ministry of Health memo, 6 Feb. 1934; A. S. MacNalty, Analysis of Replies of MOs, 21 Mar. 1934.
[9] PRO MH55/133, Ministry of Health memo, 6 Feb. 1934.

(2) CONTROL OF MILK SUPPLIES

Another mode of infection was through the consumption of meat or milk from tuberculous cattle. In the 1930s, almost 30 per cent of all non-pulmonary tuberculosis deaths and 2 per cent of pulmonary tuberculosis deaths in the British Isles were due to infection of bovine origin. Thirty per cent of cases of tuberculous meningitis (which was invariably fatal) were of bovine origin. Tuberculosis of bovine origin was, moreover, considered especially important as it struck primarily at children who drank infected milk. The Ministry of Health pointed out in 1931 that over 1,000 children under 15 died of tuberculosis of bovine origin in England and Wales each year; many more were crippled.[10]

Methods of dealing with the problem of bovine infection included the wholesale slaughter of tuberculous cattle with suitable compensation for the farmers, licensing and grading of certain types of milk so as to place consumer pressure on farmers to produce milk of the highest quality, and pasteurization of milk for consumption. While all three methods were attempted in Britain, the second was foremost, based as it was on persuasion and market incentives rather than extensive state intervention and compulsion.

The limited success of the early twentieth-century attempts to control milk supplies has already been discussed. In 1915 the Milk and Dairies (Consolidation) Act had made each local authority responsible for the control of milk supplies in its own area. But enforcement had been postponed on account of the First World War, and it was in fact left in abeyance until the Milk and Dairies Order of 1926. Under the Order of 1926, local authorities were permitted to inspect cattle and forbid the sale of milk from those found to be infected. However, it was pointed out in the report of the Reorganisation Commission for Milk appointed by the Ministry of Agriculture and Fisheries in 1933 (the Grigg Report) that inspection was not carried out very systematically.[11]

A rigorous policy to eliminate bovine tuberculosis had been adopted in some other countries including the USA. In the latter country, starting in 1917, the Bureau of Animal Industry administered a

[10] Ministry of Health, *A Memorandum on Bovine Tuberculosis in Man with Special Reference to Infection by Milk* (63; London, 1931), 23.
[11] *Grigg Report* (1933), 52.

tuberculin test to all cattle, and reactors were slaughtered. The total number of tuberculin tests administered from 1917 to 1940 was around 300 million, of which approximately 4 million reacted. Provision was made for indemnities to owners of cattle which reacted to the tuberculin test and were slaughtered, amounting to almost $27 million for the year 1935 alone. By 1940 all counties in the USA apart from two in California were scheduled as 'modified accredited' areas which meant that not more than 0.5 per cent of the milch cows in those areas were tuberculin reactors.[12]

In Britain, by the Ministry of Agriculture and Fisheries Tuberculosis Order of 1925, notification of tuberculous cattle was introduced together with a system of compensation for the slaughter of cattle found to be tuberculous. However, it was later pointed out that farmers had no incentive to notify early as compensation would be paid even when the disease was far advanced.[13] The amount of compensation offered was clearly not considered an adequate inducement. The total destruction of all reactors was said to be impossible economically for the Government at that time. It was suggested in the *EMJ* that a solution would be found if farmers could be induced to undertake a voluntary effort in respect of their herds, and that the stimulus might be considerable if there was sufficient public demand for tubercle-free milk: 'Both the farmer and the public need to be educated.'[14]

A system of licensing types of milk for sale was introduced in Britain by the 1922 Milk and Dairies (Amendment) Act and the 1923 Milk (Special Designations) Order. There were three grades of milk under this scheme—'Certified', 'Grade A (Tuberculin-Tested)', and 'Grade A', as well as two grades of pasteurized milk—'Grade A, Pasteurized' and 'Pasteurized'. For 'Certified' and 'Grade A (TT)', the cattle had been clinically examined and tuberculin-tested every six months and all reactors removed, and 'Grade A' milk came from cattle which were not tuberculin-tested but were clinically examined every three months and diseased animals removed.[15] There was evidence of some abuse of the tuberculin test, with animals being sold under a false guarantee of freedom from tuberculosis, but nevertheless by 1932 only 1,105 farms

---

[12] J. A. Myers, *Man's Greatest Victory over Tuberculosis* (Springfield and Baltimore, 1940).
[13] Ministry of Health, *Bovine Tuberculosis*, p. 14.　　　　　　[14] *EMJ* 38 (1931), 224.
[15] *Grigg Report*, p. 54. The difference between Grade A (TT) and Certified, according to the NAPT, was that the latter was not required to be bottled on the farm: NAPT Pamphlet 3, 'Milk and Tuberculosis' (1930); *EMJ* 31/3 (1924), 184.

had licenses for one of the first three grades.[16] Moreover, the expense of the higher grades of milk was such that, according to a doctor from Huddersfield, it was 'a mockery to advise poor people to buy tubercle-free milk'.[17] Similarly, in Newcastle, the high cost meant that, despite a practically unlimited supply of tuberculin-tested milk, only 7 per cent of milk sold came into that category.[18] Pasteurization had been introduced into some parts of the USA in the early twentieth century. For example, pasteurization of all except 'certified' milk became compulsory in Chicago in 1908, in Massachusetts in 1910, and in New York City in 1912. This measure, together with the slaughter of tuberculous cattle, was held responsible for the subsequent decrease in the death-rates from non-pulmonary tuberculosis. The death-rate in New York City decreased by almost two-thirds from 1910 to 1925, and in Massachusetts by a full 92 per cent from 1910 to 1935.[19]

Pasteurization was by no means universally accepted as the best method of making milk safe for human consumption. An economic objection to pasteurization was that small producers could not afford a pasteurizing plant, but medical objections were also raised. Some doctors, for example Clive Rivière, even advocated the drinking of milk containing bovine tubercle bacilli as a way of obtaining some immunity against tuberculosis.[20] The MRC's Tuberculin Committee wrote to the Ministry of Health in 1926 that it strongly deprecated the suggestion which was current in some quarters that children who drank milk containing bovine tubercle bacilli benefited in that way by obtaining some immunity against tuberculosis. The committee believed that even if some degree of immunity were thus obtained, such a method of random and uncontrolled immunization, that carried with it grave risks of producing serious and even fatal disease, was indefensible.[21] Sir Robert Philip did not favour pasteurization. He argued that the nutritional value of pasteurized milk was not as great as fresh milk, but his greatest objection was that it would be 'whitewashing

[16] MRC 205/2, F. Knight (secretary, National Veterinary Medical Association of Great Britain and Ireland) wrote to Ministry of Health of 'evidence of an extensive and far reaching system of fraud by unscrupulous persons interested in the sale of animals sold under guarantee of freedom from tuberculosis', 9 Aug. 1927; *Grigg Report*, p. 54.
[17] *15 NAPT 1929*, p. 35.
[18] Ibid., p. 27; see also *EMJ* 31/1 (1924), 185, and ibid., 38 (1931), 222–3.
[19] H. D. Chadwick and A. S. Pope, *The Modern Attack on Tuberculosis* (New York, 1942), 5; Myers, *Man's Greatest Victory*, pp. 238, 253, 331, 334; *EMJ* 41 (1934), 191.
[20] C. Rivière, *Tuberculosis and How to Avoid It* (London, 1917), 49.
[21] MRC 205/2, III, MacNalty to Ministry of Health, 4 Nov. 1926 and 9 Nov. 1926.

dirtiness and mess and encouraging at every turn slackness on the part of the producer'.[22]

In its 1931 report on bovine tuberculosis, the Ministry of Health pronounced in favour of pasteurization as rendering the milk completely safe and not impairing its nutritive and commercial value.[23] Sir Arthur Newsholme wrote in 1935 that it was generally accepted as the best method of ensuring tubercle-free milk.[24] G. S. (later Sir Graham) Wilson, professor of bacteriology at the London School of Hygiene and Tropical Medicine, analysed medical objections to pasteurization in 1942. These objections were that it diminished the nutritive value of the milk, predisposed to dental caries, lowered resistance to the disease, and favoured the development of pulmonary tuberculosis in adult life. Further objections analysed by Wilson were that it was often inefficient, that it removed the incentive to clean milk production and to the eradication of diseased animals from milking herds, and imparted a cooked flavour to the milk. Wilson concluded that, 'no serious objection has so far been raised which rests on a firm basis of fact, and which can be weighed in the scales against the immense demonstrable advantage of a safe milk supply conferred by pasteurization.'[25]

The NAPT became involved in the campaign for a clean milk supply. It did not, however, advocate universal pasteurization, but rather, in accordance with its liberal, individualistic precepts, pressed for a clearer definition of the different grades of milk so that the public were aware of the choices.[26] In fact, the designations were confusing as was pointed out by the Grigg Report. People not conversant with the conditions prescribed were frequently under the impression that 'Grade A' was milk of the highest quality because the title contained no qualifications, 'Grade A Tuberculin-Tested' of lower quality by virtue of the qualifications added to the previous designation, and 'Certified' the lowest of the three grades. The proper order was thus reversed. The reason for this situation was that the designation 'Grade A' had been introduced during the First World War to distinguish it as milk of high hygienic quality. The other grades were subsequently introduced, leaving 'Grade A' as the lowest, although still widely

[22] *EMJ* 22/5 (1925), 100.
[23] Ministry of Health, *Bovine Tuberculosis*, pp. 21, 23.
[24] A. Newsholme, *Fifty Years in Public Health* (London, 1935), 239.
[25] G. S. Wilson, *The Pasteurization of Milk* (London, 1942), 179, 185, 186.
[26] NAPT Council Annual Report 1936, p. 6; NAPT Council Minutes, 26 Nov. 1928; ibid., 17 Feb. 1934, p. 231; ibid., 18 May 1936, p. 263.

regarded as the highest. According to the Grigg Report, 'It is not unnatural that those at present selling milk under this designation have a sense of vested interest with which they desire no interference.'[27]

The licensing of milk in the 1920s did little to reduce the problem of infection from bovine tuberculosis. The Ministry of Health estimated in 1931 that 40 per cent of the cows in the country were infected with tuberculosis, although admittedly not more than 2 per cent gave tubercle bacilli in their milk. In 1934 it was further estimated that 6 per cent of all farms were sending out milk containing tubercle bacilli, and that consequently all bulked milk was probably infected.[28]

Further attempts to eradicate tuberculosis infection from cattle were made in the 1930s. By the Milk (Special Designations) Order of 1936, four new categories of milk were introduced–'Tuberculin-Tested', subsuming the first two grades of the former system ('Certified' and 'Grade A (TT)'), 'Accredited', meaning the cattle had been tuberculin-tested originally, all reactors removed and no reactors added, 'Tuberculin-Tested (Pasteurized)', and 'Pasteurized'.

In 1935 the Ministry of Agriculture and Fisheries introduced a Tuberculosis (Attested Herds) Scheme, under which the owners of a herd could apply to the Ministry for an official tuberculin test of their herd. If no reactors were found, they would be entitled to a 'certificate of attestation' and thus have their herd entered in a register of attested herds, kept and published by the Ministry. The slaughter of cattle was remunerated by the Milk Marketing Board, and a bonus paid for milk from an attested herd. The following year the National Farmers' Union pointed out that the Attested Herd Scheme, together with premiums for milk from tuberculin tested herds which had been introduced following the 1933 Ministry of Agriculture and Fisheries Report, had encouraged some farmers to test cattle and to slaughter those which reacted. But they believed that the majority of farmers did not consider the grants adequate; where there was a substantial percentage of reactors, the loss involved during the process of building up a healthy herd would be more than the average farmer could stand. By 1939 approximately 3 per cent of the dairy farms in the country had

---

[27] *Grigg Report*, p. 55.
[28] Ministry of Health, *Bovine Tuberculosis*, pp. 9, 11, 23; Ministry of Agriculture and Fisheries, Economic Advisory Committee, *Report of Committee on Animal Diseases* (1934), quoted in MRC, *Report of the Committee on Tuberculosis in War-time* (SRS 246; London, 1942), 10, 11.

had their herds attested. In Scotland by 1943, 6.5 per cent of the cattle had been attested.[29]

Nor had pasteurization become universal by 1941. While 93 per cent of the milk in London was pasteurized, the amount pasteurized in a few county boroughs was not more than 10 per cent. Less than 50 per cent of the milk distributed in all counties was pasteurized at that time, and about 15 per cent heat-treated in some other way. In smaller towns much less was pasteurized and in rural areas practically none.[30]

(3) BCG VACCINATION

In 1931 a statement appeared in the Press that, following experiments on cattle carried out by Ministry of Agriculture veterinary surgeons, arrangements would shortly be made for the distribution of the BCG vaccine to doctors in Britain for inoculating children against tuberculosis. It was pointed out that the vaccine had been successfully administered to more than one million persons in other countries, and that 'in the opinion of leading doctors, the "white man's scourge" [that is tuberculosis] will be wiped out within the next ten years'. It was further pointed out that the only countries in Europe which had not adopted the vaccine to a greater or lesser extent at this time were Austria, Portugal, and Britain.[31]

BCG (Bacillus Calmette-Guérin) was discovered by Leon C. A. Calmette and Camille Guérin at the Pasteur Institute in Paris. In 1908, Calmette and Guérin were growing a virulent bovine strain of the tubercle bacillus on a glycerine-bile-potato medium to obtain a homogeneous suspension of the culture in saline solution, when they observed that repeated passage in this medium produced a rapid loss of virulence. This led them to consider the possibility of producing a safe strain of the bacillus for the purpose of vaccination. They continued to work on the culture until 1921, by which time it was definitely shown that the attenuated bacillus did not produce tuberculosis in cattle. In that year they named their vaccine BCG, and in 1922 it was given orally to infants in Paris with apparently successful

---

[29] MRC, *Tuberculosis in War-time*, pp. 10–11; PRO MH55/1219, National Farmers' Union, Welsh Branch, 24 Jan. 1938; *EMJ* 50 (1943), 224.

[30] MRC, *Tuberculosis in War-time*, p. 11.

[31] *Daily Express*, 12 Jan. 1931 (MRC, 1319, vol. iii). The Netherlands and Iceland could have been added to this list.

results. No controlled trials on human beings were carried out, but vaccination was introduced into France on a large scale, and to a lesser degree in Germany in 1925. Following a disaster in Lübeck, Germany, in 1930, when 73 infants out of a group of 249 vaccinated died as a direct result of being given the vaccine, enthusiasm for BCG waned in France and Germany, despite the fact that the vaccine itself was later exonerated of responsibility for the deaths. Enthusiasm did not, however, wane in Scandinavia where BCG had also been adopted.[32]

The Scandinavian countries administered the vaccine intracutaneously rather than orally. In 1927 Johannes Heimbeck began an experiment with BCG at Ulleval Hospital, Oslo, on student nurses. BCG was offered to student nurses who gave a negative reaction to a tuberculin test, while those who refused it were studied as controls. The tuberculosis morbidity rate among the non-vaccinated tuberculin-negative nurses during their training period was six times higher than the vaccinated group and the mortality rate was seven times higher. Intracutaneous vaccination was also introduced in 1927 in Göteborg, Sweden, by Arvid Johan Wallgren, professor of paediatrics, and subsequently became general practice in Sweden. The mortality rate from tuberculosis in Sweden from 1922–1926 was 0.34 per cent, dropping to 0.05 per cent in the period 1933–7, a more dramatic decline than most European countries, and unlike some other countries, the downward trend was sustained in the 1939–41 period. The sharp drop in Sweden was generally attributed to the use of BCG.[33]

Despite the enthusiastic report in the British Press in 1931, the introduction of BCG was not imminent in Britain. When one tuberculosis specialist, B. E. Schlesinger, applied for support from the Ministry of Health in that year to import the vaccine, which was necessary under the 1925 Therapeutic Substances Act, such support was not forthcoming.[34]

Discussing the lack of interest in BCG in Britain, Bardswell (now a medical officer for the LCC) explained that, drawing from his experience as an administrative officer, vaccination would be 'extraordinarily difficult to carry out, in view of the known repugnance, even

[32] C. Guérin, in S. R. Rosenthal (ed.), *BCG Vaccine: Tuberculosis–Cancer*, 2nd edn. (Littleton, Mass., 1980), 35–8.

[33] *NAPT Bulletin*, 7/3 (1945), 7, 8; F. R. G. Heaf and N. L. Rusby, *Recent Advances in Pulmonary Tuberculosis*, 4th edn. (London, 1948), 55.

[34] MRC 1319, BCG, MacNalty to Newman, 18 June 1931.

hostility, of the less educated classes to vaccination, or what they call "putting things into the child" in any sort of way'.[35] Sir George Buchanan, chairman of the Ministry of Health's Immunisation Committee set up in 1931, explained to Calmette that there was much opposition to smallpox vaccination and he did not believe that BCG would be readily accepted by the public.[36] Indeed, an anti-vaccination campaign had been waged and won in the late nineteenth and early twentieth centuries in regard to smallpox,[37] and few spoke out in favour of anti-tuberculosis vaccination before the Second World War. However, the extent to which the public was responsible for the lack of interest must be queried. Opposition to anti-typhoid vaccine for the troops in the First World War had been anticipated, but to the great surprise of the administrators, little opposition had been encountered, and, although voluntary, 97 per cent of the troops had been vaccinated by the second year of the war.[38] In 1948, when some administrators and scientists still opposed the introduction of BCG, the general feeling was, according to the NAPT, very much in favour of it.[39]

Little support for the vaccine was forthcoming from British scientists in the inter-war period. When a meeting was convened by the Health Committee of the League of Nations on BCG in 1928, it was decided by the MRC not to send any delegates, for 'it would not be satisfactory or particularly desirable for British scientific credit merely to send an officer who could not participate in the discussion and only acted as an observer'.[40] In the 1920s, the MRC supported its own candidate who was developing a tuberculosis vaccine, Georges Dreyer, professor of pathology at Oxford, who directed the Dunn School of Pathology set up in Oxford by the MRC in 1922. Great hopes were held out for his work in 1923, but by 1924 the results were proving disappointing. In 1926 the MRC commissioned Stanley Griffith of Cambridge University to research into BCG; Griffith was also being funded by the Empire Marketing Board to research tuberculosis in cattle. His research did not confirm Calmette's conclusions.[41] Stanley Griffith himself may have contributed to the

[35] *17 NAPT 1931*, p. 106. [36] *Lancet* 1 (1933), 654.
[37] R. M. McLeod, 'Law, Medicine and Public Opinion in the Resistance to Compulsory Health Legislation 1870–1907', *Public Law* (Summer 1967), 107–28, ibid. (Autumn 1967), 181–211; J. Swan, *The Vaccination Problem* (London, 1936).
[38] W. G . Macpherson, W. B. Leishman, and S. L. Cummins, *History of the Great War. Medical Services. Pathology* (London, 1923), 250.
[39] *NAPT Bulletin*, 10/5 (1948), 156.
[40] PRO MH55/150, G. Buchanan, 11 Oct. 1928.
[41] *MRC Annual Report 1927–8*, Cmd. 3276 (1929), 100.

lack of enthusiasm for BCG in Britain; he was described in 1929 as 'veering on the side of extreme caution and scepticism'.[42] In 1930, Dreyer, now also working on BCG, reported that, contrary to much research on the Continent, their own results supported their previous conclusions that vaccines of BCG were not necessarily safe for use in the preventive inoculation of man.[43] The Lübeck disaster served to reinforce their reservations. Sir George Buchanan asserted in 1933, 'One is not justified at the best in claiming more for the inoculation of BCG than that there is some *prima-facie* evidence to show that it is a useful temporary precaution to take.'[44] Moreover, Greenwood was critical of the figures quoted by Calmette and others in favour of the BCG results.[45] Thus the Ministry of Health rejected Schlesinger's request to import BCG in 1931, 'in the light of Stanley Griffith's experiments'.[46]

Administrative objections were possibly more important in the non-adoption of BCG in Britain than lack of scientific verification of its efficacy. According to Buchanan, 'assuming that the power to confer this protection were definitely proved, and not merely a plausible assumption, there would still be considerable limitation in applying it in practice.' His arguments against its introduction were first that the vaccine took four weeks to confer immunity, during which time new-born infants who were vaccinated should be kept apart from their families or else the vaccination might be rendered useless. Second, it had not yet been established how long the immunity lasted and revaccination might be necessary. Third, Britain had an active preventive policy involving isolation of infected cases and hygienic measures as well as a well-developed curative service, which the introduction of BCG might interfere with. Moreover, he added that tuberculosis was rapidly declining in any case in Britain without the aid of the vaccine (the number of deaths under 1 year of age from all forms of tuberculosis declined from 1,311 in 1921 to 585 in 1930).[47]

Calmette replied to Buchanan's arguments, 'to me it is rather

[42] MRC 1319, III, BCG, Fletcher to Middleton, 22 Jan. 1929.
[43] *MRC Annual Report 1929–30*, Cmd. 3785 (1931), 84.
[44] *Lancet* 1 (1933), 654.
[45] *BMJ* 1 (1928), 793; Calmette and Guérin were not particularly meticulous in their record-keeping: see W. D. Foster, *A History of Medical Bacteriology and Immunology* (London, 1970), 157.
[46] MRC 1319, BCG, MacNalty to Newman, 18 June 1931; MRC, Stanley Griffith, *Studies of Protection against Tuberculosis: Results with BCG Vaccine in Monkeys* (SRS 152; London, 1931), 48.
[47] *Lancet* 1 (1933), 654.

Utopian to believe in the possibility of eradicating tuberculosis by measures of hygiene only'. He claimed that even if the four-week separation were not enforced, 'we learn from an experience of thousands of cases all over the world that BCG nearly always yields sufficient protection'. He also pointed out that they did not know for how long immunity resulted from smallpox vaccination and yet that did not stop them from using it. Calmette suggested that it was the authorities in Britain and not the public who opposed the introduction of BCG.[48]

Tuberculosis specialists and medical superintendents, known in other respects for their conservatism, also showed little interest in the vaccine in the inter-war period. L. S. T. Burrell, physician to the Brompton Hospital, was not alone in his remark that 'we shall not find salvation in inoculation'.[49] It seemed odd to the author of the history of the BTA in 1978 that BCG, so widely used on the Continent in the 1920s, should not have been discussed at a TA meeting until 1935.[50] K. Neville Irvine, a GP who made BCG the subject of his DM thesis in 1934, argued that there was little doubt that the vaccine did produce a definite increase in resistance to the disease. He claimed,

today we are one of the few civilised countries who have not explored its possibilities. One of the main barriers to its use in this country has been the mistaken idea that it would mean the entire reorganisation of our present scheme for fighting tuberculosis; the necessary isolation of the child before and after inoculation would seem to be fraught with financial difficulties.[51]

Sir Wilson Jameson, the Chief Medical Officer of the Ministry of Health, admitted during the Second World War that official opposition rested mainly on administrative grounds.[52] The slow adoption of BCG can be paralleled with that of the anti-diphtheria vaccine.[53]

(4) EDUCATION

Attempts to isolate tuberculous patients, to prevent people suffering from tuberculosis from working in food trades, and to control the milk

[48] *Lancet* I (1933), 655.
[49] *17 NAPT 1931*, p. 149; *21 NAPT 1935*, p. 16.
[50] *British Thoracic Association (The First Fifty Years)* (London, 1978), 14.
[51] *21 NAPT 1935*, p. 88.
[52] MRC 1319/1, Tytler to Mellanby, 16 May 1944.
[53] On the delay in implementation of diphtheria vaccine, see Foster, *A History of Bacteriology*, pp. 148–52.

supply were at best half-hearted, while vaccination as a preventive measure was not given serious consideration. Rather, emphasis was placed on raising the resistance of the individual naturally against infection or disease. Major Greenwood believed this could only be done by improving economic conditions; he wrote in 1935, 'It is not scientific or modern-minded or anything but foolish to try to believe that any other prophylaxis of this particular crowd disease [*tuberculosis*] is so important as raising the economic level and increasing the *commoda vitae* of the crowd.'[54] Ellen Wilkinson believed that the case which Bradbury allowed to be built up with the figures of his survey on Tyneside—that overcrowding, undernourishment, and insanitary conditions were the main causal factors of the high tuberculosis rate in Jarrow—seemed unanswerable. Yet, she noted, when Bradbury came to his practical suggestions for reducing the disease, his proposal regarding the food problem on which his report laid such stress was:

In view of the apparent importance of undernourishment as a predisposing cause of tuberculosis, it appears desirable that *something should be done* to improve the defences of poor families against tuberculosis by the *issuing of information* by Local Authorities on the subject of better housekeeping—particularly in the matter of providing adequate and balanced diets at the cheapest possible rates.

Wilkinson added, 'The italics are mine and comment seems unnecessary.'[55]

The 1925 Public Health (Prevention of Tuberculosis) Act empowered local authorities to spend part of their tuberculosis funds on educational propaganda, although MacNalty noted in 1932 that little work in this area was done by English authorities.[56] While in Wales the WNMA had an active educational programme, in England and Scotland the work was left almost entirely in the hands of the NAPT.

The NAPT claimed in 1930 that its propaganda was on such a scale that 'it represents possibly the largest effort to mould public opinion ever made by a voluntary organisation in this country'.[57] Following a successful appeal in 1926 raising £17,000, the propaganda campaign of the NAPT was stepped up. William Brand, TO for Camberwell, was

[54] M. Greenwood, *Epidemics and Crowd-Diseases: An Introduction to the Study of Epidemiology* (London, 1935), 358.
[55] E. Wilkinson, *The Town that was Murdered. The Life-history of Jarrow* (London, 1939), 243, 244.
[56] Ministry of Health, MacNalty, *A Report on Tuberculosis*, p. 62.
[57] NAPT Council Annual Report 1929, p. 2.

employed temporarily to tour the country and give lectures. In 1927 two motor caravans were purchased and equipped with exhibitions, films, and lantern slides, and two assistants were appointed in 1928. At the suggestion of Sir Robert Philip, J. Harley Williams, MOH for the Island of Lewis and TO for the Lewis Red Cross Society, was appointed medical commissioner in 1927 to tour Scotland and give lectures. Two nurse commissioners from the Queen's Nurses were appointed to assist him. On the termination of Brand's appointment in 1929, Harley Williams became the medical commissioner for the NAPT. In 1933, Harley Williams maintained, 'I think there is almost no kind of human group or organisation in the country that we have not reached.' Lectures had been held in 'Hyde Park, schools, a monastery, hospitals, women's institutes, market squares, a great many annual meetings of care committees, town halls, health exhibitions', as well as offices, shops, and factories.[58]

The two nurse commissioners continued to tour Scotland in the 1930s. One of them, Miss Weir, described a visit to Lewis Island in April 1939. She had paid many private visits but claimed that it was impossible to arrange public meetings, 'for at this time of the year the people are busy with the peat and the men are at the fishing'. She also described a religious revival which was spreading over the island at that time:

In this connection meetings are held in the homes of the people commencing at 10 p.m. and often continuing until 4 or 5 a.m. This naturally has a very bad effect on the health of the people who crowd into a small room with unopen windows, and many of them faint. The children too are affected, as they are pale from want of sleep and at school are unable to attend to their lessons.[59]

Harley Williams later maintained that the lectures given in the north of Scotland in particular owed their success to the opening of people's minds to a theme which was strongly repressed: 'Often, members of the audience fainted, and there were angry questions at the end.' (It is assumed these meetings were not held in small rooms with unopened windows.)[60]

The NAPT annual conferences were also designed as an educational medium, held in various cities and attended by several hundred

[58] *19 NAPT 1933*, pp. 157, 209; ibid., p. 209.
[59] NAPT Council Minutes, 19 June 1939, p. 5.
[60] J. H. Williams, *Requiem for a Great Killer: The Story of Tuberculosis* (London, 1973), 48.

delegates incuding non-medical local councillors. Sometimes the conferences became a forum for political discussion. For example, Councillor T. W. Brown from Shoreditch Borough Council spoke out against the cuts in unemployment insurance in 1931: 'When you have the Report on the Royal Commission on Unemployment Insurance, where it is suggested that a family of five should live on 29 shillings a week and pay rent, how do you think you are going to prevent tuberculosis?'[61] Political discussion was not, however, the direction encouraged by the conference organizers, as will be discussed later.

During the 1924 annual conference held in Birmingham, a short popular lecture on tuberculosis was broadcast by Sir Robert Philip from the local radio station. The NAPT council reported that it was the first lecture on tuberculosis to be given by this method in Britain and that it was interesting to note that the BBC was arranging in the near future to broadcast health talks.[62]

In 1935 the NAPT decided to launch a press campaign. A Fleet Street publicity firm was appointed for eight months at a cost of £1,000, following which the Association set up its own publicity department. This department reported in 1939 that stories and articles were sent out regularly, contact being maintained with some 900 newspapers throughout the country, embracing the national and provincial daily papers and all important weekly journals.[63]

Films were another important medium for propaganda adopted by the NAPT. Twelve films on tuberculosis had been produced by the Association by 1944, starting with 'The Story of John M'Neil', produced at the Royal Victoria Hospital, Edinburgh, by Halliday Sutherland in 1911. An NAPT film produced in 1935, 'Makers of Men', on Burrow Hill Tuberculosis Colony, was selected by the British Film Institute to be shown at an international film exhibition organized by the League of Nations at Geneva in 1935 as the best British production of the year with regard to propaganda and technique.[64] The council of the Association wrote in 1936, 'In Great Britain, over 20 million persons attend the Picture Theatres every

[61] *17 NAPT 1931*, p. 113.
[62] NAPT Council Annual Report 1923, p. 5.
[63] NAPT Council Minutes, Publicity Sub-committee Report, 20 May 1935, p. 176; ibid., 15 Mar. 1937, p. 357; ibid., 40th AGM, 29 June 1939, p. 12.
[64] NAPT Council Minutes, Propaganda Sub-committee Report, 21 Jan. 1935, p. 130. Chest, Heart and Stroke Association Propaganda Literature; letter by F. Stickland (NAPT secretary), Sept. 1935 (Radcliffe Science Library, Bodleian Library, Oxford).

week. What a field for education in Health!'[65] Yet, most cinemas preferred to show entertaining 'shorts', which is why in 1935 the Association produced a film that was designed to be 'both didactic and entertaining'.[66] Much of the viewing probably took place at meetings arranged by the Association or from their caravans, rather than in cinemas. Harley Williams later described the difficulties of the caravan tours in the north of Scotland, where 'the cinema projector had to be transported over rocks and by boats from small harbours'. In some of these localities, the cinema was considered definitely sinful and some of the stricter Presbyterians would not attend.[67]

What was the ideological stance of the NAPT? A perusal of the proceedings of the annual conferences gives a clear indication. At the 1935 conference, the suggestion of Councillor Mrs Olive Bennett from Greenwich Metropolitan Borough Council that if they wanted to abolish tuberculosis they would have to abolish poverty caused some mirth among the delegates for its naïvety. Alderman Kinley from Bootle supported her, however: 'If you are not prepared to undertake seriously the consideration of the abolition of poverty then you had better close down your Association at once, because you are wasting the whole of your time.' The chairman, Sir Robert Philip, intercepted, 'I think we must keep a little nearer to the subject at hand . . . "How may the child be safeguarded against human infection?"'[68] The Marchioness of Titchfield (later chairman of the NAPT) said at the 1928 conference, 'The masses must be instructed in the very elements of the science of living, the virtue of fresh air, cleanliness, exercise, the general sanitation of their homes and surroundings; the desire for right living must be inculcated and a public feeling in these matters must be aroused to intensity.'[69] Edith McGaw, who played a large part in NAPT activities (and later married Robert Philip), said in 1934, 'It is sound statesmanship to teach men and women how very much the eradication of tuberculosis lies within their own grasp.' She believed it a 'pathetic fact' that although the business of homemaking was essentially a woman's job, few had any real training for it.[70] A press report on the proceedings of the 1937 conference of the NAPT stated, 'Undoubtedly the most revolutionary discovery is that tuberculosis is an acquired disease which can be kept at bay by observing the rules of

[65] NAPT Council Annual Report 1935, p. 10.   [66] Ibid., pp. 10–11.
[67] Williams, *Requiem for a Great Killer*, p. 48.
[68] *21 NAPT 1935*, pp. 25, 27, 28.
[69] *14 NAPT 1928*, p. 71.   [70] *20 NAPT 1934*, pp. 136, 138.

healthy living.'[71] Self-responsibility was the emphasis of the NAPT propaganda.

The film 'The Invisible Enemy', produced in 1925, was, according to the council of the NAPT, 'of great value in bringing home the lessons which the Association has striven to teach since its foundation'.[72] The film was particularly in line with NAPT ideology as it showed that tuberculosis was not confined to the poor—the victim of the disease was heir to a beautiful estate—and stressed maternal responsibility. The mother asked at the death of her son from tuberculosis what she had done to deserve this. A dark figure symbolizing death, as in medieval morality plays, replied, 'It is just the ignorance of millions like yourself that causes the miseries of mankind—it is through ignorance that people daily commit crimes of which the victims are their own children.' Not only did she allow the child contact with the germs in his early years, she was also responsible for his failure to build up adequate resistance as she did not prevent him from working too hard at his homework and did not insist on his eating a healthy diet rather than sweets. He finally broke down after cycling with a friend, overdoing his strength by 'dashing along dusty roads', and stopping to smoke a cigarette.

The didactic film concluded with the black figure instructing:

Teach them the benefits of open air and the consequences of bad habits. Teach them to protect themselves from dirt. Hygiene in living, hygiene in the house. Air, light, cleanliness—the human flower is of all flowers the one that needs the sun the most. Give your children health, that most precious of possessions! It is a social duty from the point of view of national interest and general wellbeing. Prevention is better than cure. Remember those words, 'Too late,' for then the science of medicine is powerless.

Go and teach the truth: 'The Fate of Each Man is in his own Hands.'[73]

The emphasis in the educational propaganda of the WNMA was also on maternal responsibility, for they believed 'biologically the education of the mothers of the race in their maternal duties transcends all things in importance'.[74] Following H. D. Chalke's report revealing high tuberculosis rates and poor living conditions in Gwyrfai, the WNMA held a conference to consider preventive measures. This

---

[71] *Western Daily Press*, 3 July 1937 (PRO MH55/1179).
[72] NAPT Historical Sketch 1898–1926 (1926), 33.
[73] NAPT Council Annual Report 1924, pp. 29–31. There was no suggestion that smoking was causative, it was merely indicative of licentious behaviour.
[74] WNMA Annual Report 1937, p. 45.

resulted in the drawing up of an exemplary budget for housewives and the appointment of two health visitors in the area to supervise the homes of the tuberculous and to advise on domestic arrangements.[75]

(5) OPEN-AIR SCHOOLS AND THE BOARDING OUT OF CHILDREN

Another preventive measure which the NAPT became involved in promoting was the removal of supposedly susceptible children to a healthier environment in an attempt to build up their resistance. The Oxfordshire branch of the NAPT stated in their annual report for 1918 that 'the most important of all measures of prevention [is] the care of delicate and predisposed children who do not strictly come under any tuberculosis scheme, but who may form the consumptive population in the future'. They believed that such children could often be tided over the 'delicate years of growth' if they were ensured occasional months of country life or kept away from infected families until the danger had passed. They had 2 small country homes, accommodating 8 children, and sent others to convalescent homes or camps.[76]

By 1937 there were 96 open-air day schools in England and 53 open-air residential schools, with 11,409 and 3,985 pupils respectively. There were also 36 sanatorium schools for children with pulmonary tuberculosis, accommodating 2,451 children, and 65 schools for children with non-pulmonary tuberculosis.[77] The NAPT noted the presence (or absence) of open-air schools in each area in its *Handbook of Tuberculosis Schemes*. It recorded in 1927, for example, that Cambridgeshire had no open-air schools specifically for tuberculous cases, but that the Cambridge Borough Education Committee admitted 'pre-tubercular' cases to day open-air schools, while the Cambridgeshire Education Committee sent 'pre-tubercular' children to residential open-air schools managed by the Invalid Children's Aid Association and the Ogilvie Charity (where 10 places were reserved for such cases). In the warmer months, open-air classes were held in

[75] PRO MH96/1056, Conference of WNMA with local authorities and insurance committees, Caernarfon, 11 Nov. 1933.
[76] NAPT Oxfordshire Branch Annual Report (1918), 7; ibid. (1920), 8; ibid. (1931), 16.
[77] *23 NAPT 1937*, pp. 62–3.

almost half the elementary schools' playgrounds.[78] Other local authorities also organized open-air classes in their schools. Forty out of 221 schools in Glasgow, as well as portions of 21 others, had been constructed on 'open-air principles', with classrooms designed with open verandahs and sliding doors; it was reported in 1935 that all new schools were being constructed in this way. Glasgow also had two 'preventoria' for children 'with the stigmata of tuberculosis'.[79] The open-air movement, encouraged by the NAPT, exerted an influence on the architecture of schools in the inter-war period, causing the demise of the central-hall building and its replacement by more spacious and airy pavilion schools. The 1918 Education Act enabled local authorities to provide school camps, and school lessons in the countryside were encouraged. However, the developments were permissive, with great variation from area to area.[80]

The NAPT attempted to popularize open-air schools through a film produced in 1921 called 'Air and Sun'. The NAPT council summed up the film as showing 'the benefit to be derived from air and sun, not only as a means of special treatment for the diseased, but generally in strengthening and hardening the delicate and weakly, by a return for a time to a natural life, which, owing to the restrictions of modern conditions has been largely lost'.[81] The film was set in an open-air school in Switzerland, although the methods were said to be equally applicable to Britain. We are told, 'A child finds its proper place in the midst of Nature! Learning is no effort there—his mind is clearer than in the stuffy air of a class room.' The girls are shown at 'nature work', the boys doing 'useful work'. In winter the boys are seen ice-skating, wearing only shorts: 'By direct contact with Air and Sunlight, the skin which clothing has made tender like a hothouse plant, recovers its natural functions. By systematic training the children become so hardened that even in the depth of winter they can play naked in the sun. Their bronzed skin is a natural clothing.'[82]

The film shows the influence of Auguste Rollier, who set up a clinic

---

[78] *NAPT Handbook of Tuberculosis Schemes in Great Britain and Ireland*, 5th edn. (London, 1927), 6.

[79] *NAPT Handbook*, 8th edn. (1935), 95; *EMJ* 38 (1931), 157.

[80] M. Seaborne and R. Lowe, *The English School—its Architecture and Organization*, ii, 1870–1970 (London, 1977), 81, 83; Charles Webster, 'The Health of the School Child during the Depression', in N. Parry and D. McNair (eds.), *The Fitness of the Nation* (Leicester, 1983), 74–5, 76.

[81] NAPT Historical Sketch (1926), 32.

[82] British Film Institute Archives, 'Air and Sun' (1921).

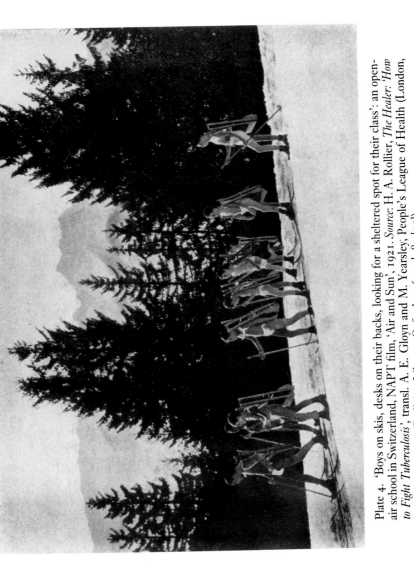

Plate 4. 'Boys on skis, desks on their backs, looking for a sheltered spot for their class': an open-air school in Switzerland, NAPT film, 'Air and Sun', 1921. *Source:* H. A. Rollier, *The Healer: 'How to Fight Tuberculosis'*, transl. A. E. Gloyn and M. Yearsley; People's League of Health (London, 1924), after p. 15 (Bodleian Library, Oxford, 15697 d. 82 [15]).

at Leysin, Switzerland, in 1903 for the systematic treatment of tuberculosis by the Alpine sun, and perhaps more directly of L. E. (later Sir Leonard) Hill, director of the department of applied physiology at the National Institute for Medical Research. In a report for the MRC in 1919, Hill described an open-air school for children taken from slum tenements. At this school, unless there was a bitter wind, the children were more or less uncovered, summer and winter, and slept in canvas shelters. According to Hill, they never showed discomfort from cold, nor did they suffer from catarrhs, and came to regard going inside as a punishment. He wrote that as they were fed to meet their energy demands, they did extraordinarily well, but that going back to the slums they would relapse again, becoming thin and pale from the caged life and ill-feeding.[83]

An alternative to open-air schools was the boarding out of children in foster-homes in the country. This was a scheme proposed for children who were exposed to an active case of tuberculosis but who did not have tuberculosis themselves. It was modelled on a French system which had been introduced by Professor Grancher in the early twentieth century. The so-called Grancher system was part of the particularly well-developed child welfare campaign in France in the early twentieth century, related to the concern for the declining birth-rate in France and the high infant mortality.[84] The popularity of the Grancher system in Britain (where it was often favourably commented on) stemmed from the belief in the desirability of caring for children within a family rather than an institutional environment, a firmly entrenched belief in the inter-war years.[85] A few local authorities financed such a scheme, such as the LCC and Surrey CC. In other places, voluntary after-care committees became involved, such as in Plymouth and Hastings. The tuberculosis after-care committee for the Borough of Hastings had an inflated view of the advantages of such a scheme; they claimed, 'Treated in this way these children almost invariably do well, but if left to themselves, it is estimated that at least 60 per cent of them die of tuberculosis'.[86] However, the Grancher

[83] August Rollier, trans. A. E. Gloyn and M. Yearsley, *The Healer, How to Fight against Tuberculosis* (London, 1925), 6; MRC, L. E. Hill, *The Science of Ventilation and Open-air Treatment* (SRS 52, Part II; London, 1920), 200.

[84] *International Congress on Tuberculosis 1905: Report of C. Theodore Williams and H. Timbrell Bulstode*, Cd. 2898 (1906), 11. See also John Guy, in C. W. Hutt and H. H. Thomson (eds.), *Principles and Practice of Preventive Medicine* i (London, 1935), 349.

[85] See P. Thane, *The Foundations of the Welfare State* (London, 1982), 200.

[86] Annual Report of Tuberculosis Care Committee for Hastings 1920–1, pp. 5, 6.

system was said to be less successful in England than in France as there were fewer smallholders in England, and a rural environment was considered essential. Another problem, according to one commentator, was the reluctance of parents to let their children go away, perhaps indicative of the growing child-centredness of the twentieth-century family.[87]

(6) PHYSICAL CULTURE

Fresh air and healthy leisure pursuits formed the theme of the Association's first sound film, produced in 1935, 'Stand up and Breathe'. The NAPT was not alone in stressing the positive effects on health of physical education and outdoor recreation. It was almost becoming a national obsession, though always carefully distinguished from the Hitler Youth Movement. By the 1930s physical education dominated the school medical service. Camping was becoming the enduring symbol of the Scouting movement which had grown up in the early twentieth century. The Youth Hostel Association was formed in 1930 and the Ramblers' Association followed, fostering a love for the countryside.

The NAPT applauded the Government's scheme for 'physical culture' introduced in 1936, which included plans for new playing fields, and led to the Physical Training and Recreation Act of 1937. It expressed satisfaction that the time had come when Parliament could turn its attention to general aspects of national fitness 'which have always been part of this Association's programme'. Yet a note of caution was added: 'Schemes of physical training must be adapted to the capacity of the individual, and the Council trust that due attention will be paid to avoid the over-fatigue which, particularly in adolescence, is among the contributory causes of tuberculosis.' Nevertheless, in the view of the NAPT, fresh air and leisure pursuits were more important than economic factors in prevention, and it applauded the Factory Act of 1937 for its restrictions on working hours of women and adolescents.[88]

The NAPT council commented on the film, 'Stand up and

---

[87] A. M. Hewat (Senior MO, LCC), *14 NAPT 1928*, p. 65. See also M. S. Rice, *Working-class Wives* (London, 1939), 15 n. 1.
[88] NAPT Council Annual Report 1936, pp. 8–9. See also WNMA Annual Report 1937–8; on the Physical Training and Recreation Act 1937, see C. Webster in Parry and McNair (eds.), *The Fitness of the Nation*, pp. 73–4.

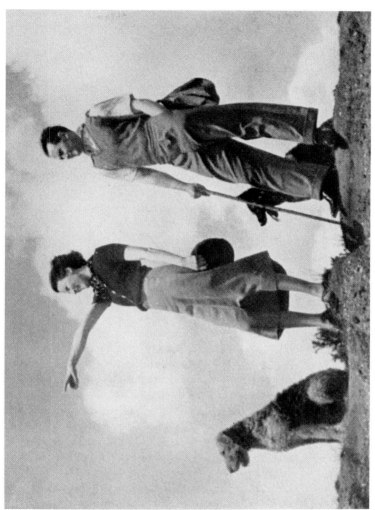

Plate 5. 'Stand up and Breathe', NAPT film, 1935.
Source: NAPT Annual Report of Council 1935, p. 11.

Breathe': 'While no formal reference is made to tuberculosis, the essential laws of prevention, the use of open-air exercise and sunshine, are illustrated in an admirable way.'[89] This film epitomizes the change in the emphasis of the NAPT propaganda which had taken place since the early twentieth century, a movement away from presenting 'a cabinet of horrors' to focusing on health education in which the word 'tuberculosis' rarely appeared. While some of its propaganda continued to stress the need for early examination to detect tuberculosis or directly concerned sanatorium life and tuberculosis nursing, much concentrated on health to the exclusion of the disease. The council stated in 1940, 'In teaching children it is not wise to stress the morbid side of the subject, and good anti-tuberculosis propaganda can be given without undue emphasis on the disease.'[90] The change was already evident in 1932 when it was reported that films and slides, shown at the popular lectures, were judiciously interpreted, with care being taken not to cause alarm or indoctrinate the public with an exaggerated fear of infection.[91] Thus there was some attempt to undo the damage of its early propaganda, which had been largely based on scare tactics, causing a widespread fear of the disease and its victims.

The change of emphasis was encapsulated in the title of a conference organized by the NAPT in 1947: the Commonwealth and Empire Health and Tuberculosis Conference. Not only were they now focusing their attention beyond Britain, but the editor of the *NAPT Bulletin* pointed to 'Health' as the operative word: 'Was it not time that we expressed in the title and style of our meeting that we believe Health is more important than disease, and that the positive outlook will get us further in preventing tuberculosis than any more negative and specialised preoccupation with ill-health?'[92]

Pamphlet literature in the 1930s showed the same shift away from specific reference to tuberculosis. The pamphlet, *Hints on the management of children from one to five years of age*, which appeared in 1930, devoted only seven lines out of fifteen pages specifically to tuberculosis. *Hints on the care of children at school age* followed, which stressed the strains involved in school life. A poster, 'The application of the idea of open-air to modern life', was produced for display in the areas of some 300 local health authorities in 1936.[93]

[89] NAPT Council Annual Report 1935, pp. 10–11.
[90] Ibid., 1939, p. 7.   [91] Ibid. 1931, p. 2.
[92] *NAPT Bulletin*, 10/1 (1947), 17.
[93] NAPT Pamphlet Literature, 1930–48 (Radcliffe Science Library, Bodleian Library, Oxford); NAPT Council Annual Report 1935, p. 12.

The NAPT thus envisaged its field of reference extending beyond the world of tuberculosis to encompass health maintenance in general. Not only can parallels be drawn with the school medical service and its open-air emphasis, but much of the NAPT propaganda was also similar to that issued by the National Council for Combating Venereal Diseases (British Social Hygiene Council after 1925). One of the latter's slogans was 'Fresh Air, Exercise, and Chastity/Win the Goal of Health'.[94] While it subscribed to the same ideology, the NAPT resisted the advances of the Council to organize joint health campaigns.[95] Tuberculosis may have been viewed as a moral failing of the people preventable by healthy living, but the Association did not want it tainted by an association with venereal disease. Nor did it encourage a link with the temperance movement.[96] Anti-alcohol propaganda was not prominent in the Association's campaigns. However, it did maintain close contact with other health organizations. In 1921 the Association participated in a National Efficiency Exhibition organized by the *Daily Mail* at Olympia, London. Representatives were sent to all conferences considered relevant, such as those held by the Women's Imperial Health Association and the Invalid Children's Aid Association, as well as Rural Community conferences, Royal Sanitary Institute congresses, National Maternity and Child Welfare conferences, and conferences of the Central Council for Health Education. The Central Council for Health Education, formed in 1927 by the SMOH, invited Sir Robert Philip and the medical commissioner, W. Brand, to attend its first conference in 1928. In 1929 the NAPT decided to contribute £125 per annum towards the cost of the Central Council's journal, *Better Health*. When the Central Council became incorporated in 1935, the NAPT was granted affiliation, and the medical commissioner was elected as one of the four representatives of voluntary organizations to serve on the council. In 1935 the newly formed Association of Open-air Schools was affiliated to the NAPT. In the same year the medical commissioner was authorized to co-operate in any way in his power with the National Federation of Personal Health Associations.[97]

The focus of preventive work carried out by the NAPT was summed

[94] National Council for Combating Venereal Diseases, Educational and Propaganda Material: Poster, *c.*1924 (records at the Wellcome Unit for the History of Medicine, Oxford; reference supplied by J. Austoker).

[95] NAPT Council Minutes, 28 Feb. 1921, p. 6; ibid., 27 Mar. 1922, p. 4.

[96] Ibid., 28 Apr. 1914, p. 2.   [97] Ibid., 15 Nov. 1935, p. 53.

up by the propaganda committee of the Association in 1937 when it stated, 'we need to convince every member of the community that the eradication of tuberculosis is his own affair'.[98] The emphasis was placed specifically on open-air leisure pursuits rather than on an attempt to reform living and working conditions.

[98] NAPT Council Annual Report 1936, p. 3.

6

Work Versus Collapse Therapy

FOLLOWING the First World War, work therapy which had grown up in the early twentieth century remained the dominant treatment practised in tuberculosis institutions. In particular, belief in the therapeutic value of open-air treatment persisted. It will be seen that the rise of surgical intervention in the 1930s, challenging work therapy or 'conservative treatment', had more to do with professional interests, and economic and social pressures than with any inherent superiority of surgery over conservative treatment. It will also be seen that despite the widespread advocacy of surgery, conservative treatment remained paramount throughout this period, in Britain at least, even in the 1940s when surgery was at its peak. Nor did chemotherapy pose any real threat to conservative treatment at this time.

(1) WORK THERAPY

In the immediate post-war years, tuberculosis specialists were placed on the defensive owing to the poor results of sanatorium treatment during the last two decades. They did not, however, abandon this form of treatment. Sir George Newman reflected the dominant view among tuberculosis specialists when he asserted in 1927 that sanatorium treatment was 'absolutely sound'.[1] The problem, in the view of the specialists, was the temporary nature of such treatment. Relapses would occur when patients returned to the environment and lifestyle under which the disease had been contracted. The ideal solution was therefore to place the patients in a village settlement where they would be permanently supervised and would live under the healthiest possible conditions. Thus, Sir James Kingston Fowler suggested in 1923 that in the future treatment of tuberculosis, 'settlement treatment' should replace 'sanatorium treatment' just as 'sanatorium treatment' had replaced 'open-air treatment'.[2] The MRC recommended in 1920 that

[1] 9th CMOH Annual Report 1927 (1928), p. 59.
[2] J. K. Fowler, Problems in Tuberculosis (London, 1923), 43.

any institution for the treatment of tuberculosis should include a village settlement.[3] Two Government committees set up in 1919, the Barlow Committee and the Murray Committee, also favoured the development of village settlements for the tuberculous.[4]

Papworth Village Settlement, founded in 1917 by P. J. (later Sir Pendrill) Varrier-Jones with the support of Sir German Sims Woodhead, professor of pathology at Cambridge University, was held up as the model. It consisted of a hospital, sanatorium, and village settlement with industries attached. Patients were first received in the hospital section, then transferred to the sanatorium section, when they would work in the industries, and finally they could apply to live in the village settlement with their families and work in the industries at trade-union rates of pay. For unmarried men there was a hostel. A hostel was also set up for single women in 1927. By 1938 Papworth Village Settlement had a population of over 1,000 people, including patients, families, and staff. There were 142 cottages, all occupied, with a total of 368 children, in the village.[5]

Papworth Village Settlement was planned as a 'Garden City', inspired by the writings of Ebenezer Howard and the product of his ideas, Letchworth Garden City. Like Letchworth, Papworth was 'to combine as far as is practicable the benefits and amenities of rural life with the social and industrial advantages of urban existence so devised as to promote the healthiest possible conditions of life'. Howard himself approved the application of the Garden City movement to tuberculosis institutions.[6]

The idea of a village settlement for the tuberculous had added appeal in that it involved their permanent segregation from society, important now that the infectious nature of the disease was popular knowledge. For example, J. E. Esselmont, medical superintendent of Home Sanatorium, Bournemouth, who published a brochure entitled 'Garden Cities for Consumptives: a National Scheme Outline' in 1913, considered this its prime attraction.[7] To Varrier-Jones, however,

---

[3] MRC MB4, Sub-committee on Phthisis in Relation to Occupation, Minutes of meeting, and letter to London Society of Compositors, 15 Nov. 1920.

[4] *Barlow Report*, p. 12; PRO MH55/169, Murray Report, p. 4.

[5] L. Bryder, 'Papworth Village Settlement: A Unique Experiment in the Treatment and Care of the Tuberculous?', *Medical History*, 28/4 (1984), 372–90.

[6] H. H. Thomson, *Tuberculosis and National Health* (London, 1939), 103; E. Howard, *Garden Cities of Tomorrow*, 2nd edn. (London, 1902). See also A. Sutcliffe (ed.), *British Town Planning: The Formative Years* (Leicester, 1981); T. N. Kelynack (ed.), *Tuberculosis Yearbook and Sanatoria Annual*, i, *1913–14* (London, 1914), 83 n.

[7] Kelynack (ed.), *Tuberculosis Yearbook 1913–14*, p. 84; *BJT* 12 (1918), 76.

Papworth was not a 'leper' colony, nor was it merely an attempt to create a favourable environment for 'arrested' cases of tuberculosis. It was an institution for the treatment of tuberculosis in all its phases. Those in the village were still regarded as patients in need of supervision, for Varrier-Jones did not believe that tuberculosis could be cured.

Treatment at Papworth was based on a holistic approach to medicine. Explaining the scheme in 1935, Varrier-Jones wrote that he and Woodhead 'were sure that our scheme would have to aim at treating the whole man or woman, and not merely the diseased portion of that man or woman, and on that basis the Village Settlement scheme has been built'.[8] Inspecting Papworth in 1920, A. S. MacNalty and N. Raw noted approvingly, 'At Papworth the individual case is studied, temperamentally, psychologically, physically, and socially, and there is no mere academic classification of the patient according to his pulmonary physical signs.'[9] On the subject of treatment, Varrier-Jones advised in 1920:

Treat the patient, the whole patient, and his environment as well, and he and his body fluids will conquer his distemper far more surely than any quantity of medical, surgical and X-ray apparatus . . . I have used the word person advisedly, for . . . we are dealing with persons, not cases, and with this firmly fixed in our minds we shall be more likely to find a solution. In reality these considerations should often have the first place in our minds and the medical picture the second.[10]

Varrier-Jones believed in the importance of raising the general resistance of the patient by providing fresh air, good food, and exercise. But he also believed that psychological factors played a large part in raising resistance, if not the major role. A psychological clinic was established at Papworth in 1928, to which Varrier-Jones attached great importance in treatment.[11]

Work was an important part of the scheme. Varrier-Jones explained that some persons working in the factories at Papworth with large tuberculous lesions would soon 'throw up the sponge' if they were treated as permanent invalids. Furthermore, in his opinion, the work usually imposed in sanatoria, consisting of maintenance and 'odd jobs',

---

[8] *Tubercle* 17 (1936), 529.
[9] PRO MH52/1, Report by MacNalty and Raw, 20 Apr. 1920, p. 16.
[10] *Lancet*, 1 (1941), 368; P. J. Varrier-Jones, *Papers of Pioneer*, collected by P. Fraser (London, 1943), 27, 28.
[11] Papworth Annual Report 1930, p. 14.

would cause the patients to feel exploited for the benefit of the institution and would have a detrimental psychological effect on them. The work which he was to impose would be useful work paid for at trade-union rates of pay. The industries established at Papworth included carpentry, joinery, cabinet-making, bootmaking and repairing, tailoring, portmanteau and attaché-case making, printing, sign writing, and jewellery making. While poultry farming and horticulture were also included, Varrier-Jones did not believe that work in the open air was essential for tuberculous patients. For psychological as well as economic reasons, Varrier-Jones aimed to make the industries of Papworth a commercial enterprise and not dependent on charity. Papworth Industries were to become a very successful enterprise indeed, expanding from a turnover of £400 in 1918 to over £130,000 in 1937.[12]

Treatment at Papworth was not confined to work therapy. Family and community also played an important role. Varrier-Jones opposed institutions, claiming that they had a detrimental psychological effect on the patient. In his opinion, 'institutional treatment, separating the patients as it did from their families, and imposing upon them utterly unnatural restrictions' was wrong. He believed that the advantages of settling a patient in a village settlement with his family were immense:

He can look the future in the face; he has hope; he has independence; he has position; he has authority. The environment is his home—a wonderful thought; home with all its associations, something to work for, not an institution in which he is 'placed' or to which he is 'sent'. He has a sense of security . . . I am convinced that it is his mental outlook . . . that makes for success, nay, is success.[13]

The family model Varrier-Jones envisaged for his village settlement was patriarchal—a tuberculous man, his wife, and children. His ideology was firmly rooted in the cult of domesticity. The private sphere was important, that 'privacy . . . so dear to the heart of an Englishman'.[14] The cottages at Papworth were semi-detached, two-storeyed, with three bedrooms, a verandah on the first floor for the

---

[12] Ibid., 1923, pp. 14, 16; ibid., 1935, p. 19; see also *BJT* 34 (1940), 93; *NAPT Bulletin*, 7/3 (1945), 30. Varrier-Jones also received a great deal of charitable support in building up the Industries, earning him the reputation of being 'one of the biggest beggars in England': *British Thoracic Association (The First Fifty Years)* (London, 1978), 54.

[13] *The National Insurance Gazette*, 11 Oct. 1919, (Papworth Archives); *BJT* 20 (1926), 15.

[14] *Lancet*, 2 (1918), 136.

tuberculous patient, and windows almost permanently opened. Ornaments and wallpaper were forbidden as they collected germs. Each cottage had its own garden.

The community of Papworth by the 1930s included a school house, a post office, a parish church and nonconformist chapel, two stores, a public house, a village hall with recreation rooms and cinema, and an open-air swimming pool. Referring to the social activities of the settlement in his 1923 report, Varrier-Jones wrote,

I am again faced with the impossibility of describing adequately the life and times of a small country town. Sports clubs (tennis, cricket, and golf), social activities such as Amateur Dramatics and Horticultural Society, . . . Women's Institute, Boy Scouts, educational and religious activities, all have their own workers, secretaries, and committees . . .[15]

The *Daily Mail* reported in 1926 that the community at Papworth enjoyed 'the simple pleasures of country life'.[16]

In stressing the importance of family and community in health restoration and maintenance, Varrier-Jones shared views with G. Scott Williamson and Innes Pearse, who founded Peckham Health Centre in 1926.[17] One major difference was that the latter couched their beliefs in biological terms, whereas Varrier-Jones was not concerned with biological theories. His interest lay in sociological and psychological theories; he believed that health was to be promoted by favourable social as well as psychological conditions; the patient's mental attitude was of chief importance.

Despite great enthusiasm for village settlements for tuberculous patients, there was also an awareness that the lack of financial resources and an unwillingness on the part of some patients to live in such a controlled environment, were inhibiting factors in their large-scale development. Even at Papworth only 123, or 6.9 per cent of the admissions in the first ten years, became settlers.[18] Training colonies were also advocated as a solution to the inadequacy of 'ordinary' sanatorium treatment. In training colonies, patients were to receive instruction in trades considered suitable to their condition, such as gardening, leatherwork, or carpentry, to prevent relapse following discharge. Training colonies were in effect an extension of sanatoria;

---

[15] Papworth Annual Report 1923, p. 24.
[16] *Daily Mail*, 15 July 1926 (PRO MH52/2).
[17] J. Lewis, 'The Peckham Health Centre: "An Inquiry into the Nature of Living"', *SSHM Bulletin*, 30 and 31 (1982), 39–43.
[18] *BJT* 24 (1930), 86.

they were discussed jointly by the Ministry of Health in 1920, 'since neither can function satisfactorily without the other'.[19] As already noted, the Ministry of Pensions financed a scheme of 'treatment and training' of ex-servicemen in 1920. Asked to prepare guidelines for the scheme, the Ministry of Health recommended that all patients should receive instruction in the lighter kinds of gardening and allotment work in addition to instruction in special occupations. This would enable them to supplement their earnings by their produce and to secure healthy exercise in the open air. It would also induce them to live on the outskirts rather than in the centre of a town and so counteract the tendency for them to spend too much time in crowded places.[20]

Training in gardening as a supplementary activity was not provided, but the persistence of the idea that market gardening was the most suitable occupation for people who had contracted tuberculosis can be seen by the number recommended by tuberculosis officers for the course in market gardening, which had only 62 places; by 1922, 400 had been recommended for it. Coutts suggested that in selecting candidates, account should be taken of physical condition ('curable' afebrile cases only), temperament and suitability, experience of country life, and the amount of capital at their disposal.[21]

By 1924, when the Ministry of Pensions' scheme was brought to an end, 900 had passed through it. Tuberculosis care committees in London discovered it 'not uncommon to be faced with the necessity of dealing with ex-servicemen returning home after a period of training and not following the trade in which they had received prolonged training at considerable public expense'.[22] Varrier-Jones had argued that the scheme could not possibly succeed. First, he claimed that they were 'attempting to cure a disease which is incurable'. Second, he did not believe that the man would be able to follow the trade he had learnt because under existing conditions neither employers nor trade unions would accept a partially-trained worker.[23] Sir Robert Morant, Permanent Secretary to the Ministry of Health, similarly thought that, while the provision of organized training in a suitable occupation was one of the most important elements in any sound scheme of

[19] PRO MH55/139, Ministry of Health memo, 30 June 1921, p. 26.
[20] PRO MH55/132, Ministry of Health memo, Jan. 1920, pp. 3–5.
[21] PRO MH55/165, Ministry of Health Circular 307, and Conference 2 Aug. 1922 (originally there were only 14 places in this course); see also *Tubercle* 3 (1922), 468.
[22] *Local Government Journal*, 9 Feb. 1924 (PRO MH96/1030).
[23] PRO MH55/164, Varrier-Jones to R. L. Morant, 10 Dec. 1919.

institutional treatment of tuberculous ex-servicemen, it would be unwise for the Government to finance such a scheme without providing village settlements as well. He explained that it had been proved beyond doubt that large numbers could not hope to survive in the ordinary competitive world, and that the only way sanatorium ex-patients could hope to avoid the prospect of relapse was to live in a village settlement.[24]

Summarizing the scheme in 1930, Bardswell noted that it had been carried out on a scale never previously attempted, well organized, generously administered and efficiently staffed, but that, judging by the number of men who subsequently adopted the occupations in which they were trained, failure could scarcely be more complete.[25] Even for those patients trained in farming, who could subsequently afford to carry on the occupation, there might have arisen the situation described in the novel, *The Land of Green Ginger*, whereby the wife of the tuberculous man had to bear the burden of the maintenance of the farm owing to his physical weakness.[26]

The training had not, however, been imposed entirely with a view to future specific employment. Rather, it was considered of therapeutic, not to mention moral, value in itself, as earlier in the century. A. H. MacPherson, superintendent of Burrow Hill Colony, set up by the NAPT and the Ministry of Pensions as part of the scheme in 1921, said in 1923, 'It becomes daily more evident that the longer the convalescent tuberculous subject, capable of work, remains unemployed, the more difficult does it become to discover initiative in a large percentage of them.'[27] It was also seen as a solution to the indiscipline problem so widespread among tuberculous ex-servicemen in sanatoria, which was thought to arise from their boredom.

Outdoor work was also the basis of treatment at Preston Hall, a tuberculosis institution near Maidstone, Kent, opened in 1919, for 300 ex-servicemen. The institution was situated in 98 acres of gardens and 287 acres of woodland. According to Nathan Raw who inspected the site in 1919, it was ideal for a sanatorium, situated in the 'Garden of England', and the proposed scheme was 'most complete'. It involved the admission of 150 'early' cases of tuberculosis who were to be given

[24] PRO MH55/141, Morant to G. R. Maclachlan, 24 Dec. 1919.
[25] N. D. Bardswell, *Urban Work Centres for the Tuberculous: The Experience of the Spero Firewood Factory, London* (London, 1930), 35.
[26] W. Holtby, *The Land of Green Ginger* (London, 1927).
[27] NAPT Council Minutes, Report of Medical Superintendent, Burrow Hill Colony, 26 Nov. 1923, p. 3.

prolonged training in high-class gardening and poultry farming, and, for the less intelligent, green keeping, laying of golf courses and bowling greens, agricultural tractor work, general smallholding work, and boat building. The only medical person on the management committee was E. H. T. Nash (formerly MOH for the Borough of Wimbledon) who believed that outdoor work was essential for tuberculous patients.[28]

Outlining the scheme for Preston Hall, Raw noted that leisure activities, such as golf and bowls, were also to be included. The staff were to be RAMC orderlies who had been bandsmen, with the idea of creating a band to which the patients would also contribute. There were to be organized lectures in the evenings, music, whist drives, billiards, and a theatre. The men were to be kept busy during the day and entertained in the evenings, so that they would not have time to think of their illness.[29] That conventional medical concerns were not paramount is clear from an advertisement for an assistant medical officer. Among the qualifications required was ability to play association football. Coutts objected that this game was too strenuous for tuberculous patients, but it was pointed out that the staff, not the patients, were to play.[30]

When L. G. (later Sir Laurence) Brock visited the institution in 1920 on behalf of the National Relief Fund, he noted that there were 25 gardeners and that any attempt to use patient labour had led to trouble among the regular gardeners. In his opinion, 'it is impossible . . . to visit Preston Hall without coming to the conclusion that a deplorable waste of money and of time is largely due to the slackness of Dr Nash'.[31] Nash received a salary of £1,500, double the average salary for medical superintendents of tuberculosis institutions at that time.[32] Nash resigned in 1920 and was followed by three other medical superintendents, until 1925 when the British Legion took over Preston Hall and requisitioned Varrier-Jones to reorganize the institution along the lines of Papworth. Varrier-Jones was made honorary medical

[28] PRO MH52/66, Kent CC, Preston Hall Sanatorium, Raw, 10 July 1919, p. 3; PRO MH52/66, Chapman, 23 July 1919.
[29] PRO MH52/67, Report by Oldham Insurance Committee after visit to Preston Hall, 26 Feb. 1921, p. 3.
[30] PRO MH52/67, Coutts, to medical superintendent Reeves-Smith, 29 Sept. 1921; Reeves-Smith to Coutts, 20 Oct. 1921.
[31] PRO MH52/66, L. G. Brock, 14 Oct. 1920.
[32] For example, WNMA medical superintendents earned £600 rising to £875 plus board and lodging: PRO MH96/1036, Returns as to staff of WNMA, May 1926, pp. 4, 5.

director, and a medical officer from Papworth, Edgar Obermer, was appointed resident medical superintendent until 1927, when Varrier-Jones and Obermer were replaced by J. B. McDougall, formerly medical superintendent of Wooley Sanatorium, Northumberland. Thus Preston Hall became the second tuberculosis village settlement in Britain. Like Varrier-Jones, McDougall believed that successful work in the industries should be complemented by a well-organized social life in the village.[33] By 1937 the community of Preston Hall numbered 1,110 people. A major difference between Papworth and Preston Hall was that residence in the village of Preston Hall was based on a five-year tenancy (except for key persons in the industries who were permitted to remain permanently), thus destroying a major ingredient of a village settlement according to Varrier-Jones—security.

Another 'treatment and training colony' was Wrenbury Hall, Cheshire, donated by the Cheshire branch of the British Red Cross Society to the Cheshire CC in 1922 for 22 ex-servicemen with early tuberculosis. Once again, agricultural work was the central concern, until 1926 when the medical superintendent, J. G. M. Sloane, was persuaded by J. E. Chapman of the Ministry of Health that open-air work was not the only work suitable for tuberculous men. A woodwork department was set up, and the farm (which had been running at a loss) was taken over by healthy labour.[34] The Red Cross specified that patients admitted to Wrenbury Hall were to be early cases of tuberculosis judged to be 'intellectually and temperamentally capable of learning a new mode of living'. It advised further that the accommodation provided for the colonists should be in separate rooms or 'chalets' rather than in wards, where patients would be taught how to live hygienically under conditions 'obtainable in the home of ordinary industrial workers'.[35] Occupational training was therefore not the only consideration.

Even when organized training was not provided, patients in tuberculosis institutions in the 1920s were generally not idle. Most medical superintendents subscribed to the belief which had grown up in early twentieth-century sanatoria that idleness was 'the worst of

---

[33] Preston Hall, Council of Management Minutes, Report by Medical Director, Mar. 1927.
[34] PRO MH52/11, Peyton, 30 Mar. 1920, p. 20; PRO MH52/11, Chapman, Conference, Wrenbury Hall, 10 Nov. 1926, pp. 3, 5.
[35] PRO MH52/11, Provisional Report of Cheshire Branch of British Red Cross Society, Proposed Training Colony, 21 May 1919, pp. 3, 5; Report by TO, 30 Mar. 1920, p. 19.

curses for the sanatorium patient'. In 1920, Newman outlined the 'true sanatorium principle', in which he believed exercise, suitably alternating with rest, played an important part. In his opinion, games were an inappropriate form of exercise as they could cause strenuous exertion and competition leading to undue stress. Walking exercise alone was apt to be either too monotonous or incapable of sufficient gradation under the close supervision of the resident medical officer, and tended to the formation of 'loafing' habits. He believed that the provision of training at every sanatorium was essential, for without occupation of the mind and body there would be physical and moral deterioration.[36] Setting the patients to work was moreover convenient in the many newly established institutions. The estimate of the cost of establishing a Surrey County Council sanatorium in 1920 for 200 patients, included the costs only for such roads and paths as were necessary for access to the buildings; all other roads and paths and the general laying-out of the grounds were left to the patients after the institution was opened.[37]

R. C. Wingfield, medical superintendent of Frimley from 1920 to 1945, continued the routine in that institution laid down by Marcus Paterson, albeit not so rigorously. He explained in 1924:

I do not feel disposed to follow or to endorse the arguments on which Paterson based the rationale of his system of treatment. I prefer to regard its value as a fact, empirical if you like, in the light of my experience of its use. But whatever may be its use on the physical side, the value of its moral effect, both for the individual and the sanatorium community as a whole, cannot be overestimated.

He quoted the 'famous remark' of Surgeon-General Bushnell of the US Army which he said lay at the basis of all tuberculosis treatment: 'For tuberculosis we prescribe not medicine, but a mode of life.' In Wingfield's opinion this was a confession of failure, a confession that as yet there was no specific cure for tuberculosis. But he also thought that it showed a realization that in a large proportion of cases the disease was due to, or exacerbated by, a faulty mode of life, and that if that mode of life were altered this would be giving the correct treatment in some measure. He defined faulty modes of life as 'overwork, overplay, overworry, undernourishment, lack of necessary

[36] *2nd CMOH Annual Report 1920* (1921), 96.
[37] PRO MH52/126, Surrey County Council Sanatorium, Milford, Architect's Descriptive Report upon Plans, 23 June 1920.

sunshine and fresh air, or chronic intemperance in any form'.[38]

A public inquiry into the administration of the West Wales Sanatorium accommodating 45 women and children, carried out in 1923–4 as a result of a complaint sent to the Carmarthenshire CC, reveals much concerning the nature of treatment at that institution. It was alleged that the patients were forced to do hard physical labour and that this resulted in the death of at least one patient. In defence, the medical superintendent, Isobel Ferguson, pointed out that the methods used at the institution were not unique but were those set out in Dr Paterson's book, and which she believed were practised in sanatoria throughout the country.[39]

Maud Morris, whose uncle Alderman Tom Morris registered the complaint in 1923 shortly before her death from tuberculosis, claimed that the girls were compelled to work on their knees in the snow sawing trees. A witness at the inquiry, held after Maud Morris's death, assured her examiners that she took no objection to the work, which she regarded as part of the general routine, and, as far as she was aware, nor did any of the other girls. She pointed out that the medical superintendent took part in the sawing of the trees herself.

Morris had described other activities they were required to perform, such as digging and carrying potatoes and manure, and claimed that she did not always feel strong enough, but was forced to carry on. The carting of manure was described as 'nasty work' by a witness at the inquiry, who also claimed that the superintendent was a hard taskmaster. Inside the house, patients were required to clean brass, scrub potatoes, wash floors and walls, sweep the hall, polish furniture, wash bed-patients' dishes, and clean the dispensary; the children cut firewood.

The *Western Mail* explained the system in 1924 following the wide publicity given to the sanatorium:

The life of a patient in a sanatorium is controlled both as to diet and movements. The restraint may seem a little hard at first, until he realises that the object of the discipline is to benefit his health and aid his recovery . . . It is now agreed that a system of graduated walking and some form of manual work has proved of great benefit to tuberculous patients who are free from fever . . .

---

[38] R. C. Wingfield, *Modern Methods in the Diagnosis and Treatment of Pulmonary Tuberculosis* (London, 1924), 41, 43, 57.

[39] *Western Mail*, 6 Feb. 1924 (PRO MH96/980); PRO MH96/980, West Wales (Llanybyther, Alltymynydd) Sanatorium, Evidence of M. Morris before T. Haydn Jones, Examiner, Llwynderi, Garnant, 3 Aug. 1923.

Manual work in the snow, which would naturally raise the heat of the body, can be very pleasant.[40]

D. Llewellyn Williams (Senior MO of the Welsh Board of Health) wrote a report for the inquiry. He did not believe that there was any medical objection to the type of work carried out at this institution, but thought that certain operations, such as taking manure from the pigsties to the garden and digging this into the earth, were scarcely suitable for women patients. While the medical basis of the treatment was not questioned, the competence of the medical superintendent in applying the method was discussed. Charles Lloyd, tuberculosis physician for Cardiganshire, who had attended the sanatorium during Ferguson's holiday, had taken a number of patients off graded exercise and placed them in bed. Williams pointed out that the decision to place Miss Morris on Grade V was based on inadequate data as there were no regular records of the patient's pulse-rates and weight. The physical condition of the patient did not seem to justify the decision, but Ferguson indicated that she had deliberately balanced physical and psychological considerations and arrived at the conclusion that the work was suitable. The result had proved an error of judgement which, according to Williams, did not warrant severe reprimand as Morris was 'a difficult case, a type which rarely did well', which was also the opinion of S. Lyle Cummins, professor of tuberculosis at the Welsh National School of Medicine.

Referring to statements made by Alderman Morris, Williams wrote that it was 'wrong and contrary to the evidence to say that most of the patients were taken away from the sanatorium in a worse condition than when they had arrived'. Alderman Morris, he said, was 'dealing with a highly technical subject, and one difficult to grasp in all its different bearings by a layman not familiar with medical practice'.[41]

Graduated labour in sanatoria for women usually took the form of domestic work. Paterson had pointed out that such work was beneficial in that it gave an opportunity for testing the capacities of the patients in this direction while they were under supervision, and that it was work which the patients usually preferred as they were accustomed to it.[42] At Rufford Hall, Lancashire, a sanatorium for women, patients were

---

[40] *Western Mail*, 1 May 1924 (PRO MH96/980).
[41] PRO MH96/980, Report by D. L. Williams, 9 Apr. 1924, 13–23; Report by T. W. Wade, 26 Apr. 1923; *Western Mail*, 1 May 1924.
[42] PRO MH96/980, WNMA, 'The Treatment of Pulmonary Tuberculosis, Words of Advice and Explanation to Patients entering a Sanatorium', 25–6.

'prescribed' potato peeling, silver cleaning, light brasswork, and sewing.[43] F. R. G. Heaf (professor of tuberculosis at the Welsh National School of Medicine) described 'an interesting experiment' carried out at the North Wales Sanatorium for women, where the medical superintendent, Dan Powell, had set up cottages to train women in housekeeping. They were given a weekly sum of money and had to keep house in a suitable manner for a tuberculous person to live in. This was, in Heaf's opinion, one of the best methods of rehabilitating women in the art in which they all should be trained, namely housewifery. The scheme was widely commended. The *Cambrian News* described how the women patients were placed in cottages 'such as would make a sanitary inspector weep', cottages 'equipped with every drawback, crammed with furniture and replete with all the gadgets beloved of the sanitary defective', which they were then taught to make habitable.[44] The Cheshire Joint Sanatorium established a similar scheme in the 1930s.

One disadvantage of work therapy, from the perspective of the medical superintendents, was that it did little to enhance their professional standing. Faced with being classified as an industrial administrator, McDougall asserted,

. . . it seems clear that any successful village settlement must always insist that medical principles shall take precedence over every other factor in the life of the community. I should prefer to go even further and say that the work which is taking place from day to day in any of the departments of a village settlement is a specialised form of treatment . . .[45]

Like Varrier-Jones, he explained that the settlers were really patients, that they were all examined at regular intervals for signs and carefully interrogated as to symptoms.[46] He equated the knowledge required by physicians practising occupational therapy with that required for surgical operations: 'Occupational therapy is a form of treatment, it is not a business . . . What is required . . . is a thorough grasp of the principles underlying occupational therapy, and in this respect occupational therapy differs in no way from any other form of treatment for tuberculosis or any other disease.'[47]

[43] PRO MH52/78, Inspection by D. J. Williamson, 10 Sept. 1926, p. 3.
[44] F. R. G. Heaf (ed.), *Symposium of Tuberculosis* (London, 1957), 711; *Cambrian News*, 2 May 1924 (PRO MH96/982).
[45] *BJT* 31/3 (1937), 203–4.
[46] Preston Hall Annual Report 1929–30, p. 12.
[47] *BJT* 21/2 (1927), 86, 87.

The problems perceived by medical superintendents of tuberculosis institutions such as McDougall can be compared with the mental asylum medical superintendents in the nineteenth century practising 'moral therapy'. If cures could be effected by non-medical means, then the administrators were reduced to mere custodians of the patients, and their status and very existence were threatened. Medical superintendents of sanatoria, as of asylums, required means of justifying their place in the institution as purveyors of essential medical expertise.[48] The medical superintendent of Wrenbury Hall from 1922 to 1927, J. G. M. Sloane, did little to contribute to the medical prestige of the superintendents of tuberculosis institutions. Sloane, who qualified as a medical practitioner in Canada in 1895, had had no special experience in tuberculosis work before coming to Wrenbury, and, according to Chapman, the medical work and records showed evidence of his lack of special experience. Chapman described Sloane as 'first a farmer and second a doctor'. He believed, however, that as the majority of the patients were early cases of tuberculosis requiring little special medical treatment, Sloane's lack of experience was of relatively little importance, compensated for by his excellence in other respects and his enthusiasm. During the winter of 1924–5, the patients had built a recreation room under Sloane's direction.[49]

Nursing in tuberculosis institutions also had dubious professional standing at this time, which was thought to be one of the main reasons for the difficulty tuberculosis institutions constantly experienced in attracting nursing staff. Training in tuberculosis nursing was not approved for State registration. In 1919 the Nurses Registration Act had established a State Register for nurses and the General Nursing Council had been set up to administer the examinations for entry to the Register. The Register consisted of six parts, and included fever nursing, mental nursing, and the nursing of children, in supplementary registers, but not tuberculosis nursing. Not only did the absence of tuberculosis nursing on the Register affect the intake of probationer nurses, it also meant that the posts of staff nurses and sisters carried less prestige than in an approved training school. This was pointed out by the Lancet Commission on Nursing which reported in 1932. The

---

[48] See R. Cooter, 'Phrenology and British Alienists', in A. Scull (ed.), *Madhouses, Mad-doctors and Madmen: The Social History of Psychiatry in the Victorian Era*, (London, 1981), 76.
[49] PRO MH52/11, J. E. Chapman, 31 July 1925, pp. 3–7.

Commission also maintained that the anomaly involved in the refusal of recognition was emphasized by the fact that, under the Local Government (Qualification of Medical Officers and Health Visitors) Regulations of 1930, experience in tuberculosis nursing was recognized by statute as a qualification for appointment as a tuberculosis visitor in Local Government service. However, the General Nursing Council pursued a policy of 'one portal' entry into the profession, fearing that a supplementary register for tuberculosis nurses would provide a 'back door entry into the nursing profession', and so resisted attempts to set up such a register.[50]

Tuberculosis nurses did have a form of specialized training, started by the Society of Medical Superintendents of Tuberculosis Institutions in 1920 and conducted by it until 1928, and thereafter by the Tuberculosis Association. The course lasted two years, consisting of two examinations, one equivalent to the State preliminary examination and the other specializing in tuberculosis; State-trained nurses could qualify in one year, taking only the second examination. By 1927, 210 nurses had the certificate, and by 1944, over 3,000.[51]

Tuberculosis nursing, nevertheless, did not require highly specialized skills. The early British sanatoria were modelled on Otto Walther's sanatorium in Nordrach, and Walther was known to eschew all nurses.[52] Jane Walker pointed out in 1904 that while 'people of the regular serving class' should not be employed as nurses in sanatoria, little nursing skill was required.[53] Nor had the situation changed noticeably by the 1920s. The staffing arrangements at Wrenbury Hall were based on no pretence of professionalism of tuberculosis nursing: in 1924, the wife of the medical superintendent replaced the matron as 'lady housekeeper', an arrangement reminiscent of Poor Law institutions prior to the twentieth century, which had often been managed by a married couple.[54] In an investigation of Poor Law infirmaries in London in 1924, it was discovered that a nurse with a certificate from Brompton Hospital was not nursing on a tuberculosis ward; when consulted, the matron claimed that the nurses she had allocated to the

---

[50] *Lancet Report*, Sect. 9 (London, 1932), 142, 143; see also B. Abel-Smith, *A History of the Nursing Profession* (London, 1960), 148–60, 173.
[51] *NAPT Bulletin*, 6/6 (1944), 7; *Tubercle*, 32 (1950), 41. For syllabus, see J. H. Walker, *The Modern Nursing of Consumption*, 2nd edn. (London, 1924), Appendix.
[52] S. V. Pearson, *Men, Medicine, and Myself* (London, 1946), 37.
[53] J. H. Walker, *The Modern Nursing of Consumption*, 1st edn. (London, 1904), 21.
[54] PRO MH52/11, Cheshire CC to Ministry of Health, 7 Aug. 1924; J. E. Chapman, Report, 31 July 1925, p. 7.

ward were just as good, even though they had no training in tuberculosis nursing.[55] Other factors apart from the lack of professionalism contributed to the shortage of nurses in tuberculosis institutions, such as long hours, poor living conditions, poor pay, and the isolated location of many of the institutions. Nor did 'such unusual privileges as . . . permission to keep a dog' compensate for the disadvantages.[56] In order to alleviate the shortage, male orderlies were often employed. For example, Highland Moors, opened in 1931 with a female medical superintendent, Marion Owen-Morris, was staffed by male orderlies. At Preston Hall, the matron reported that male nurses and orderlies were employed as a result of the inability to attract female nurses. She maintained in 1937 that the institution was having increasing difficulty in obtaining the 'right type' of orderly. As a result of a concern for the standard of male nursing, a series of lectures followed by an examination was started at Preston Hall to grade orderlies into three groups differentiated by rates of pay.[57]

Most of the male labour at Preston Hall was in fact probably recruited from the ex-patient population, for recruitment among ex-patients, males and females, was a common solution to the staffing problems of many of the sanatoria. McDougall estimated in 1938 that there were probably 450 ex-patients employed in the largest sanatoria in the country.[58] Sometimes a third or more of the regular staff were recruited from ex-patients.

Instructors were also often appointed from among patients or ex-patients. Occupational therapy as a separate paramedical profession (which was being instituted in the inter-war period) had not yet made an impression on sanatoria.[59] Indeed, being a patient or an ex-patient seemed to be the best qualification for the job. Varrier-Jones explained in 1926,

No healthy man can realize the condition of the consumptive. No amount of teaching can bring home to him the differences between incapacity for work and shirking or malingering. But if the instructor has himself suffered from the

[55] PRO MH55/145, LCC Public Health Committee Report 528, E. P. Manby and F. R. Seymour, Mar. 1923, p. 4.
[56] *Lancet Report*, pp. 142, 145 (paras. 288, 289).
[57] Preston Hall, Minutes of Council Management, Reports by Medical Director and Matron, 25 Jan. 1937.
[58] Preston Hall Annual Report 1933, p. 10.
[59] L. Bryder, 'Occupational Therapy and Tuberculosis Sanatoria', *SSHM Bulletin* 40 (1987), 64–6.

peculiar nervous or physical fatigue produced by the disease, and has by a course of treatment known how to recover from it he is ready to appreciate the phenomenon when he next meets it.[60]

Similarly, the Ministry of Health recommended that in the treatment and training schemes financed by the Ministry of Pensions, instructors should be chosen from ex-patients, as they possessed 'a better appreciation of the needs and difficulties of tuberculous patients'.[61]

Thus, work therapy did little to enhance the professional status of its administrators; it required minimal technology and professional training of medical officers, nurses, and occupational therapists.

(2) COLLAPSE THERAPY

Conservative treatment, based on a holistic approach to medicine, was challenged as the dominant therapy for tuberculosis in the 1930s and 40s by surgical intervention, which can be seen as an attempt to bring tuberculosis treatment more into line with the orthodox medical treatment of the twentieth century. In 1938 MacNalty reported, 'The sanatorium has at length become a specialised hospital.'[62] The specialism referred to was collapse therapy.

Collapse therapy was based on the idea that by collapsing and thereby resting the lung, the tuberculous lesion would have more chance of healing. Collapsing the lung to treat pulmonary tuberculosis had been suggested by a Liverpool physician, James Carson, in 1821, but it was not until 1882 that the method of 'artificial pneumothorax' was devised by Carlo Forlanini, an Italian doctor. He carried it out successfully in 1892 and reported his results to an international congress on tuberculosis in 1894. The purpose was to admit air into the pleural cavity so as to collapse the diseased lung. When air was introduced between the two layers of the pleura, the adhesive force which held the layers together was destroyed and the lung contracted by virtue of its elasticity (see Fig. 6). The air was inserted with a needle, and in 1904 a type of water manometer to record the air pressure was invented by Chr. Saugman at Vejlefjord Sanatorium, Denmark. Subsequently other types of manometer were designed,

---

[60] *BJT* 20 (1926), 16.
[61] PRO MH55/132, Ministry of Health, Training Sections for ex-servicemen at sanatoria, Jan. 1920, pp. 3–5
[62] *20th CMOH Annual Report 1938* (1939), 131.

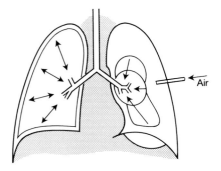

Fig. 6. Principle of artificial pneumothorax. Lung is held out to the chest wall by the negative pressure of the pleural cavity. If this pressure is released by letting air into the pleural sac the elastic lung will contract down.

Source: L. E. Houghton and T. H. Sellors, *Aids to Tuberculosis Nursing* (London, 1949), 123.

making the procedure simpler. The air had to be inserted periodically as the lung regained its normal functions. These 'refills' were carried out at weekly intervals, then monthly, and finally six-monthly, up to a period of five years, or until the tuberculous lesion had healed. One possible complication was air embolism, which was due to the needle having penetrated the lung, which might cause sudden unconsciousness or death, or 'less dramatic[ally] . . . faintness, giddiness, and the development of paralysis, blindness, or other nervous symptoms. Death may take place at any stage during the first week, or the patient may recover without the persistence of symptoms.'[63]

The method was introduced into Britain by Claude Lillingston in 1910. He had contracted tuberculosis while on his honeymoon in Norway in 1907 and received the treatment there at Mesnalien Sanatorium, near Lillehammer, with apparent success. Returning to England in 1910, he induced an artificial pneumothorax on a patient at Mundesley Sanatorium. By this time the number of reported cases who had received the treatment in Europe and the USA exceeded 400. In a lecture on the treatment, Forlanini did not state how many of his patients were cured, but, according to Lillingston, the whole tenor of the lecture suggested that the results were eminently satisfactory. In

[63] E. A. Underwood, *A Manual of Tuberculosis, Clinical and Administrative*, 3rd edn. (Edinburgh, 1945), 247.

Lillingston's view, it was striking to find so few articles on the subject in the English medical press compared with other countries, and he pointed out that the lack of interest in the treatment had the ludicrous effect that English pneumothorax patients at Davos in Switzerland were unable to return to England owing to the inability to find anyone in this country to continue the injections.[64]

In the following years, however, the method was adopted in Britain with great enthusiasm. Clive Rivière wrote in 1917, 'No more hopeful ray of sunshine has ever come to illuminate the dark kingdom of disease than that introduced into the path of the consumptive through the discovery of artificial pneumothorax.'[65] In a report for the MRC in 1922, L. S. T. Burrell and A. S. MacNalty recorded that, of 150 cases in which pneumothorax was successfully induced, 62 per cent had improved (they did not give the number of unsuccessful inductions). They claimed to know of no one who had tried the treatment seriously and then discarded it, but added that too little was known about it in this country.[66] In 1927 Newman encouraged local authorities to install facilities for artificial pneumothorax at their tuberculosis institutions. In his opinion, this form of treatment which he stressed held few risks, should be available for all suitable patients under the local authorities' schemes.[67]

By the 1930s, artificial pneumothorax was offered in many British sanatoria. However, there was still a difficulty in finding tuberculosis dispensaries where the treatment could be carried on. When treatment was carried out at dispensaries, it was often without the assistance of X-rays. X-rays were considered an essential accessory to monitor the progress of the pneumothorax (in particular to check for intra-pleural adhesions). It amazed Vere Pearson, one of the earliest practitioners of artificial pneumothorax in Britain, to remember that he had performed his first artificial pneumothorax without the assistance of X-ray apparatus.[68] In 1939, George Day maintained that, while the days of the blind performance of the appendicectomy were over,

the scandalous thing is that the day of the blind Tuberculosis Officer is still here. Do you know how many tuberculosis dispensaries are yet unequipped

---

[64] *Lancet*, 2 (1911), 145, 149.
[65] C. Rivière, *The Pneumothorax Treatment of Pulmonary Tuberculosis* (London, 1917), 1.
[66] MRC, L. S. T. Burrell and A. S. MacNalty, *Report on Artificial Pneumothorax* (SRS 67; London, 1922), 7, 55.
[67] *9th CMOH Annual Report 1927* (1928), 66–7.
[68] Pearson, *Men, Medicine, and Myself*, p. 96.

with X-ray plant? [He did not provide the answer] . . . Very often Tuberculosis Officers are staunch unbelievers in this form of therapy [artificial pneumothorax] and write quoting from personal experience how disappointing and dangerous they have found it. And no wonder![69]

In a discussion on the architecture of dispensaries, F. R. G. Heaf said that every dispensary should have a back door whereby collapsed patients could be removed, for, 'In all places where pneumothorax treatment is done tragedies occur.'[70]

Artificial pneumothorax was sometimes described as positively dangerous. In one of the last clinical papers on artificial pneumothorax in 1959, an unidentified authority was quoted to the effect that the pneumothorax needle was 'the most dangerous weapon ever placed in the hands of a physician'.[71] There are, however, no figures on fatalities as a result of accidents related to collapse therapy.

While McDougall and Bardswell claimed in 1935 that the advent of artificial pneumothorax had, without a doubt, been the most epoch-making event in the history of treatment during the last 50 years, they believed that it was 'sometimes pursued with a vigour that was more enthusiastic than informed, and that its injudicious use further darkened the already gloomy prospect of the phthisical patient'.[72] F. J. Bentley estimated that approximately 10 per cent of all patients undergoing residential treatment for pulmonary tuberculosis in 1934 under the LCC scheme were suitable for receiving it. By his calculations, if the degree of improvement then ascertained were doubled, the method would raise the level of results as judged by survival after 5 years in all pulmonary tuberculosis patients under treatment by approximately 4 per cent.[73]

Artificial pneumothorax generated a voluminous literature. Yet in 1941 a study of 2,100 papers published from 1929 to 1939 revealed that only 4.7 per cent of them were concerned with the results of the treatment. Further, 99 papers were analysed featuring results taken from 18 countries from 1918 to 1939, from which it was concluded

[69] *25 NAPT 1939*, p. 58; Even in 1950 it was reported that many tuberculosis dispensaries had no X-ray equipment, *BMJ* 2 (1950), 1382. One out of 26 London boroughs possessed X-ray equipment in 1935: *21 NAPT 1935*, p. 126.

[70] *25 NAPT 1939*, p. 157.

[71] *Diseases of the Chest*, 35/1 (1959), 1.

[72] *Tubercle*, 16 (1935), 267.

[73] MRC, F. J. Bentley, *Artificial Pneumothorax: Experience of the London County Council*, (SRS 215; 1936), Preface and p. 91.

that only 34 per cent adopted acceptable standards of assessment in the reviewers' opinion.[74]

Despite its limitations, known and unknown, pneumothorax was pursued enthusiastically by the 1930s, and was increasingly accompanied by thoracic surgery. It was pointed out that a third of the suitable cases for artificial pneumothorax failed on account of pleural adhesions, and would benefit by a thoracoplastic operation, the collapsing of the lung permanently by rib resection.[75] Other thoracic operations included 'phrenicectomy' or 'phrenic evulsion' (the removal of a portion of the phrenic nerve, causing permanent elevation of that side of the diaphragm and partial collapse of the corresponding lung), and 'apicolysis' (performed during the thoracoplastic operation, involving the dissection of the lung apex so that the site of the disease would collapse downwards as well as inwards).

The first thoracoplastic operation for tuberculosis in Britain was performed in 1912 at University College Hospital by H. Morriston Davies, later described as 'one of the world's outstanding thoracic surgeons'.[76] Thoracic surgery at Brompton Hospital developed following the appointments of two thoracic surgeons, J. E. H. Roberts and A. Tudor Edwards, in 1919 and 1922 respectively. The first two-stage thoracoplasty at Brompton Hospital was performed in 1922; and in 1924, 21 thoracoplasties were recorded.[77]

By the 1930s, Britain still had few qualified thoracic surgeons. Morriston Davies claimed in 1931 that during the last two years he had been looking out for suitable young men (*sic*) to train up as thoracic surgeons, but had been unsuccessful. He pointed out that all the sanatoria he worked with, whether in England or Wales, were finding it difficult to recruit really suitable candidates.[78] There were, according to McDougall, only 6 or 8 qualified thoracic surgeons in Britain.[79] In

[74] *Journal of Thoracic Surgery*, 10 (1941), 310; *Tubercle*, 38 (1957), 21.

[75] C. Rivière, *The Pneumothorax Treatment of Pulmonary Tuberculosis*, 2nd edn. (Oxford, 1927), 251.

[76] *Tubercle*, 53 (1972), 229: G. M. Meade, delivering the Morriston Davies Memorial Lecture, related how Davies permanently lost the use of his operating right hand through infection and moved to a country sanatorium in north Wales where he learned to operate with his left hand, becoming an outstanding thoracic surgeon.

[77] *Tubercle*, 58 (1977), 48; J. R. Bignall, *Frimley: The Biography of a Sanatorium* (London, 1979), 103.

[78] MRC 1615, II, Davies to Fletcher, 17 June 1931; see also H. M. Davies, *Pulmonary Tuberculosis: Medical and Surgical Treatment* (London, 1933).

[79] Preston Hall, Minutes of Council Management, Report of Medical Director, 24 July 1934, p. 116.

1935 Morriston Davies again expressed concern regarding the slow progress being made in Britain in thoracic surgery: 'For example, apart from Brompton, there is really no place . . . which is properly and adequately equipped for the treatment [of patients by] all forms of thoracic surgery.'[80]

The years from 1939 to 1945 have been described as the era of the hospital treatment of pulmonary tuberculosis as opposed to the sanatorium era. The new era involved all the facilities and many of the characteristics of sanatorium treatment; the tuberculosis hospital was 'in many ways simply a very up-to-date sanatorium'.[81] The major difference was the addition of surgical facilities.

What were the reasons for surgical intervention to all appearances gaining precedence over more conservative methods? One reason was that conservative treatment was most suited to early afebrile cases of tuberculosis, and such cases rarely presented themselves for treatment. Before the First World War, it had been believed that with increased education, more early cases would come forward, but not surprisingly this did not happen. In 1931 Powell pointed out that the provision made by the WNMA for the 'sanatorium type of pulmonary case, the early or ambulant, afebrile type whose condition was such that he could be restored to full working capacity after six to nine months' treatment', had always been fairly adequate owing to the comparative rarity of this kind of case.[82]

McDougall and Bardswell considered the enthusiasm for collapse therapy hardly surprising in the face of results of conservative treatment—for example, of the 3,000 patients discharged after sanatorium treatment under the LCC in 1927, it was recorded in 1932 that 2,280 or 76 per cent were dead. They maintained, 'To be in a position to say that "something more can be done" is in itself a tremendous fillip to the patient who has failed to respond to the usual conservative measures.'[83]

While thoracic surgery required surgical specialists, artificial pneumothorax as well as 'pneumoperitoneum' (the reinforcement of the collapse by inserting air into the abdominal peritoneal cavity to force up the diaphragm, developed in the 1930s) could be, and were, performed by tuberculosis physicians. It is clear that collapse therapy

[80] PRO MH96/1042, Davies to MacNalty, 24 June 1935.
[81] Underwood, *A Manual of Tuberculosis*, pp. 160, 171.
[82] PRO MH96/1040, memo by Powell, Proposed New Hospital, 1 Apr. 1931.
[83] *Tubercle*, 16 (1935), 267, 269.

was an attractive treatment to tuberculosis specialists as it increased the range of treatments under their purview, and was more scientific than practising work therapy. Requiring specialized skill, it enhanced their professional status. The medical superintendent of the South Wales Sanatorium noted in 1930 that medical officers seemed to prefer such treatment judging by the amount of time spent on it.[84] Professional pressure was exerted on tuberculosis practitioners to learn the technique. McDougall wrote in 1930, 'No tuberculosis physician can pose as an expert unless he has at his command the technique of the induction of pulmonary collapse.'[85] Tattersall thought that no tuberculosis officer should be regarded as fit for his appointment who had no experience in collapse therapy.[86] With improving methods of diagnosis and the introduction of artificial pneumothorax, it was being suggested that there should be a change in the designation of tuberculosis officers to chest physicians, and dispensaries to chest clinics, enhancing their specialist status.

Surgery was also seen as a way of making tuberculosis institutions more attractive to nurses. The Lancet Commission believed that the monotony of tuberculosis nursing was likely to diminish in the future owing to developments in thoracic surgery.[87] One nurse who began working in a sanatorium during the Second World War wrote of the excitement she experienced when she first attended a thoracoplastic operation and another rare operation: 'This indeed was a thrill and I was one of the lucky few, able to go to the theatre as a spectator.'[88] Several textbooks on tuberculosis nursing appeared in the 1940s, the main aim of which seemed to be to point out that tuberculosis nursing was interesting and required specialist knowledge.[89]

Patients also had been educated in the supremacy of mechanistic medicine. Heaf spoke in 1939 of a feeling among patients that when they were not receiving artificial pneumothorax they were receiving no treatment at all.[90] McDougall reported in 1934 that there was little difficulty in obtaining the permission of the patients for operations.[91]

---

[84] PRO MH96/987, visit by Wade, 22 Apr. 1930 (Report, 30 Apr. 1930).
[85] Preston Hall Annual Report 1930–1, p. 12.
[86] *Tubercle*, 12 (1931), 377.
[87] *Lancet Report*, pp. 146–7 (para. 302).   [88] *NAPT Bulletin*, 6/6 (1944), 16.
[89] L. E. Houghton and T. H. Sellors, *Aids to Tuberculosis Nursing*, 1st edn. (London, 1945); J. G. Eyre, *Tuberculosis Nursing*, 1st edn. (London, 1949); G. S. Erwin, *Tuberculosis and Chest Diseases for Nurses* (London, 1946).
[90] *25 NAPT 1939*, p. 60.
[91] Preston Hall, Minutes of Council of Management, Medical Director Report, 31 Jan. 1934.

Alan Dick, describing his experiences in a sanatorium in 1939, commented on the curious medical snobberies among the patients as a result of surgery: 'Thoracoplastic cases looked down unchallenged from the height of their surgical experience. Extra-pleurals considered themselves a cut above the plain A.P. People with A.P.s placed phrenics in the apprentice stakes. All who were having active treatment gazed with disdain upon those on gold and rest.'[92] G. S. Erwin, medical superintendent of Liverpool Sanatorium, in discussing the causes of premature self-discharge, wrote:

Patients with a vague notion of the treatment of disease in general and with perhaps a little knowledge of the more sensational treatments now available for a few diseases, are often disappointed that no such dramatisation of their own case is possible. Not infrequently they feel that no treatment is being undertaken, and discharge themselves on the pretext that they can get plenty of food and fresh air at home.[93]

Collapse therapy was therefore one way of keeping the patients in the institutions.

In the case of Preston Hall and Papworth an important factor in the adoption of collapse therapy was the need to attract voluntary support and patients. They were competing for patients with local authority institutions which were often cheaper, and therefore had to 'modernize' to make their institutions as appealing as possible.

Preston Hall was having trouble filling its beds in the late 1920s; in 1927 McDougall feared that the position might shortly become acute.[94] It was an institution for ex-servicemen which was one factor in the dwindling number of admissions, but the extension in 1928 of the qualification for admission to include dependants of ex-servicemen did not lead to an increase in admissions, even though the qualification was not in any case interpreted very strictly—on inquiry in 1934 several patients did not know whether they were dependent upon ex-servicemen.[95] Thoracic surgery was developed in the early 1930s; McDougall reported that this development was receiving wide notice and simultaneously that the number of patients in residence had doubled from 151 in 1927 to 301 in 1934.[96]

[92] A. Dick, *A Walking Miracle* (London, 1942), 68. (For 'gold' treatment see Chapter 6, Section 5.)
[93] G. S. Erwin, *A Guide for the Tuberculous Patient* (London, 1944), 57.
[94] Preston Hall Report 1925–8, p. 38; Minutes of Council of Management, Medical Director Report, 29 Sept. 1927, Oct. 1927; Preston Hall Annual Report 1933–4, p. 75.
[95] Preston Hall, Minutes of Council of Management, Medical Director Report, 22 Nov. 1934, addendum.   [96] Ibid., 31 Jan. and 29 May 1934.

The medical prestige of Preston Hall was further enhanced by being the first institution in Britain to install a tomograph. The tomograph, first seen by McDougall while visiting the Sauerbruch clinic in Berlin, was a device perfected by Dr Grossman and Professor Chaoul which enabled the lungs to be viewed without any of the details being obscured by the normal bone markings of the ribs. In this way the position and size of the cavity could be determined in terms of length, breadth, and depth in a precise way which had previously been impossible. A tomograph was purchased from Germany and installed at Preston Hall in 1936. McDougall reported in May 1936, 'At no time in the history of Preston Hall has there been such a demand on the bed accommodation. Enquiries are coming in from London, Kent, Essex, Middlesex and Surrey in particular and we are hard put to it to obtain the accommodation which is required.' In September of the same year he wrote, 'We keep nearly 400 beds constantly occupied, even in days when each Local Authority has its own institution, and when there is a tendency to keep patients for treatment within their own Local Authority boundaries. There is no doubt that the advent of the Tomograph has been responsible for much additional interest in Preston Hall and the recent annual report has received wide recognition in the medical press.'[97]

Surgical intervention initially formed no part of Varrier-Jones's scheme at Papworth. As already noted, Varrier-Jones firmly believed in a holistic approach to medicine. Surgical intervention, which immobilized the patient, interfered with the graduated labour routine. Moreover, according to the matron, Varrier-Jones considered surgery cruel.[98] Yet, when Varrier-Jones opposed surgical intervention in the 1920s, he found himself involved in a conflict with Cambridgeshire CC which accused him of negligence.[99] One patient complained in 1920 that at Papworth no treatment 'in any real sense of the word' was given.[100] Papworth, like Preston Hall, was a voluntary institution competing with the often cheaper local authority institutions for patients. Therefore Varrier-Jones was forced to modify his own beliefs and keep up with modern trends in treatment. In his 1933 report, he boasted that when the thoracic surgery unit was completed, Papworth

[97] Ibid., 25 May and 25 Sept. 1936.
[98] R. Parker, *On the Road, The Papworth Story* (Cambridge, 1977), 149.
[99] PRO MH52/5, Cambridgeshire CC memo, 2 Mar. 1926.
[100] PRO MH52/5, letter to Ministry of Pensions, East Midlands Region, Nottingham, 13 Aug. 1921.

would possess 'what is believed to be the most complete scheme for the treatment of tuberculosis that exists anywhere'.[101] MacNalty reported in 1934 that Varrier-Jones hoped Papworth would in the future become the centre for the surgical treatment of pulmonary disease for the midland and eastern counties of England.[102] The operating theatre was formally opened in 1936.

Burrow Hill Colony, administered by the NAPT, was constantly having problems filling its beds. One reason may have been that, on the insistence of Sir Robert Philip, neither thoracic surgery nor even artificial pneumothorax was performed there, and nor were patients admitted who had already had artificial pneumothorax operations and required refills. This institution was forced to close down in 1943.[103]

Rivalry between institutions, local authorities, and organizations was therefore an important factor. McDougall was determined that Preston Hall would be the first institution in Britain to install a tomograph. The WNMA wanted Sully Hospital, a new tuberculosis hospital in south Wales opened in 1936, to be seen as the most progressive in Britain, despite the expressed need for accommodation for advanced cases of pulmonary tuberculosis in the area (who were accommodated in the Public Assistance institution, the City Lodge). Reporting the results of an architectural competition to design Sully Hospital, the *Western Mail* anticipated that 'when this scheme is carried out it will result in the possession by Wales of one of the finest tuberculosis hospitals in Europe'.[104]

Thus, apart from any inherent value of surgical methods, there were other factors favouring their adoption. Specialists preferred treatment which required more specialist skill and enhanced their professional status. Surgery was seen as a way of making tuberculosis institutions more attractive to nurses. Patients, who would not present themselves for treatment early enough to make conservative treatment effective in any case, also preferred more interventionist medicine; and institutions vied with one another to be the most progressive, to be equipped with the latest technology.

There was moreover a feeling that if artificial pneumothorax and thoracic surgery were not developed, Britain would fall behind other Western countries in the treatment of pulmonary tuberculosis. Sir

---

[101] *Tubercle*, 16 (1935), 182.
[102] PRO MH52/3, MacNalty, 16 Apr. 1934, p. 4.
[103] PRO MH55/156, MacNalty, 4 Feb. 1935; PRO MH55/1181.
[104] *Western Mail*, 14 Nov. 1931 (PRO MH96/1041).

Walter Fletcher, secretary of the MRC, wrote to Morriston Davies in 1931 that Britain had been behind others in the adoption of artificial pneumothorax and was now lagging behind just as badly in the development of thoracoplasty. He referred specifically to progress being made in Germany and America which, he said, had been inadequately followed in Britain.[105] Thoracic surgeons in Britain generally studied abroad. Lawrence O'Shaughnessy, Hunterian Professor of the Royal College of Surgeons, consultant to the LCC on chest surgery and appointed consultant to Preston Hall in 1934, had studied under Ferdinand Sauerbruch in Berlin. H. P. Nelson, appointed thoracic surgeon to Papworth in 1935, had studied under John Alexander at Ann Arbor, Michigan, USA. Nelson stated a decided preference for the methods used in America over Germany: 'I think on the whole English surgery is nearer to that of America than to that of the Germanic countries, and some of the drastic procedures that emanate from Sauerbruch's clinic are rather revolting to the English mind.'[106] Morriston Davies travelled to the USA and Canada in 1935 and returned to Britain 'with a still greater feeling of despair at the backwardness of this country'.[107]

Britain may be described as 'backward' in the adoption of thoracic surgery, but there is in fact little evidence to suggest the superiority of such treatment over other methods in any case. Bignall believed that on balance it may have saved a few lives and pointed to the speeding up of the decline in mortality, from 2 per cent per annum at the end of the nineteenth century to 4.5 per cent in the late 1930s—hardly a revolutionary change, and there is no evidence that it was related to collapse therapy.[108] In a study of the after-histories of 1,192 cases in the County Borough of Reading from 1914 to 1940, it was found that only 15 (8.5 per cent) of the 178 still surviving patients had had any form of collapse therapy, and it was therefore concluded that the operation could have had little influence on survival rates.[109]

Morriston Davies himself was later disillusioned. R. R. Trail quoted results of thoracoplasty published by Davies in 1953, showing that both breakdown and death from tuberculosis were postponed for only

[105] MRC 1615, II, Fletcher to Davies, 16 June 1931.
[106] Liddall Hart Collection, Nelson to Varrier-Jones, 4 May 1934, 27 Jan. 1936. Nelson's tragic death in 1936 at the age of 34 after contracting septicaemia while conducting an operation was widely reported in the Press at the time (Mrs K. Liddall Hart collection).
[107] PRO MH96/1042, Davies to MacNalty, 24 June 1935.
[108] Bignall, *Frimley*, p. 105.   [109] *Tubercle*, 28 (1947), 85, 92.

some two years as against the effects of sanatorium regime alone. Trail pointed out, 'Moreover, we have known for some time that roughly 50 per cent of cases rendered negative by thoracoplasty in days prior to antibiotics were again positive in five years.' He claimed that there were now more papers against than for pneumothorax and pneumoperitoneum, 'their possible complications in a large percentage of patients having assumed such importance as to bar their usefulness for any patients'.[110]

(3) REST VERSUS WORK THERAPY

The growing use of artificial pneumothorax and thoracic surgery, starting in the 1930s, altered the nature of sanatorium treatment. Operations required longer periods of rest. Rest was increasingly prescribed even when surgery was not involved. H. Batty Shaw of the Brompton Hospital claimed in 1933 that it was a singular fact that patients who had been sent to a sanatorium to rest their lungs were allowed to use them hard once they got there, and believed that by more adequate rest of infected lungs the terrific tuberculosis mortality would be materially reduced.[111]

American tuberculosis specialists had not evinced the same enthusiasm for work therapy. Lawrence Flick, president of the (American) National Tuberculosis Association, maintained in 1914 that false notions connecting consumption in some way with inactivity had resulted in wrong conceptions about the treatment of the disease, which were shared by the medical profession and laity alike. He wrote that, 'Exercise as part of the treatment is insisted on under any and all circumstances . . . Frequently poor consumptives exercise themselves into the grave. The worst of it is that they do it under advice from the doctor and for the purpose of recovery.'[112] Allen K. Krause of the Johns Hopkins Medical School and editor of the *American Review of Tuberculosis*, asked in 1919, '. . . who is there among us that would not sooner put his money on the tuberculosis patient living at perfect rest—physical and mental rest—in a close room rather than on a

---

[110] *Chemotherapy in the Treatment of Tuberculosis, NAPT Conference Papers, Cambridge 1953* (London, 1954), 6.

[111] *Tubercle*, 15 (1933), 233.

[112] L. Flick, *Consumption: A Curable and Preventable Disease: What a Layman Should Know*, 7th edn. (London, 1914), 230–2.

similar individual wielding a pick and shovel beyond his capacity in all outdoors?'[113] Gerald Webb, another president of the NTA, wrote in 1936 that Brehmer had advocated rest in bed and in the open air, but that unfortunately many physicians, while partly adopting the rest regime, also advocated 'la cure de travail' and the clock was set back.[114] Paterson, the main advocate of 'la cure de travail' in Britain, was not described by tuberculosis specialists in Britain in the inter-war period as 'setting the clock back' but as 'the great master'.[115] The tuberculosis specialist and medical historian, E. Ashworth Underwood, claimed that Paterson's principle of auto-inoculation was of great importance in the development of modern methods.[116] Following a visit to Canada and America in 1930, McDougall reported,

Some are of the opinion that Sanatoria in this country in which occupational therapy and settlement work are carried on are not, in fact, practising the most orthodox forms of treatment, which is REST of the diseased organ. We feel it is our duty to remove this apprehension and say that we regard rest as the very foundation upon which the whole fabric of occupational therapy and vocational training is built . . .

We have even heard of Dr Marcus Paterson's original methods of exercising patients at Frimley Sanatorium in pre-war days being criticised when, in fact, rest was the prime factor in his scheme of treatment.[117]

Paterson did advocate rest, but only for a very short period. Webb maintained in 1936 that it had been found that at least four years of rest, whatever the method applied, were usually necessary for healing pulmonary tuberculosis.[118]

J. R. Dingley, medical superintendent of Darvell Hall, also believed that rest was unnecessarily prolonged in American and Canadian tuberculosis institutions which he visited in 1930. He found no patients there doing 'grade work', and discovered only one attempt to practise 'after-care', at the Altro Workshop in New York. The Altro managers told him that patients turned out of American sanatoria were too nervous to work, and that it took the Altro management a long time

[113] *Tubercle*, 1 (1920), 242.
[114] G. B. Webb, *Clio Medica: Tuberculosis* (New York, 1936), 164.
[115] For example, W. E. Snell (medical superintendent, Colindale Hospital, 1938–67), interview, 27 June 1983. See also P. Ellman, *Chest Diseases in General Practice with Special Reference to Pulmonary Tuberculosis* (London, 1932) 195–7. (Dedicated to M. Paterson.)
[116] Underwood, *A Manual of Tuberculosis*, p. 158. Paterson himself was reported to say in 1920 that open-air work had been 'proved a farce': *Tubercle* 1 (1920), 252.
[117] Preston Hall Annual Report 1929–30, pp. 10, 12.
[118] Webb, *Clio Medica: Tuberculosis*, p. 167.

to convince these patients of the curative value of regular employment and financial independence. Dingley was not surprised by this 'in view of what we had seen on the tour [of the sanatoria]'.[119]

Possibly part of the reason for the difference between Britain and America (that is work versus rest therapy) lies in the more competitive ethos in America. While some free treatment for tuberculosis was provided in America, it was not developed to the same extent as in Britain. American doctors, competing in an open market and concerned with their own professional status, were possibly more concerned with technological advances. Rest therapy was a corollary of surgical intervention. In Britain, tuberculosis physicians were not paid for each artificial pneumothorax performed, and thus there was no financial incentive to perform more operations.[120] Moreover, paying patients could not be persuaded so easily to undertake labour which was the form most of the occupational therapy took, even in the interests of their own health—patients paid to go to hospital to have treatment carried out on them.

One observer, D. Melville Dunlop, described what he considered excessive surgical intervention in America:

I saw one man at Philadelphia who had had a large cavity, for which he had received phrenic evulsion and scalemiotomy, then pneumothorax, then division of adhesions under the thoracoscope, then posterior thoracoplasty, and then, the rigid walls of the cavity being still undefeated, a localized anterior thoracoplasty . . . When I saw him, the cavity was closed, and the man was in wonderfully good shape . . . whether because of or in spite of treatment it would be difficult to say. I quote this simply as one of the many examples of the pertinacity with which the cavity is chased.[121]

Bilateral pneumothorax was not unusual in America; in Britain, active disease in both lungs was generally regarded as a contra-indication of pneumothorax. It was recorded in 1942 that 70 per cent of the patients discharged from the Massachusetts sanatoria had had some form of collapse therapy, whereas in Britain in the 1930s it was estimated that the treatment was given to no more than 10 per cent of the patients.[122]

---

[119] East Sussex County Record Office, HH10/7, 'Sun Life' Scholarship Tour, Canada and USA, 1930, Darvell Hall Sanatorium, Report by Medical Superintendent, 1930.

[120] As has been shown with hysterectomies, when the physician was paid per operation performed, the number of such operations increased: R. Taylor, *Medicine out of Control: The Anatomy of a Malignant Technology* (Sydney 1979), 157, 162–3.

[121] *EMJ* 41 (1934), 192; Underwood, *A Manual of Tuberculosis*, p. 241.

[122] H. D. Chadwick and A. S. Pope, *The Modern Attack on Tuberculosis* (New York, 1942), 45; *British Thoracic Association*, p. 16.

In Britain, even when thoracic surgery was at its height, there are indications that many tuberculosis specialists continued to prefer conservative methods of treatment. The medical superintendent of the Cheshire Joint Sanatorium, P. W. Edwards, reported in 1946 that routine sanatorium treatment was fairly rigorously practised at his sanatorium, and that despite the amount of operative work undertaken, it would be wrong to attribute the results of the sanatorium to the use of the knife and needle: 'Rest, an abundance of air, an all-round diet, and education in a mode of life are the foundations of treatment . . . After strict rest comes work.' He regarded his scheme to train women patients in housewifery as 'one of the notable advances in sanatorium work'. In 1943 he stated that sanatorium life was 'a life of treatment but need not, and should not, be for the great proportion of patients an idle existence', echoing Sir Robert Philip thirty years previously. In 1945, Edwards claimed it was very important that tuberculous patients should not be turned into idle loafers.[123]

Others shared his views. H. G. Trayer of Baguley Sanatorium reported in 1947, 'Whilst all modern forms of therapy are used in suitable cases, routine sanatorium treatment is extensively practised and remains . . . the basis for all treatment.'[124] At Colindale Hospital it was reported in 1947 that the general principles of sanatorium treatment were carried out.[125] E. A. Spriggs wrote in 1960 that a sanatorium with which he had recently been connected avoided, 'interestingly enough', the twentieth-century vogue for rest. Its medical superintendent from 1918 to 1955, C. G. R. Goodwin, did not keep his patients in bed once they were afebrile. At two or three months many of his patients were walking eight miles a day, and he employed some on heavy labour as Marcus Paterson had done at Frimley. His results were reported to be as good as those from other sanatoria.[126] In 1944, G. S. Erwin, medical superintendent of Liverpool Sanatorium, described his regime which included graded work of a useful character such as dusting and sweeping the wards, cleaning, gardening, and woodcutting.[127] In 1954 it was pointed out at Frimley Sanatorium that 'the prescription of physical work has been a feature of the treatment at Frimley since the days of Marcus Paterson

[123] *Tubercle*, 24 (1943), 59; ibid., 26 (1945), 30; ibid., 27 (1946), 101.
[124] Ibid., 28 (1947), 125.
[125] Ibid., 28 (1947), 58.
[126] Ibid., 41 (1960), 461.
[127] G. S. Erwin, *A Guide for the Tuberculous Patient* (London, 1944), 54.

. . . and it still proves its value.'[128] A medical textbook published in 1947 also referred to the system of 'graduated exercise' which Paterson had instituted at the Frimley Sanatorium, which 'has proved of great value'.[129] In 1955 George Day, medical superintendent of Mundesley Sanatorium, spoke in favour of graduated exercise and the discipline it involved: '[The patient] may have to evolve a new set of values, putting away ambition and contenting himself with what lies within his reach. If these spiritual changes are not wrought within him, if he does not leave the sanatorium a wiser man, the sanatorium treatment has failed to achieve complete victory.'[130]

(4) SUNLIGHT THERAPY

In the inter-war period, conservative methods came to dominate treatment of what was commonly known as 'surgical tuberculosis' or non-pulmonary tuberculosis (mainly tuberculosis of the bones and joints, the lymphatic glands, the abdomen, and the skin [lupus vulgaris]). In the early twentieth century, orthopaedic surgeons such as Sir Robert Jones were advocating open-air treatment for these conditions.[131] In 1925, Sir Henry Gauvain, medical superintendent of Lord Mayor Treloar's Home for Crippled Children, Alton, explained how the old theory which regarded a tuberculous joint as a lesion to be excised, 'a procedure which practised systematically resulted in high direct or subsequent mortality, in much suffering through added sepsis and in deplorable and unavoidable crippling' had been abandoned. He claimed that it was now recognized that 'surgical tuberculosis' was a general disease or a generalized infection, and that lesions were merely special manifestations. This conception of the disease led to general treatment: 'climatic, hygienic, dietetic, drug, educational, and other general measures'. In his opinion, the locality of the hospital was important; essential requirements included remoteness from towns and absence of interference from outside visitors, 'a flat littoral with absence of cliffs, and an extensive sandy beach with wide tidal excursion'.[132]

[128] Pamphlet, Brompton Hospital Sanatorium Jubilee Garden Party, 4 Sept. 1954.
[129] F. W. Price (ed.), *A Textbook on the Practice of Medicine*, 7th edn. (Oxford, 1947), 1229.
[130] *Tubercle*, 36 (1955), 54.
[131] See R. Cooter, *The Making of Modern Orthopaedics: A Social History of Orthopaedics 1881–1945* (forthcoming). [132] 11 *NAPT 1925*, pp. 109–11.

Heliotherapy or sunlight therapy was regarded by Gauvain as a valuable adjunct to the general treatment of non-pulmonary tuberculosis. Such treatment had been popularized by Auguste Rollier and his famous clinic in Leysin 'for the systematic treatment of tuberculosis by the Alpine sun'. This treatment was widely adopted for non-pulmonary tuberculosis in British sanatoria. However, the treatment did require a suitable climate, which despite the claims of the early twentieth-century advertisements for the sanatoria, was not aways available.

Reporting on outdoor treatment in Scotland, the Scottish Board of Health wrote in 1927:

It would probably come as a surprise to many to learn that, in spite of the rigours of our Scottish climate, it is found possible during even the colder months of spring and autumn to allow the children at some sanatoria to spend the greater part of the day in an almost nude state, so ensuring to them the maximum benefit from sunlight and fresh air.[133]

However, the application of direct sunshine was another matter. In 1924, the Scottish Board of Health pointed out that light therapy was practised in its institutions, but that since the summer of 1921 the possibilities in this direction had been limited owing to the dearth of sunshine. They noted that in Scotland even in favourable summer weather, the duration of sunshine was apt to be too uncertain for continuous treatment.[134] For example, it was reported from Robroyston Hospital, Glasgow, in 1926, that heliotherapy was difficult to carry out because of the fitful appearance of the sun and the relatively weak actinic value of its rays, coming from grey skies and blotted out by clouds of smoke. Thus, in 1925, the systematic treatment of tuberculosis by artificial sunlight was introduced at Robroyston.[135]

Artificial light therapy was, according to MacNalty, 'a weapon that advanced civilisation [had] provided to diminish by some degree some of its own defects'. These defects included 'increasing urbanisation, the smoke-pall over cities, darkness and dirt'.[136] An artificial substitute for heliotherapy in the form of carbon arc lamps had been developed by Niels Ryberg Finsen in Denmark in the 1890s, who successfully treated lupus vulgaris by this method. Finsen was awarded a Nobel

[133] *Scottish Board of Health Annual Report 1927*, Cmd. 3112 (1928), 100.
[134] *Scottish Board of Health Annual Report 1924*, Cmd. 2416 (1925), 58.
[135] *12 NAPT 1926*, p. 114.
[136] Ministry of Health, A. S. MacNalty, *Report on Tuberculosis* (Reports on Public Health and Medical Subjects, 64; London, 1932), 138–9.

prize for his work in 1903, and a Finsen Institute was set up in Copenhagen. 'Finsen–Reyn' lamps (Professor Reyn was a director of the Institute) were purchased and installed in some British tuberculosis institutions in the 1920s which reported favourable results, particularly for cases of lupus. Such a light department with Finsen–Reyn lamps at the cost of £1,250 was donated in 1927 to Glan Ely Hospital in Wales by the local freemasons as a memorial to the late Sir David Evans, first director of the WNMA and Deputy Provincial Grand Master of the Masons in the Province of South Wales (Eastern District).[137] In the 1930s, with the decline of non-pulmonary tuberculosis among children, many of the institutions, for example the Liverpool Open-air Hospital for Children, Leasowe, broadened their categories to include children suffering from other disabilities.[138] Surgery in the treatment of non-pulmonary tuberculosis was not, however, totally abandoned, and splints were devised to rest infected parts. X-ray therapy was developed for tuberculous adenitis in the 1930s.

(5) CHEMOTHERAPY

Tuberculous meningitis was invariably fatal, with patients often dying within three to six weeks of diagnosis, and therefore claims of treatment could not be sustained. This was not the case for pulmonary tuberculosis, for which the course of the disease was very unpredictable, with occasional cases which were apparently advanced making miraculous recoveries. As a result, it provided a prime subject for the exploitation of all sorts of medications.[139] Requests were constantly sent to the Ministry of Health to investigate 'this or that wonderful cure for tuberculosis'.[140]

The search for a chemotherapeutic cure for tuberculosis had been given impetus by the success of chemotherapy in the treatment of syphilis in 1909 when Paul Ehrlich discovered salvarsan. The famous tuberculosis specialist in the USA, who founded the first tuberculosis sanatorium there, Edward Livingstone Trudeau, for example, saw 'no

---

[137] PRO MH96/967.
[138] *Tubercle*, 16 (1935), 181.
[139] A. L. Thomson, *Medical Research Council: Half a Century of Medical Research*, ii, *The Programme of the Medical Research Council (UK)* (London, 1975), 9; see also F. B. Smith, 'Gullible's Travails: Tuberculosis and Quackery 1890–1930', *Journal of Contemporary History*, 20 (1985), 733–56.
[140] PRO MH55/148, Coutts, 14 Aug. 1919.

reason why what had been accomplished in the treatment of syphilis should not be attained in tuberculosis'.[141] However, H. H. (later Sir Henry) Dale of the National Institute for Medical Research admitted in 1921 that there appeared at that time to be no real starting point for research in the chemotherapy of tuberculosis. Nor did Dale discover much progress being made at the Henry Phipps Institute for tuberculosis research in Philadelphia, which he had recently visited.[142]

A more popular field for research in tuberculosis as in many other diseases at this time was the exploration of a therapy developed through bacteriology or immunology. For tuberculosis, variants of Koch's tuberculin were explored. The Tuberculin Dispensary League under Camac Wilkinson continued to advocate the use of tuberculin. The MRC showed little interest in tuberculin as a potential cure, rejecting successive requests by the League for an investigation.[143] Wilkinson was not, however, alone in advocating tuberculin. Sir Robert Philip was among the most persistent practitioners of tuberculin—he was reported still to be using it in the treatment of tuberculosis in 1927.[144] C. J. Campbell Faill, TO for Bristol, maintained in 1937 that tuberculin had been greatly neglected in recent years, and that it had in his own experience proved invaluable in the treatment of admittedly carefully selected cases.[145] Writing in 1935, Halliday Sutherland also regarded tuberculin as 'our greatest asset of the diagnosis and treatment of tuberculosis'. Like Wilkinson, he believed that it might effectively replace sanatorium treatment.[146] In 1962 it was claimed that tuberculin had been used until comparatively recently in a few special types of tuberculosis.[147]

Another treatment based on microbial products which caused a great deal of excitement was the Spahlinger treatment, discovered in 1912 by Henri Spahlinger, a Swiss bacteriologist without medical

---

[141] *BJT*, 10/1 (1916), 30.

[142] MRC 205/1, MacNalty, Conference on the Future of Tuberculosis Work of the MRC, 5 Mar. 1921, p. 9.

[143] *Lancet*, 2 (1923), 984–8; MRC 141/3, Tuberculin Dispensary League Committee, Inquiry, 30 July 1919, and the work of the Tuberculin League, Chelsea, 6 Oct. 1923; W. C. Wilkinson, *The Tuberculin Dispensary for the Poor* (London, 1923). See also MRC, N. Bardswell and J. H. R. Thompson, *Pulmonary Tuberculosis: Mortality after Sanatorium Treatment* (SRS 33; 1919), 52.

[144] MRC 205/2, III, Tuberculin Sub-committee, 28 July 1927.

[145] *23 NAPT 1937*, p. 146.

[146] H. G. Sutherland, *The Tuberculin Handbook* (Oxford, 1936), Review, *Tubercle*, 17 (1936), 369; G. N. Meachen, *A Short History of Tuberculosis* (London, 1936), 33.

[147] C. Singer and E. A. Underwood, *A Short History of Medicine*, 2nd edn. (Oxford, 1962), 424.

qualifications who had set up the Spahlinger Institute on his family estate at Caroque, Geneva. This treatment was an anti-tuberculosis serum derived from the blood of black horses, although the substance of the treatment was kept a secret. It was reported enthusiastically in Britain in 1920 and 1921, and MacNalty was impressed when he visited the institute in 1922. Several appeals were conducted in Britain in the 1920s to help Spahlinger financially, for his financial problems were alleged to be the reason for the unavailability of the serum for a large-scale inquiry. Remaining sceptical throughout, Fletcher claimed in 1931 that Arthur Stanley had wasted a lot of Red Cross money on Spahlinger, and that J. B. Buxton (professor of animal pathology at Cambridge University) was now wasting money on him. Spahlinger's popularity was never great among the British tuberculosis specialists themselves, and by the 1930s his popularity was beginning to wane in general, although some loyal supporters claimed that he had never been given a fair trial.[148]

For the development of an 'improved Tuberculin', the MRC had its own candidate, of whom great expectations were held. These expectations seemed to be realized in 1923. In a report on the work of Georges Dreyer, MacNalty claimed that Dreyer's remedies were of far-reaching importance and, if confirmed and maintained, were calculated in the near future to revolutionize not only the treatment of tuberculosis but that of other bacterial diseases such as pneumonia and septicaemia (see also Chapter 5, Section 3). According to an MRC report, the results of the treatment in over 80 cases of tuberculosis of various kinds were 'extremely favourable and . . . frankly astonished all the workers concerned'. The early results were not confirmed however, and in November 1924 it was concluded that it was not more efficacious in the treatment of tuberculosis than other forms of tuberculin.[149]

Some tuberculosis specialists were very sceptical of any cures for tuberculosis. Varrier-Jones had conveyed his own scepticism so

---

[148] *Lancet*, 1 (1921), 550. *Hansard*, 5th Series, 138 (1921), 974, 1821; ibid., 139 (1921), 432; ibid., 141 (1921), 662–3; PRO MH55/153, MacNalty, 22 Jan. 1923; MRC 1381/2, IV, Fletcher to Lord Mildmay, 16 Feb. 1931; PRO MH55/155, William Bulloch, 14 Apr. 1932; *Observer*, 6 May 1934 (MRC 1381/2); L. Macassey and C. W. Saleeby (eds.), *Spahlinger 'contra' Tuberculosis 1908–1934: An International Tribute* (London, 1934). See also Smith, *Journal of Contemporary History*, 20 (1985), 733–56.

[149] MRC 1220, I, Report by MacNalty, 23 May 1923; MRC 1220 I, Report for Members MRC only, 11 June 1923; MRC 205/2 II, Final Report on Diaplyte Vaccine, 21 Nov. 1924.

convincingly to his patients that when Dreyer's antigen was available in 1923 following much favourable publicity, 'most of the colonists refuse to have it and prefer . . . to wait and see'.[150] He was asked to carry out a clinical trial of the serum; he reported that it had no influence on the course of the disease but that he had taken the opportunity to carry out simultaneously a useful psychological investigation. Other medical superintendents also advised their patients against 'miracle cures' for tuberculosis.[151]

In 1923 a significant development occurred in the chemotherapy of tuberculosis—Holger Moellgaard, professor of animal physiology at Copenhagen University, discovered sanocrysin or sodium aurothiosulphate, with a gold content of 37 per cent, and thus inaugurated the 'gold decade' in tuberculosis treatment.[152] The MRC began a trial on sanocrysin in 1924, concluding in 1926 that sanocrysin was of benefit in a limited number of cases.[153] S. Lyle Cummins was very optimistic about it in 1926, while L. S. T. Burrell, writing in 1929, was not so optimistic. Burrell estimated, in fact, that at first almost 16 per cent had died as a direct result of the treatment either from shock or acute metal poisoning. Subsequently, the size of doses was reduced, which Burrell did not think had much effect. He still believed that chronic pulmonary tuberculosis cases did improve with sanocrysin.[154] Most local authorities reported that sanocrysin was being used in their institutions in the late 1920s, but by about 1935 sanocrysin was going out of fashion, the 'gold decade' was ending. Two tuberculosis specialists wrote in 1949 that the results had not really been convincing, and that some of the complications had been alarming, such as kidney damage and severe skin rashes.[155] A questionnaire on sanocrysin was sent to 364 specialists in 1940. Only about a third replied which suggested to the investigators, who had designed the

[150] MRC 1220/5, Varrier-Jones to Fletcher, 13 Sept. 1923.

[151] For example, R. C. Wingfield, *A Textbook of Pulmonary Tuberculosis for Students* (London, 1929), 225; G. S. Erwin, *A Guide for the Tuberculous Patient* (London, 1944), 1; McDougall, Preston Hall Annual Report 1933, p. 6; East Sussex County Record Office, HH14/8, J. R. Dingley, Darvell Hall Magazine (1937).

[152] F. R. G. Heaf and N. L. Rusby, *Recent Advances in Pulmonary Tuberculosis*, 4th edn. (London, 1948), 122; D'Arcy Hart, *BMJ* 2 (1946), 808.

[153] MRC 1380/3, sanocrysin trials, 1924: Maclean (St Thomas's Hospital), to Fletcher; *MRC Annual Report 1926–7* Cmd. 3013 (1928), 94–5; *9th CMOH Annual Report 1927* (1928), 69.

[154] MRC 1380/3, S. L. Cummins, notes on sanocrysin, 15 Jan. 1926, p. 17; L. S. T. Burrell, *Recent Advances in Pulmonary Tuberculosis* (London, 1929), 91, 92, 98.

[155] L. E. Houghton and T. H. Sellors, *Aids to Tuberculosis Nursing, A Complete Textbook for the Nurse*, 3rd edn. (London, 1949), 68–9.

questionnaire as simply as possible, that not much interest was taken in sanocrysin. The results showed that the treatment was losing favour, that those who continued to use it did so 'because one must do something' rather than because they believed in it.[156] One ex-patient from Eversfield was still reported to be 'having gold' in 1947.[157]

(6) POST-SANATORIUM TREATMENT

It was widely recommended in the early twentieth century that ex-sanatorium patients should emigrate to the colonies where the climate would be kinder to their health. The Barlow Committee considered this one possible solution to the 35,000 ex-servicemen with tuberculosis in 1919. Yet it also discovered that the colonies had already introduced restrictions on entry for those suffering from an infectious disease, incuding tuberculosis.[158] The Scottish Board of Health investigated the possibility of emigration for tuberculous patients to Australia in 1920. It reported that the Commonwealth authorities excluded immigrants in whom the disease was active, but that they were willing to admit persons in whom the disease had been arrested for at least twelve months, and if they had received a period of treatment in a sanatorium. The conditions of admission included a certificate from an expert in tuberculosis, and the Scottish Board of Health offered to pay a guinea per examination to local authorities who examined prospective emigrants.[159]

There are no statistics on the number of people classed as 'arrested' cases of tuberculosis who emigrated. Host countries were clearly not enthusiastic. One specialist from New Zealand, who described the anti-tuberculosis campaign in New Zealand in the *Tuberculosis Yearbook* in 1914, added in italics, '*New Zealand does not invite persons suffering from tuberculosis, in any form, to come to the Dominion. Therefore in no sense of the word can this Southern Britain be regarded as a health resort for the consumptive.*'[160] Yet, some tuberculosis specialists in Britain continued to advocate emigration. Wingfield suggested in 1929 that emigration to South Africa, Australia, or New Zealand might double

[156] *Tubercle*, 21 (1940), 174.
[157] East Sussex County Record Office, HH68/6, Eversfield Patient Records, H.C. (patient's initials), 25 Jan. 1947.
[158] *Barlow Report*, pp. 17–18.
[159] *Scottish Board of Health 3rd Annual Report 1921*, Cmd. 1697 (1922), 23.
[160] Kelynack (ed.), *Tuberculosis Yearbook 1913–14*, p. 114.

the chances of survival, even for the 'good case'.[161] It was explained at Burrow Hill Colony in 1924 that training was provided in all branches of farming and market gardening 'to fit them for situations on small holdings in this country or in the colonies should they choose to emigrate'.[162] The follow-up records of the Frimley Sanatorium show that emigration was not uncommon. The Eversfield Hospital authorities published in the sanatorium magazine in 1937 a letter from an ex-patient who had moved to Australia. This patient 'reports that she still works full time at Secretarial Duties and takes as much exercise in the open air as possible. She recommends the climate of Melbourne to any one who can afford to get there as the maximum of time can be spent out-of-doors, for there is an abundance of sunshine and the winters are mild.'[163]

Patients who did not emigrate continued to be supervised by their local dispensaries for up to five years after the discharge from the sanatorium. Dispensaries were advised to keep the dispensing of medicines to a minimum. Newman felt that the practice of treating patients at the dispensary on a large scale and over prolonged periods with bottles of medicine or cod-liver oil, and of giving medicines to ensure attendance of patients should be discouraged: 'Patients should rather be educated out of the belief in the efficacy of drugs, and be taught the value of personal advice and of instruction in a hygienic mode of life.'[164] It was reported from the Denbigh and Flint dispensary in 1929 that 'treatment consists of advice chiefly'.[165] The stress on advice rather than treatment in the form of medicines also helped to persuade GPs that their sphere was not being encroached upon by the dispensaries.

Nevertheless, evidence suggests that medicines, and cod-liver oil in particular, were routinely dispensed, as well as other supplementary foods. It was specified that a new dispensary (or 'tuberculosis clinic' as it was now designated) planned at the Finsbury Health Centre in 1939 was to have no facilities for the dispensing of medicines, as it was felt that the issuing of routine medicines detracted from its status as

[161] R. C. Wingfield, *A Textbook of Pulmonary Tuberculosis for Students* (London, 1929), 370.
[162] NAPT Council Report 1923, Burrow Hill Colony, Medical Superintendent Report, p. 24.
[163] Eversfield Hospital Annual Report 1937, p. 30.
[164] *2nd CMOH Annual Report 1920* (1921), 92.
[165] PRO MH96/1021, Welsh Board of Health, Arrangements for Treatment of Tuberculosis, Denbigh and Flint Area, 14 Oct. 1929.

a specialist centre, indicating that the practice was not unknown.[166] Domiciliary treatment, carried out by the dispensary staff, also consisted primarily of 'detailed advice . . . to the patient as to the regulation of his life and conduct in his own interest and in that of others'.[167] Visiting tuberculosis nurses were to educate patients and their families in the laws of hygiene, and to watch for additional cases of tuberculosis in the family. Thus the families of the patients, not just the patients themselves, were to be supervised, as in the village settlements.

The various rehousing schemes were a further attempt to maintain supervision over ex-sanatorium patients and their families. The tenancy agreement of the Sheffield rehousing scheme shows very clearly that an important element of the scheme was the control it enabled the dispensary staff to exercise over the tuberculous patients and their families. Under the agreement, no lodgers were allowed, the patient had to occupy a separate bedroom and attend the dispensary regularly, health officers were allowed access to the house for purposes of supervision, and all members of the family were to attend the dispensary when required and submit to examination at least once a year.[168]

Special workshops also facilitated further supervision over ex-sanatorium patients. At the Spero Workshop in London, for example, employees and their families were said to be 'looked after by experienced physicians and social workers'.[169] The TO for the City of London, T. H. Young, believed that the supervision of the lives of workers was an important aspect of workshops for ex-sanatorium patients.[170]

Rehousing and workshop schemes were therefore not only perceived to have economic advantages for the ex-sanatorium patients and their families, but also enabled tuberculosis specialists to retain close supervision over the lives of ex-patients. According to Varrier-Jones, the tuberculous person's 'whole life, waking, working, sleeping and all the manifold activities of existence [should] be carefully guarded and guided'. He maintained that a consumptive must learn to be a consumptive just as a blind person must learn to be blind.[171] If they could

---

[166] *25 NAPT 1939*, p. 151.   [167] *2nd CMOH Annual Report 1920*, (1921), 89.
[168] *12th CMOH Annual Report 1930* (1931), 100.
[169] *The Times*, 24 Feb. 1926 (letter to editor); *17 NAPT 1931*, p. 140.
[170] PRO MH55/140, F. H. Young, 1925.
[171] *Journal of State Medicine*, 30/5 (1922), 90; *Lancet*, 2 (1918), 133; ibid., 1 (1941), 368.

not be supervised in a village settlement then they were to be supervised in their homes and workplaces following a course of training in the correct lifestyle in a sanatorium or training colony. MacNalty wrote in 1935:

It cannot be too strongly emphasised that the benefit derived from treatment in residential institutions may be and frequently is undone and early relapse invited if the patient returns to unsatisfactory conditions of life and work. This has been demonstrated to be one of the main causes of the so-called 'failure' of sanatorium treatment. In the new concept of the fight against tuberculosis, an essential point is that the consumptive must remain under medical observation for a number of years; his is a damaged life and must be regarded as such.[172]

Wingfield similarly wrote, 'The main problem in the treatment of tuberculosis is that patients do not realise that "tuberculosis is a life sentence".'[173]

There was no indication that treatment given in 1941 was more successful than that given in 1911, according to the WNMA annual report for 1944.[174] The Brompton Hospital Research Department had reached a similar conclusion in 1935: 'The prognosis of the average case of pulmonary tuberculosis has not materially changed during the past thirty years and . . . our patients of more recent years show after-histories very similar to those of cases treated in the earlier period.'[175] Percy Stocks of the General Register Office also wrote in 1935, 'It has to be admitted by a dispassionate critic that up to the present no satisfactory statistical proof of the curative advantage of sanatorium over other forms of treatment has been produced . . .'[176] Nor did thoracic surgery alter the situation, as already noted. However, tuberculosis specialists continued to stress that the problem lay not with the nature of the treatment itself but with post-sanatorium experience. Sir Geoffrey Todd firmly believed that those who did not follow his instructions as to the mode of life they should live following sanatorium treatment, were the ones who had to be readmitted.[177] Wingfield pointed out that the chances of survival were very poor for 'the fool, the overbold, the weak-willed or the evil-doer'.[178] His

[172] *17th CMOH Annual Report 1935* (1936), 78–9.   [173] *Tubercle*, 22 (1941), 199.
[174] *Tubercle*, 26 (1945), 164–5.
[175] *17th CMOH Annual Report 1935* (1936), 91–2.
[176] P. Stocks, in C. W. Hutt and H. H. Thomson (eds.), *Principles and Practice of Preventive Medicine* (London, 1935), ii. 1561.
[177] Sir Geoffrey Todd, interview, 25 Aug. 1983.
[178] R. C. Wingfield, *Modern Methods in the Diagnosis and Treatment of Pulmonary Tuberculosis* (London, 1924), 120.

predecessor at Frimley, W. O. Meek, had pointed out that there was a number of individuals among the admissions to a public sanatorium whose treatment was 'foredoomed to failure on account of their habits, lack of will-power or intelligence', adding that such persons formed 'an appreciable percentage of the total admissions'.[179] Other more socially conscious commentators, such as the tuberculosis officers of Kent, West Riding, and Oxfordshire, stressed the economic difficulties faced by ex-patients.[180] This was the point taken up by the social surveyor, Seebohm Rowntree, who argued that ex-sanatorium patients had little chance of survival given the economic conditions to which they often had to return.[181] A councillor of Glamorgan believed that good work was being done by the WNMA, 'but we are living in a madhouse paying a 7*d*. rate in order to give health to the people, and when they have regained it forcing them back to live under conditions which make them ill again—no extra food, no warm beds and often no shelter'.[182]

Whether they blamed personal behaviour or economic circumstances, the focus was on post-sanatorium experience. Thus, after-care assumed a greater importance by the late 1930s—as an attempt to supervise the life of the ex-patients, or improve their material circumstances, or both. The JTC in 1942 maintained that 'care work should proceed as regularly and systematically as the provision of treatment and prevention, from which it cannot be separated. It follows that it should be an integral part of every scheme for dealing with tuberculosis and not just associated with it.'[183] After-care work still varied greatly, however, from one area to another, largely dependent on the initiative of the local councils, tuberculosis officers, or voluntary organizations.

---

[179] *Lancet*, 2 (1917), 786.
[180] West Riding TO (B. Mann), *Tubercle*, 23 (1942), 72; Oxfordshire TO (F. H. Pearce), NAPT, Oxfordshire Branch Annual Report 1926–7, p. 6; Kent TO, Papworth, Sims-Woodhead Memorial Laboratory Research Bulletin 1940, p. 25.
[181] S. Rowntree, *Poverty and Progress: A Second Social Survey of York* (London, 1941), 84.
[182] *Manchester Guardian*, 8 Feb. 1936 (PRO MH96/1030).
[183] *Tubercle*, 23 (1942), 92.

7

The Patient's View

In 1823 and 1824 . . . it was the fashion to suffer from the lungs;
everybody was consumptive, poets especially; it was good form to
spit blood after each emotion that was at all sensational, and to
die before reaching the age of thirty.

Duma's *Memoirs*, quoted in R. and J. Dubos, *The White Plague:
Tuberculosis, Man and Society* (London, 1953), 58–9.

NINETEENTH-CENTURY literature romanticized the experience of
suffering from tuberculosis. This genre was disappearing by the early
twentieth century, with the spreading knowledge of the infectious
nature of tuberculosis. The NAPT and its 'cabinet of horrors',
stressing the unpleasantness and infectiousness of the disease (see
Chapter 1, Section 1), aided this process. Yet for the post-1950
generation the romantic view has resurfaced, as a result of a retreating
memory of the reality of the disease, and the endurance of the
nineteenth-century romantic novels together with the impressive list of
famous victims of tuberculosis of the past (including Balzac, the
Brontë sisters, Chekhov, Chopin, Dostoevsky, Kafka, Keats, D. H.
Lawrence, Katherine Mansfield, Edgar Allan Poe, Joseph Priestly, Sir
Walter Scott, Shelley—who drowned, but was believed to be suffering
from tuberculosis—R. L. Stevenson, and Voltaire, among others).[1]
The romantic view of tuberculosis has been perpetuated further by
Susan Sontag in her book *Illness as Metaphor*, where she drew upon
nineteenth-century novels and yet claimed that the romantic associations of tuberculosis disappeared only when the disease was finally
brought under control in the Western world in the 1950s.[2] In his
history of tuberculosis, J. Harley Williams similarly perpetuated the
myth of the romance of the disease. He did so first by singling out

[1] H. D. Chalke, 'The Impact of Tuberculosis in Literature, History and Art', *Medical
History*, 6 (1962), 301–18 and 'Some Historical Aspects of Tuberculosis', *Public Health*,
74/3 (1959), 83–95.
[2] S. Sontag, *Illness as Metaphor* (New York, 1977; Harmondsworth, 1983), 38–9.

Thomas Mann's novel, *The Magic Mountain*, which depicted a sanatorium in the Swiss Alps as a setting for philosophical reflections and discussions, as 'the best insight into the sanatorium idea'.³ This was despite his own experience of sanatoria, and his admission forty years earlier that people regarded such an institution as 'a kind of centre of plague'.⁴ Secondly in his history of tuberculosis, he stated his aim to be not merely to present the history of tuberculosis as a series of theoretical discoveries and administrative acts but 'as a great catalyser in a human being's life'.⁵ This he aimed to achieve by discussing the experiences of famous people who suffered from tuberculosis. While he provided an interesting account of the experiences of these people, by focusing exclusively on famous artistic people, he helped to advance the image of the disease as being somehow related to creativity and artistic genius and in this way romantic. Moreover, one is left to wonder about the experiences of the millions of 'ordinary' sufferers from the disease.

(1) THE 'TOTAL INSTITUTION'

Despite the advertisements and descriptions of British sanatoria in the early twentieth century as idyllic, there was little romance in the reality of the sanatoria. Indeed, twentieth-century British sanatoria conformed very closely to Erving Goffman's model of a 'total institution', sharing features with other institutions such as prisons, schools, lunatic asylums, and hospitals.⁶

In a crucial sense, tuberculosis institutions resembled Goffman's total or all-encompassing institution with its characteristic isolation from wider society. While they were not separated from the outside world by physical barriers, tuberculosis institutions were isolated both geographically and socially. There is much evidence to suggest that inmates of sanatoria felt estranged from the outside world. Not only did their geographical isolation make visits difficult and therefore infrequent, but social attitudes accentuated that isolation. In a book

---

³ T. Mann, *The Magic Mountain* (1924, trans. H. T. Lowe-Porter, 2 vols. (London, 1927; repr. Harmondsworth, 1979); J. H. Williams, *Requiem for a Great Killer: The Story of Tuberculosis* (London, 1973), 35.

⁴ *23 NAPT 1937*, p. 12.

⁵ Williams, *Requiem for a Great Killer*, p. 14.

⁶ E. Goffman, *Asylums: Essays on the Social Situation of Mental Patients and other Inmates* (Harmondsworth, 1961), 15, 16.

describing a patient's experiences at Frimley Sanatorium around 1940, the author wrote of a fellow patient:

It was said that he had never had a visitor all the time he had been there. He wrote occasionally to a younger sister, but I believe theirs were step parents and I have the impression that, in his diseased state of health, he was looked on by them as a social pariah, best forgotten; not too uncommon an attitude at that time.[7]

Joan McCarthy, relating her experiences in the Cheshire Joint Sanatorium in 1950, described her husband's visits:

My husband will tell of ghastly journeys from Birkenhead in a 'Charabanc'. Most of his fellow travellers were women, and they viewed the visiting as if they were entering a leper colony. Few men visited, perhaps they remained home to care for the family, but I suspect the implications of the disease kept them away . . . The obvious despair in the eyes of the patients whose husband, or loved one failed to visit, was an acknowledgement of the rejection they felt, and the fear that their relationship may never be re-established.[8]

Rejection was indeed the experience of Mary Hewin's sister when she contracted tuberculosis after the First World War: 'As soon as he knew, Frank Pollitt, soon as he knew she'd got it, he gave her up . . . She was broken-hearted. She'd been going with him three years, but he never came round again, when he heard she'd got TB.'[9]

Nor did surrounding communities look kindly upon tuberculosis institutions. Mrs Stockford, who moved into Preston Hall in 1923 with her husband who had tuberculosis, said, 'We were regarded like a leper colony.'[10] The *County Times* wrote of patients at Machynlleth Hospital, Montgomeryshire, in 1931, '. . . once a patient went to the hospital all his movements in the town were watched with interest, everyone being very careful to see where he went when he went into the town'.[11]

Local reaction to the siting of a sanatorium in the neighbourhood is indicative of a widespread aversion to such institutions. In 1923 the siting of a 'surgical tuberculosis' (non-pulmonary) hospital at Ascot aroused protest. Although it was explained to the local residents that surgical tuberculosis was not infectious in the ordinary sense, the

[7] G. A. Cook, *A Hackney Memory Chest* (London, 1983), 44–5.
[8] J. M. McCarthy, '"Tuberculosis" Before and After Waksman', unpublished dissertation, BA (General) Health and Community Studies, Chester College, 1986, p. 42.
[9] A. Hewins, *Mary, After the Queen: Memories of a Working Girl* (Oxford, 1986), p. 35.
[10] Mrs Stockford, interview, 22 June 1983.
[11] *The County Times* (Montgomeryshire), 24 Oct. 1931 (PRO MH96/1019).

authorities had to promise to omit the word 'tuberculosis' from the name of the hospital.[12] Surrey CC encountered similar opposition when it planned a sanatorium at Milford in 1923; a deputation was sent to the Minister of Health in 1924 to register the protest, claiming that the sanatorium would be a danger to the locality.[13] In 1920 the *Tubercle* commented on the 'selfish viciousness' of residents in a locality opposing the etablishment of a new sanatorium.[14] The *Lancet* believed such opposition to be very common, and gave an example of a medical officer who argued against the establishment of such an institution in the locality by painting 'a most lugubrious picture' of local climatic conditions.[15] The WNMA also encountered protests when planning to open a sanatorium for children at Highland Moors in the spa district of Llandrindod Wells in 1931. A local doctor was concerned that Llandrindod might be prejudiced by having an institution which was labelled a tuberculosis hospital. He wanted to avoid even the suspicion of any association of the name of Llandrindod Wells with an infectious disease. The Association promised to omit the word 'tuberculosis' from the name of the hospital, and also promised not to send children with active tuberculosis, although in the event active cases were sent.[16] Again in 1935, when the Association was planning to establish an institution in Swansea, local residents protested to the Ministry of Health. The Vicar of Sketty described the scheme as 'the most absurd suggestion ever made by a competent authority' and as a 'suicidal policy'.[17] When a dispensary was being planned in Cardiff in 1931, the neighbours registered a protest. They replied to a letter from the Association: 'We are obliged for your offer for us to inspect other dispensaries, but we think no useful purpose would be served by our doing so. The point is that the public in general have a fear of anything in connection with a Tuberculosis Hospital.'[18]

A neighbour of Papworth Village Settlement sold his farm 'solely because the patients would insist on mixing with other people'. When the union of the village settlement parish church with the neighbouring

[12] PRO MH52/96, Coutts, The Heatherwood Hospital, Ascot, 4 June 1923.
[13] PRO MH52/126, A. S. MacNalty and R. C. Hetherington, Surrey, Report on Inspection of Sanatorium Site, 16 Jan. 1925.
[14] *Tubercle*, 1 (1920), 386.   [15] *Lancet*, 1 (1920), 398.
[16] J. Murray, *Brecon and Radnor Express*, 23 July 1931 (PRO MH96/1055). PRO MH96/1055, Public Inquiry, 16 July 1931, Report by T. W. Wade, 22 July 1931.
[17] PRO MH96/1008, Swansea CC to Ministry of Health, 16 Aug. 1935. *Western Mail*, 2 Oct. 1935 (PRO MH96/1008).
[18] PRO MH96/1060, Linton & Sons, Solicitors, Pontypridd, to WNMA, 28 Sept. 1931.

parish, Papworth St Agnes, was being contemplated in 1921, every adult member of St Agnes signed a petition in protest. One woman said she refrained from attending church after finding seven members of the colony sitting in her pew. A resident of Papworth recalled that 'some of the more ignorant of the local inhabitants would by-pass the village, rather than pass through it, . . . a fact that did not go unnoticed by the villagers'. But she believed that 'this attitude only tended to greatly increase the spirit of community and togetherness, and this was all to the good of the village'.[19] The ostracism which the inmates experienced thus enhanced the all-encompassing character of the institution.

Not only were Papworth and Preston Hall 'all-encompassing' communities with their village settlements, but other institutions, while providing fewer community facilities, were also fairly self-contained; for example Midhurst, described, under the pseudonym of Cranston, by Alan Dick.[20] W. A. Murray, who became medical superintendent of East Fortune Sanatorium, Scotland, said that as medical superintendent he learned the art of being—not just a doctor—but the leader of a community or provost of a small village.[21]

The structure of the sanatorium was strictly hierarchical with the medical superintendent at the head of the household. Otto Walther of Nordrach Sanatorium had been described as a patriarchal figure; according to Vere Pearson, his patients stood a good deal in awe of him, but loved him well, and called him affectionately 'The Old Man'.[22] R. C. Wingfield, medical superintendent of Frimley Sanatorium from 1920 to 1945, was described as 'a large formidable looking but very shy man with a military bearing . . . He was a strict disciplinarian, autocratic like Marcus Paterson, essentially very kind and sincere with a sense of humour'. An ex-patient remembered that they called him 'Father'.[23] The medical superintendent of 'Cranston', called Kidd, was described as 'a strict disciplinarian': a patient drew a sketch of him 'bestraddling the sanatorium like a menacing colossus . . . captioned, "The Dictator of Cranston" and presented to Kidd with love and good wishes'.[24] J. B. McDougall of Preston Hall was also described as a

---

[19] Papworth Archives, *Cambridge Weekly News*, 7 Mar. 1921, 'Enid Remembers', 2, 3.
[20] A. Dick, *A Walking Miracle* (London, 1942), 80; *Lancet*, 2 (1942), 292, identifies the sanatorium as Midhurst, which is in any case not too difficult to guess.
[21] W. A. Murray, *A Life Worth Living, Fifty Years in Medicine* (Haddington, 1981), 19.
[22] S. V. Pearson, *Men, Medicine and Myself* (London, 1946), 33.
[23] J. R. Bignall, *Frimley: The Biography of a Sanatorium* (London, 1979), 134, 158.
[24] Dick, *A Walking Miracle*, pp. 56, 109–10.

'benevolent autocrat'.[25] Varrier-Jones was known among the patients at Papworth affectionately as 'The Old Man'. He clearly saw himself as a benevolent dictator. McDougall wrote of Varrier-Jones, 'From the very inception . . . he remained in supreme control, dictating policy to the minutest detail.' The *Western Mail* reported in 1922, 'In the centre of this delightful little community village is Papworth Hall, where Dr P. C. Varrier-Jones . . . controls his little community . . . Perhaps the happiest man in the whole village is Dr Varrier-Jones, who takes tremendous pride in what may be termed his own community.'[26]

Senior staff assumed a similar disciplinary function. George Cook described the sister at Frimley as a 'fearsome figure': 'A commanding personality whose word was law . . . Like many formidable people however, she was a sheep in wolf's clothing; at heart a most kindly soul.'[27] The senior medical officer at Papworth, L. Stott, was described by a patient as a firm disciplinarian but fair: 'We feared him but we loved him.' The matron, Miss Borne, evoked a similar response from patients.[28]

W. A. Murray marvelled at the loyalty and affection inspired by senior doctors and nurses in those days as he saw the frankly dictatorial manner in which they sometimes acted. He wrote, 'Imagine the reaction today to a decision that a man, lying in a plaster case with spinal tuberculosis, who had made a complaint about the lunch served to him, would be sent home by ambulance that very afternoon. Discipline was stern in many instances but, remarkably, it seemed to work.'[29]

Joan McCarthy was told at an initial interview with the medical superintendent of Cheshire Joint Sanatorium, Peter Edwards ('The Chief'), that:

the disease was very advanced, my only hope was to obey all the rules of the Sanatorium implicitly, as I would be there for a very long time. It was a privilege to be given the opportunity for treatment, and staff were not prepared to waste time on unco-operative patients, there were plenty of other people

---

[25] Williams, *Requiem for a Great Killer*, p. 75.

[26] F. Jordan, interview, 23 Mar. 1983. Papworth Archives, G1, 'History of the Trunk Making Department 1921–59'; *Lancet*, 1 (1941), 198; *Western Mail*, 16 Aug. 1922 (PRO MH52/2).

[27] Cook, *A Hackney Memory Chest*, p. 48.

[28] Papworth Archives, G2–16, F. Durham, Personal Recollections; R. Parker, *On the Road: The Papworth Story* (Cambridge, 1977), 147; interviews, Mr and Mrs Langdon, Mr and Mrs Huffer, Papworth, 23 Mar. 1983.

[29] Murray, *A Life Worth Living*, p. 19.

who would be glad of the bed. No deviation from the stipulated routine would be tolerated, and the Time Table governed all activities . . .

She added that it was suggested that this initial interview was intentionally demoralizing, getting the patient into 'a passive and submissive state of compliance' which was necessary for the treatment to succeed.[30]

Discipline was strict 'in the interests of the health of the patients', and as such was readily accepted by the patients. G. S. Erwin, medical superintendent of the Liverpool Sanatorium, wrote that the refractory type of patient occasionally likened the sanatorium to a school: 'the comparison, though meant unkindly, is not inept, because the sanatorium is a school in which the attainment of good health is the main teaching.'[31] Alan Dick drew constant comparisons with schools in his description of sanatorium life.[32] The whole life of patients was strictly regulated by bells; sanatorium patients were in fact treated like children, incapable of making decisions for themselves, of controlling their own lives and bodies. Surgery served to increase the subordination of patients to the medical officer.

Wingfield suggested a class dimension to patient control:

The working-class patient still looks upon the doctor as a member of the 'master class' whose decisions for generations he has been accustomed to obey without questioning their wisdom or truth. He therefore surrenders himself easily to the discipline of treatment. For the rich patient the doctor may be somewhat separated by the supposed mysteries of his craft, but is in no sense a superior—he may even appear an inferior—being, and complete and protracted submission to his discipline does not come easily or naturally.[33]

This statement was, however, probably more a reflection of the attitude of the medical superintendent himself than an accurate assessment of the situation. Evidence suggests that the majority of patients, whether working-class or not, were not totally submissive. There existed in fact what Goffman has described as a 'hospital under-life' in all the institutions investigated.[34] The two greatest disciplinary problems faced by medical superintendents were familiarity with members of the opposite sex and consumption of alcohol.

[30] McCarthy, '"Tuberculosis" Before and After Waksman', p. 38.
[31] G. S. Erwin, *Tuberculosis and Chest Diseases for Nurses* (London, 1946), 51.
[32] Dick, *A Walking Miracle*, p. 116. See also Bignall, *Frimley*, p. 117.
[33] R. C. Wingfield, *A Textbook of Pulmonary Tuberculosis for Students* (London, 1929), 367.
[34] Goffman, *Asylums*, pp. 157–280.

Rules on socializing were generally strict. For example, at Eversfield Hospital the regulations specified that 'conversation between men and women patients is not allowed'.[35] Similarly at the Cheshire Joint Sanatorium, female and male patients were gathered together only for Christmas dinner.[36] Wingfield was said to be proud of the fact that not a single patient in his institution had become pregnant, suggesting that other superintendents could not make the same boast, although even at Frimley, Bignall considered it doubtful that no children were conceived in the forbidden pine-forests.[37] In 1922, analysing instances of patients discharged irregularly, McDougall noted that in one institution for 200 patients (male and female), there occurred only 6 cases of undue familiarity between the sexes leading to dismissal over a period of 15 months—which he thought was very low.[38] There was a large number of young people in sanatoria, not only because tuberculosis was a disease which struck the young, but also because institutions were more receptive to young cases who were more likely to recover than to older patients whose disease was often more chronic. Most sanatoria admitted both sexes although generally men outnumbered women 60 to 40. It was reputed to be not uncommon for nurses to marry patients suggesting that despite the prohibition, some socializing occurred there as well. Two nurses who still live at Papworth married patients there. One pointed out that, with the isolation of the sanatorium, there were few other social diversions.[39] Romances at Papworth included a suicide pact between a patient and a nurse.[40] One patient claimed to have been cured by nightly meetings with a nurse.[41] Two maids at Frimley were dismissed in 1921 for being 'too familiar with the patients', although no nurses were recorded as having been dismissed for that reason.[42]

Patients were strictly forbidden to enter public houses during the Saturday or Sunday afternoon leave from the institutions which was often granted to those who were well enough. Entering a public house, or returning to the sanatorium intoxicated, often led to instant dismissal. McDougall reported in July 1929 that three men were

[35] Eversfield Hospital Annual Report 1916, p. 35.
[36] McCarthy, '"Tuberculosis" Before and After Waksman', pp. 41–2.
[37] Bignall, *Frimley*, p. 147.
[38] *Tubercle*, 3 (1922), 442.
[39] Mrs Goozee and Mrs Langdon, interviews, Papworth, 23 Mar. 1983.
[40] *Daily Mail*, 28 May 1938 (Papworth Archives).
[41] F. Durham, Papworth, 'My Early Days', Papworth Archives, G2–16.
[42] Frimley Sanatorium, Nurses and Servants: Engagement Book.

discharged that month for returning to the sanatorium in a disorderly condition.[43] Possession of alcohol by patients was also strictly forbidden, although W. E. Snell, medical superintendent of Colindale Hospital appeared amused by the extreme lengths to which some patients went to acquire alcohol, suggesting that at least some medical superintendents turned a blind eye, which was also Dick's experience.[44] Sloane of Wrenbury Hall had his own solution to the alcohol problem. After discovering that 8 patients had spent their Saturday afternoon leave in a public house, he called a meeting of all patients to discuss the matter. He found that the majority of the patients looked on beer in moderation as good for their health (although he himself did not think so) and seemed to consider the taking of a glass of beer when he wanted it 'an inalienable right of an Englishman'. He therefore decided to allow the consumption of a restricted amount of mild ale with meals in the sanatorium to prevent such visits to public houses where they might drink unrestrictedly of any drink they fancied. As a result, he thought that discipline had improved. He added that the majority still drank tea rather than ale.[45] Papworth also had its own public house, which was under the close scrutiny of the medical officers. Sir Percival Phillips maintained in 1926 that one public house was quite sufficient for the eighty families at Papworth, 'who are usually ready for bed at the end of the day's work'.[46]

Complaints by patients in sanatoria, particularly regarding the food, were not uncommon but were generally futile, dismissed as a manifestation or symptom of the disease. Tuberculous patients were reputed to be particularly finicky about their food and therefore complaints in that direction were not taken seriously. Norman Langdon at Papworth claimed that there was no point complaining about the food; he recalled one patient who was 'sent on the bus' in 1926 for doing so.[47] Two complaints reached the Ministry of Health from patients at Papworth in 1921 concerning food and training. In an interview with MacNalty, one of the complainants apparently contradicted himself several times, which suggested instability. Moreover,

[43] Preston Hall, Minutes of Council of Management, Medical Director Report, 19 July 1929.
[44] W. E. Snell, interview, 27 June 1983; Dick, *A Walking Miracle*, p. 69; *Tubercle*, 37 (1956), 2.
[45] PRO MH52/11, Sloane to J. E. Chapman, 30 Oct. 1926.
[46] *Western Mail*, 15 July 1926 (PRO MH52/2).
[47] N. Langdon, interview, Papworth, 23 Mar. 1983. See also Dick, *A Walking Miracle*, p. 45.

according to his instructor, the gardener (who was unqualified medically but was consulted on the medical condition of the patient), he was too ill to be properly trained and had 'the warped temperament occasionally found associated with his malady which makes him impatient and discontented with institutional discipline'.[48] A patient at the West Wales Sanatorium in 1923 said that all the patients were objecting to the food. When asked why they did not repeat their complaints to the medical superintendent, who had received none, the witness said they were afraid.[49] The 1923 inquiry into the administration of the West Wales Sanatorium following complaints by Maud Morris revealed once again the futility of registering discontent. Llewellyn Williams explained concerning the evidence of Maud, 'The advanced stage of the disease at the time she gave her evidence would naturally have affected her memory and perspective.' A local doctor maintained, 'It is true that here as well as in other Institutions of different kinds, carried out at very best [*sic*], there are a certain few whose pathetically hopeless physical condition reacts upon their imagination and distorts their judgement—nothing satisfies them—though deserving every pity and consideration the truth is seldom got at by listening to [them] . . .'[50]

Another frequent cause of discontent was the total absence of heating. The *South Wales Argus* reported in 1937 that all the patients in the South Wales Sanatorium were complaining of the cold and that a visitor who was wearing an overcoat also felt cold.[51] Conditions in sanatoria were often spartan, particularly in some of the converted smallpox and isolation hospitals. Cymla Hospital in Wales was such an institution, with 20 beds in 1914 and 60 by 1924. In 1927 its two main buildings were described as very damp; the roof in one leaked. In 1936 it was reported that one of the buildings was unfit to house patients and should be demolished.[52] Glan Ely was infested with rats in 1919, and in 1936 one of its wards was described as 'a building of temporary type which has far outlasted its satisfactory life'.[53] Other institutions were

---

[48] PRO MH52/5, Report by MacNalty, 13 Sept. 1921.

[49] *Western Mail*, 25 Oct. 1923 (PRO MH96/980).

[50] PRO MH96/980, D. L. Williams, 9 Apr. 1924, sect. 3 and Dr D. D. Harris, 29 May 1923.

[51] *South Wales Argus*, 30 Oct. 1937 (PRO MH96/994).

[52] PRO MH96/947, Cymla Hospital, Report by His Majesty's Office of Works, 20 July 1927; PRO MH96/957, Public Inquiry, 17 Jan. 1936.

[53] *South Wales Echo*, 31 Oct. 1919 (PRO MH96/901); PRO MH96/957, Public Inquiry, 17 Jan. 1936.

described similarly by the 1937–9 Committee of Inquiry into the Anti-tuberculosis Service in Wales and Monmouthshire as 'cold, uncomfortable, and cheerless'.[54] At least one patient discharged herself from Harefield Sanatorium, Middlesex, in 1929 because she found it too damp.[55] In 1922, McDougall discovered that 'the severe climatic conditions during the winter months were the immediate cause of 26 premature discharges in the West Riding County Council sanatoria, chiefly on account of rheumatism'.[56] In 1923, a visitor to Cowley Road Sanatorium, Oxford, found that all the male patients on the verandah, with two exceptions, were soaked with the rain which had fallen during the night, and that without any exception the top blankets on the beds were wet. The water had reached the patients partly through the roof and partly by being driven in by the wind.[57] W. A. Murray described the conditions of a Scottish sanatorium, Glenafton, New Cumnock, Ayrshire, which, until he became medical superintendent in 1931, was totally unheated. He had heating installed, but he wrote that the rooms remained draughty as the large windows did not fit and the wind blew under the floors 'raising the linoleum in waves which made the ward round something like a trip on a roller-coaster'. Rain also came through the windows to such an extent that a patient with some skill as a cartoonist pictured Murray in the hospital magazine, doing his ward round in thigh boots while a patient sailed his toy boat round his bed.[58] Joan McCarthy described the depression she experienced on entering the Cheshire Joint Sanatorium in 1950: 'a howling gale blowing through the wide open windows behind the beds did nothing to raise my spirits'. She explained how stone hot water bottles were the only means of heating, 'no matter how inclement the weather'.[59]

The site of the sanatoria was also sometimes bleak. For example, Kensington Hospital in Wales was on a promontory facing the Atlantic and was very exposed to the elements—the 1937–9 Committee of Inquiry noted, 'We were told, and could well believe, that during stormy weather, which is frequent, healthy and vigorous persons have a hard struggle to walk up the drive from the road to the hospital.'[60]

[54] *Clement Davies Report*, pp. 261–76 (in particular, Brynseiont, Meadowslea, Sealyham, and Machynlleth Hospitals).
[55] Frimley Follow-up Records, 1928 (date of admission to Frimley), i. 165.
[56] *Tubercle*, 3 (1922), 443.
[57] *Oxford Chronicle*, 2 Nov. 1923 (Radcliffe Infirmary, Oxford).
[58] Murray, *A Life Worth Living*, p. 33.
[59] McCarthy, '"Tuberculosis" Before and After Waksman', pp. 38, 39.
[60] *Clement Davies Report*, p. 269.

While complaints were often futile, patients did ultimately have the power to leave, although Marcus Paterson's famous remark to a patient taking his own discharge, 'Tell your widow to send us a postcard', was used more than once in the following decades by medical officers of tuberculosis institutions.[61] A patient at the West Wales Sanatorium left in 1923 despite the fact that it involved a personal confrontation with the medical superintendent, Isobel Ferguson, who apparently applied physical as well as psychological pressure. The patient alleged that Dr Ferguson took hold of her by the scarf and twisted it around her throat until she was purple in the face. Ferguson, however, denied using physical force and denied telling the patient that if she left she would be a 'chronic invalid for life'.[62] Peter Edwards of the Cheshire Joint Sanatorium was said to despise those who were unable to tolerate the rigorous life and left the sanatorium, 'only to come or be carried back when the disease became more progressive; of those poor unfortunates, he [was] quoted as saying "they come crawling back on their knees, after death comes knocking at the door"'.[63] G. S. Erwin, medical superintendent of Liverpool Sanatorium, cited an American study of several thousand discharged patients—60 per cent of those normally discharged were alive five years later, but only 30 per cent of those prematurely discharged; the inference he drew was that self-discharge halved the patient's chances of survival.[64]

Few figures are available on self-discharges, but in 7 sanatoria in Lancashire, 127 out of a total of 305 patients leaving altogether in 1921–2, took premature discharges, that is almost half, which did not strike the Ministry of Health observers as extraordinary.[65] In 1922, a survey of West Riding CC sanatoria showed that out of a total of 3,205 discharges from sanatoria (2,396 men and 809 women), 44 per cent of the male and 32 per cent of the female discharges were 'irregular'. This included those who discharged themselves and those who were discharged for disciplinary reasons (24 per cent came into the latter category).[66] Similarly at Peel Hall, Lancashire, 44 out of 113 patients left for reasons other than medical, of which 39 took their own discharge and 5 were dismissed.[67]

---

[61] Suzanne Beven, interview (social worker, Brompton Hospital), 27 Sept. 1984.
[62] *Western Mail*, 25 Oct. 1923; 6 Feb. 1924 (PRO MH96/980).
[63] McCarthy, '"Tuberculosis" Before and After Waksman', p. 39.
[64] Erwin, *A Guide for the Tuberculous Patient*, p. 57.
[65] PRO MH52/75, Ministry of Health memo, 9 June 1922.
[66] *Tubercle*, 3 (1922), 441.
[67] PRO MH52/75, Ministry of Health Inspection of Peel Hall Sanatorium, Lancashire, S. Seymore, 20 July 1922, p. 6.

The high proportion of self-discharges suggests that working-class patients did not submit to the discipline and the conditions of the sanatorium regime as easily as the medical superintendents such as Wingfield hoped. Self-discharging patients were also probably primarily responsible for modifying the rigorous conditions of the institutions. Powell said in 1937 that since installing heating in some of their institutions, they had been able to keep patients longer.[68] The number of patients in tuberculosis institutions was also higher in summer months suggesting a reluctance to remain during the cold winter months.[69] Artificial pneumothorax and thoracic surgery served as an added inducement to stay. One patient was promised sanocrysin in 1930 if he stayed at Colindale Hospital.[70]

However, 'pull factors' from home were possibly most important in causing self-discharges. At least one female patient at Eversfield Hospital discharged herself prematurely without consulting the medical superintendent because her home was 'in a dreadful pickle'. She explained that her husband was unable to cope alone with the children and a dependent father.[71] H. Old of the Welsh Board of Health referred to the constant difficulty they had in persuading women (for whom there was little outside assistance available) to leave their domestic responsibilities and undertake instiutional treatment.[72] Margery Spring Rice, in her study of working-class wives in the 1930s, also noted this problem.[73]

Yet undoubtedly the experience of the sanatorium was also important. The adverse publicity following the 1923 inquiry into the West Wales Sanatorium affected patient intake (despite the fact that Ferguson resigned after the inquiry). Reports in the *Western Mail* included evidence from the uncle of Maud, who likened the sanatorium to two prisons, Wormwood Scrubs and Dartmoor. The impression of a visitor to the sanatorium was also noted: 'I was in charge of hospitals during the war . . . and had I run them as this institution was run when I visited it I would have had to serve time and would not complain either.' A Mr Edward Jones was quoted who said

[68] *News Chronicle*, 30 Oct. 1937 (PRO MH96/994).
[69] PRO MH55/145, LCC, Public Health Report 528 (Poor Law Infirmaries in London, 1923) pointed out that while the number of admissions to sanatoria declined in the winter months, the number admitted to Poor Law institutions increased.
[70] Frimley Sanatorium Follow-up Records, 1922 (date of admission to Frimley), i. 9.
[71] West Sussex Record Office, HH68/3, P.R. (patient's initials), 8 Sept. 1946.
[72] PRO MH96/1111, H. Old, Dec. 1926; PRO MH96/1034, H. Old, 26 Mar. 1928.
[73] M. S. Rice, *Working-class Wives* (London, 1939), 30–1, 14 n. 1.

he had often persuaded people suffering from consumption to go to the sanatorium, but after seeing it when he visited with the committee, he would never do so again.[74] In 1924 Charles Lloyd reported: 'every effort has . . . been made to persuade the parents of these children to allow them to be treated in the West Wales Sanatorium, even to threatening to cut off their supply of malt and oil—but to no purpose.' He maintained that the 'ill-advised course taken by the Carmarthenshire County Council to remedy supposed irregularities in the administration of the West Wales Sanatorium by broadcasting a highly coloured report of their findings through the medium of the Press, has thoroughly frightened the parents of this county'. He had found that some people looked upon the West Wales Sanatorium more as a reformatory for children than as a sanatorium, and concluded, 'Unless the County Councils of Wales entrust these investigations in the future to the Welsh Board of Health, and they are conducted in camera, the campaign against tuberculosis is going to be put back many years.'[75] Fourteen years later, J. Kenyon Davies reported concerning the West Wales Sanatorium, 'Hitherto there has always been great difficulty in some cases in persuading them to accept treatment, but during the year I was able to place 110 patients in our institution.'[76]

One method of making sanatorium life more endurable, or of increasing the 'togetherness' of the institution, was the holding of festive occasions. Most institutions had their special fêtes, flower shows, and sports days. Christmas festivities always figured prominently in the annual calendar. At Christmastime at Darvell Hall Sanatorium, for example, 'It is forbidden . . . even to mention troubles. On the contrary, all are expected to join in making mild "whoopee".'[77] As Goffman pointed out, special occasions were an important means of fostering good relations between staff and inmates in total institutions, staff often assuming the parental supervisory role.[78] When the cricket club at Papworth (where workers were paid at trade-union rates of pay) asked Dr Stott to present a cup at the prize-giving ceremony, Stott patronizingly offered to buy the cup as well.[79] Most sanatoria also issued a magazine to which patients and staff contributed.

[74] *Western Mail*, 26 Apr. 1923, 6 June 1923, 25 Oct. 1923 (PRO MH96/980).
[75] PRO MH96/1073, C. Lloyd (tuberculosis physician, Cardiganshire) to D. Evans, WNMA, 13 Feb. 1924.
[76] *Welsh Gazette*, 18 Aug. 1938 (PRO MH96/1073).
[77] *The Sussex County Herald*, 8 Jan. 1932 (East Sussex County Record Office, HH14/5).   [78] Goffman, *Asylums*, pp. 89–105.
[79] Mr Huffer, interview, Papworth, 23 Mar. 1983.

Surgery, with its greater emphasis on rest, changed the nature of the sanatorium regime. Esther Carling wrote in 1937 that the 'up-patient' had been replaced by the 'bed-patient' and that they now 'looked in vain for the garden gang, the tray carriers, the sing-song parties of former days'.[80] Yet, the continued emphasis on physical exercise discussed in Chapter 6 suggests that life in at least some of the sanatoria was far from dominated by bed-patients, even in the 1940s. Indeed, an outstanding feature of twentieth-century sanatoria was the absence of social change, possibly partly related to the long service of most medical superintendents, who typically remained in the post for thirty years or more.

Surveys indicated that there was a large number of ex-patients on the staff of the institutions, suggesting a willingness, at least on the part of some, to stay beyond the required time for treatment. A possible reason for this phenomenon was that, during the process of becoming institutionalized, they had developed a dependency on the institution, another characteristic of a total institution, accentuated in the case of tuberculosis by the social stigma attached to the disease. There may have been a fear of not being able to cope in the outside world. They were indeed alerted to this possibility by medical superintendents, perhaps further undermining their confidence. Bignall explained, 'In the competitive world outside they might have quickly relapsed, even if they could have found employment at all. It is not surprising that they were content to stay, often for the rest of their working lives, in such sheltered conditions and with such considerate employers.'[81]

Some ex-patients at Frimley remained on the sanatorium staff for long periods—four patients remained as porters from 1908 to 1929, 1912 to 1938, 1915 to 1938, and 1917 to 1932 respectively. Another patient stayed as gardener from 1919 to 1942, and a patient who became a nightwatchman stayed from 1905 to 1926.[82] Similarly at Peppard Common Sanatorium, three of the patients who came in 1903 were still on the staff in 1937, one as head maintenance officer, one as storekeeper, and one as senior male nurse.[83]

However, an examination of the Frimley 'Nurses and Servants: Engagement Book' belies the idea of a sense of permanent attachment to the institution, at least among the female patients, inducing them to

[80] *Tubercle*, 18 (1937), 454.
[81] Bignall, *Frimley*, p. 141.
[82] Ibid., p. 143.
[83] E. and H. Carling, 'A Short History of Peppard Hospital' 1938, 8.

remain long beyond their period of treatment.[84] They typically remained one or two years on the staff. It is probable that patients regarded such employment as part of the process of rehabilitation, a stepping stone to rejoining the wider society. At Fazakerley Sanatorium, Liverpool, patients were encouraged to work at the sanatorium as 'an intermediate stage between the sanatorium and the outside world'.[85] The number of ex-patients on the staff was therefore not a measure of their commitment to the institution so much as a desire to gain confidence in working ability before leaving the sanatorium, or sometimes the inability to find employment elsewhere.

Varrier-Jones gave his reasons for preferring to employ tuberculous people on the staff: that such people would be more committed to the institution, feel more part of the community than an employee who merely considered it a job. He thought this was paticularly important for foremen or instructors in the industries, but also applied to the medical staff (he exempted himself however, there is no evidence that Varrier-Jones suffered from tuberculosis).[86] In general, however, it seems clear that the overriding reason for the employment of tuberculous ex-patients was the inability to attract other labour. Esther Carling pointed out that no one apart from people who had contracted tuberculosis responded to the advertisements.[87]

(2) POST-SANATORIUM EXPERIENCE

A 'total institution' is an instrument of socialization. Wingfield was very explicit about his aims at Frimley:

When a man has pulmonary tuberculosis, if he is to be sure of surviving, his whole life must be altered. The essentials of sanatorium treatment must be followed, modified to individual conditions, for the rest of his life . . . The strict routine of sanatorium life is designed to produce this automatism, with the idea that if the patient is made to live in a certain way without variation for long enough, he will continue to do so without conscious effort . . . The conscientious performance of a sanatorium treatment entailing, as it does, continuous self-denial, self-restraint and endurance of discomfort, and the consciousness that one's attitude and actions cannot be without their effect on

[84] Frimley Sanatorium, Nurses and Servants: Engagement Book.
[85] *12th CMOH Annual Report 1930* (1931), 98.
[86] *BJT* 20 (1926), 16.
[87] *Tubercle*, 18 (1937), 456.

the other patients, is a sure and ready method of developing this most necessary possession [self-discipline].[88]

Most medical superintendents expressed similar views. To McDougall, readmission implied the patient had been 'a victim of an unaltered mode of life'.[89] The foregoing discussion of 'hospital underlife' and premature discharges suggests that the reality was different from that which Wingfield and other medical superintendents hoped to achieve, that a distinction should be made between prescription and practice. Nevertheless, it is possible that a period in a sanatorium did have a profound effect on the life of individual patients. Alan Dick maintained, 'A sanatorium gives you a physical attitude to life which it is impossible to break. So does a prison, they say.'[90] In the early twentieth century Bardswell claimed to have evidence that ex-patients from Midhurst Sanatorium did modify their lives and continue a sanatorium life in their own homes.[91] Midhurst was an expensive private sanatorium admitting patients who could perhaps afford to make such changes. Yet there is also evidence from Frimley Sanatorium that at least some patients, whose treatment was often paid for by the LCC after 1921, were influenced by what they had been taught in the sanatorium. A confectioner's assistant lived in good health for 40 years after being at Frimley. He wrote in 1929, 'Chief weapon against sickness—sobriety, good food, good rest, not forgetting a good bath frequently.' In 1932 he claimed that he took good care of himself as far as he could and tried to carry out what he had learnt at Frimley.[92] A patient discharged in 1925 wrote to the Frimley almoner in 1944 when he was still working, 'I still keep as near as possible to the lessons I received at Frimley and I must again thank all concerned at that place.' In 1948 he wrote, 'There is no doubt about it, that if persons after treatment at Frimley would follow instructions and advice given, although sometimes hard to follow, they would find themselves enjoying very much better health.'[93] It is open to question how typical this was. The MOH for the City of Aberdeen wrote in 1931, 'Those of us who have been Tuberculosis Officers know that, in

[88] R. C. Wingfield, *Modern Methods in the Diagnosis and Treatment of Pulmonary Tuberculosis* (London, 1924), 65.
[89] Preston Hall Annual Report 1933, p. 8.
[90] Dick, *A Walking Miracle*, p. 124.
[91] King Edward VII Sanatorium, Midhurst, Annual Report 1907–8, p. 47.
[92] Frimley Sanatorium Follow-up Records, 1906, p. 65.
[93] Ibid., 1925, ii. 124.

the main, these cases do not practise the hygienic methods of living that they were taught in institutions.'[94]

Ex-patients were encouraged to gain weight. One Frimley ex-patient reported proudly that she was as 'plump as a partridge'.[95] An ex-patient from Eversfield reported that his weight had increased to just over 12 stones: 'This is about as much as I can comfortably carry, though the Stroud doctors seem to regard it as only a beginning.'[96]

Not all patients, however, had such agreeable 'after-histories'. More typical appeared to be a long period of invalidity intercepted by short periods in an institution. One patient, discharged from Frimley in 1919, who was married and had ten children, was constantly from 1920 to 1925 in and out of Colindale Hospital (or 'Coffindale' Hospital, as it was known among patients because it was a hospital for advanced cases; its counterpart in South East London, Grove Park, was known as 'Grave Park[97]'). In 1925 he was reported to be fairly well but unable to find work, so that he had to stay at home and look after the children and house while his wife went out to work, which 'rather troubles him', the Frimley Sanatorium almoner recorded after inquiring into his circumstances. In 1926 he still had not found work. In 1927 he reported that he 'could have got a job but on hearing he had tuberculosis the employers had refused him'. He continued to look for work without success. By 1931 he was 'fed up with things in general'. In 1932 he reported that he had given up looking for work 'as a bad job'. In 1934 he wrote, 'I have not felt I could interest myself in anything like I used to.' In 1943 he had 'had odd jobs but had to leave as they were too heavy'. He died in 1945, 26 years after leaving Frimley.[98] Another patient, discharged from Frimley in 1922, appeared totally despondent in 1933, having been in eight different institutions in the interim, writing that he was willing to be experimented on by any doctor seeking a cure for tuberculosis.[99]

If contracting tuberculosis caused any changes in self-image, it was often in the direction of hypochondria. Some learned the lessons of the sanatorium—that they were permanent invalids needing to 'take care'—all too well, and lived a life of unnecessary invalidism. This

---

[94] *EMJ* 38 (1931), 153.

[95] Frimley Sanatorium Follow-up Records, 1906, p. 29.

[96] Eversfield Hospital Patient Records, HH68/6, H.C. (patient's initials), 10 Sept. 1948.

[97] *British Thoracic Association (The First Fifty Years)* (London, 1978), 17.

[98] Frimley Sanatorium Follow-up Records, 1919 (date of admission to Frimley), ii. 191–2.

[99] Ibid., 1922, i. 9.

attitude was encouraged further among Frimley ex-patients by the almoner's annual inquiries into their health, undertaken for medical research purposes. Frimley Sanatorium was unique in instituting a thorough follow-up study in 1920 of all patients who passed through the sanatorium. The resultant records cover approximately 15,000 patients who passed through the sanatorium from 1905 to 1957. The success rate in tracing patients was over 90 per cent, largely owing to the indefatigable efforts of the 'Lady Almoner' and her staff, who were based at Brompton Hospital.[100]

While much of the almoner's follow-up records reads like a diary of annual colds, influenzas, and other minor ailments, not all ex-Frimley patients wallowed in chronic invalidism. Some resented the annual inquiries into their health. Sometimes they simply wanted to forget their medical history, but more often than not the resentment arose from the embarrassment the inquiries caused, both professionally and socially. The Frimley follow-up records tell us a great deal about social responses to tuberculosis.

One patient, aged 27 on his discharge in 1918, answered the almoner's inquiries every year until 1952 (having had no further symptoms in the meantime) when he wrote that he was very annoyed as a letter from the almoner had been opened by one of his employees. He asked that letters in future be marked 'Private and Confidential' and that the envelope not disclose its origin.[101] Another patient, aged 22 when he was discharged in 1918, wrote in 1922 that he did not wish to be written to again. In 1923 he attended Brompton Hospital and there was no evidence of active disease. He was working as sanitary inspector for a borough council in London. In 1925 he became sanitary inspector for another borough council. As he would not reply himself, the almoner made inquiries regarding his health through the local town hall annually until 1940. In 1942 he wrote that he was very indignant that news had been received through the town hall without his knowledge. In 1946 the almoner wrote to him again. He replied that he was very annoyed, that the letter went to his place of business and might have been opened by the staff.[102]

It appears that employers were often kept in ignorance of ex-sanatorium patients' medical histories. A student discharged in 1928 who subsequently became a school teacher, wrote in 1935 that he had

[100] Frimley Follow-up Records held at the Wellcome Unit for the History of Medicine, Oxford.
[101] Frimley Follow-up Records, 1918, ii. 61.   [102] Ibid., 1918, ii. 19.

passed a medical examination at the Admiralty, that the Board of Education had told him that they no longer required reports, and asked that Brompton Hospital not write any more. He was afraid that his medical history might prevent him from attaining an appointment. He also said that he was living in 'digs' and feared that the letters might be seen. Following unanswered letters and failing other sources of information, the almoner wrote to the Board of Education who said that he was working under the Kent Education Authority. In 1938 the Board of Education wrote that they did not think that the Kent Education Authority knew of his past illness and the Board seemed to think that he was unduly sensitive about it. The Board of Education was willing to co-operate with the almoner in giving information annually as to whether he was still working under the Kent Education Authority. In 1958, the last report, he was still employed as a teacher, and as far as the Ministry of Education (successor to the Board of Education) was aware, had not yet been absent on sick leave.[103]

Many other examples can be given of ex-patients striving to keep their medical history a secret from employers—insurance agents, salesmen, and policemen figuring most prominently. Among the women who feared that their employers might discover their medical histories were domestic servants, shop assistants, a district nurse, and an assistant matron in an asylum. One patient who wrote annually from 1922, having had no further symptoms since leaving Frimley, nevertheless declined the opportunity for promotion in his job in 1956 (that is 34 years after leaving Frimley) because it required a medical examination and he feared that his employers might discover his past illness. Nor did he tell his wife when he married in 1948.[104]

There are many other examples of spouses and families being deceived. One female patient, discharged in 1918, wrote in 1948, 'If ever I am ill I will at once inform you, but I should be much obliged if you would discontinue sending the annual enquiry as I like to keep the past a secret from my family.'[105]

A male patient, discharged in 1918, wote in 1948 telling the almoner that he had had haemoptysis but that he could not rest or do anything about it as he had never told his wife who was unaware of his early breakdown. He asked the almoner to be careful how she worded any future letter.[106] The mother of a patient who was discharged in 1918 and married in 1926 sent annual reports on his health: his wife did not

---

[103] Frimley Follow-up Records, 1928, ii. 117.   [104] Ibid., 1922, i. 299.
[105] Ibid., 1918, i. 223.   [106] Ibid., 1918, i. 251.

know he had had tuberculosis.[107] The discovery of a letter in 1931 by the wife of a discharged patient in 1925 apparently caused a temporary rift in their relationship.[108] The father of a patient discharged in 1922 and married in 1930 sent annual reports until 1951 when the patient's sister took over the correspondence: his wife still did not know.[109] The mother of another patient discharged in 1923 sent annual reports; she wrote that the patient's wife did not know, and nor did his sister's husband.[110] When a patient discharged in 1924 was engaged to be married in 1934, his mother asked that no more inquiries be sent. He was married in 1935, but in 1936 he broke down and was sent to an institution, his wife being told by his mother that he had 'the flu'. In 1938 his mother wrote that she would like the almoner to visit in future in case her daughter-in-law saw the letters. When the almoner visited in 1940, he was very ill but his wife still did not know about his tuberculosis. In 1942, when he was still in bed, the almoner noted, 'Wife now knows patient was at Frimley.'[111] Visiting another ex-patient in 1935, the almoner spoke to the wife's grandmother who told her that it had once been feared that her granddaughter's husband had been 'going into consumption' but that it had proved to be 'only nerves'. The almoner noted that she herself managed to get away without saying where she had come from.[112]

Examples of wives deceiving husbands can also be found. One patient, discharged in 1922 and subsequently married, objected to the inquiries when she was traced in 1946—she said that she had never found it necessary to tell her husband what had happened twenty years earlier.[113] The mother or sister sent news of another patient discharged in 1924 and married in 1935.[114] The entry in 1940 for a patient discharged in 1925 and married in 1940 was 'Husband does not know past illness and she uses maiden name and parents' address for these reports.'[115] Possibly the most remarkable deception was that recorded in 1949 of a woman who had had a thoracoplastic operation, whose husband did not know she had had tuberculosis.[116]

Sometimes spouses knew but parents-in-law were not told. The mother of a patient discharged in 1921, subsequently married, said in 1929 that her daughter's husband knew of the illness but that 'his

---

[107] Ibid., 1918, ii. 43.
[108] Ibid., 1925, ii. 89.
[109] Ibid., 1922, i. 39.
[110] Ibid., 1923, i. 99.
[111] Ibid., 1924, i. 301.
[112] Ibid., 1924, i. 305.
[113] Ibid., 1922, ii. 101.
[114] Ibid., 1924, i. 15.
[115] Ibid., 1925, i. 149.
[116] Ibid., 1928, ii. 297.

people are inclined to make trouble'.[117] A patient discharged in 1928 and married in 1940, wrote in 1956 that she was very upset as the Brompton letter had got into the hands of her mother-in-law who had the same name and that there were embarrassing results.[118] Occasionally it was the children who were not told. The almoner received a letter in 1941 asking that correspondence cease as their daughter was very upset because her friend had just died of tuberculosis and they did not want her to find out that tuberculosis was 'in the family'.[119]

Thus ex-patient records at Frimley show concealment and subterfuge relating to tuberculosis histories within families, the most frequent being parents conspiring with ex-patients to prevent in-laws from finding out. There is no evidence to suggest that one sex was more likely to conceal the truth than the other.

Not a large proportion of ex-patients objected openly to the inquiries, only approximately 4 per cent of those admitted per annum. Nevertheless, this is a significant number when the number lost sight of is taken into account (approximately 7 per cent per annum), as well as those who died within 5 years (approximately 50 per cent) and those who could not possibly keep their condition a secret from their families or find a job in any case owing to illness. Nor is there any reason to regard ex-Frimley patients as unrepresentative of ex-sanatorium patients in general, except that, being chosen as convalescents from Brompton Hospital, they possibly had longer survival rates or 'after-histories' than patients from many other institutions, and that they were energetically pursued by the very conscientious 'Lady Almoner' (Miss Marx, from 1918 to 1943) and her staff, whose extreme diligence was clearly unappreciated. One patient discharged in 1918, wrote in 1932 that he regretted that he was still 'hounded' with Brompton Hospital letters: 'If letters are sent they will be ignored and if any callers come I shall not show them even common decency.'[120] Ex-patients were indeed hounded. Even 'escaping' to Australia did not exempt them, as one patient was to find. Discharged in 1923, he wrote in 1927 from Australia that the Commonwealth Repatriation Commission had written to him on behalf of Brompton regarding his state of health: 'To say that I am exceedingly annoyed and consider whoever is responsible as being guilty of colossal impudence, is to put it very mildly . . . Am I to be annoyed and sought after as though a common

[117] Frimley Follow-up Records, 1921, i. 69.   [118] Ibid., 1928, ii. 333.
[119] Ibid., 1922, i. 31.   [120] Ibid., 1918. i. 317.

felon?'[121] Frimley indeed boasted that patients were traced as far as the Arctic Circle.[122] Another ex-patient pointed out that Frimley would be doing a much greater service were it to establish contact with an employment bureau rather than merely recording the ex-patient's condition for the benefit of medical science.[123] At least one patient wrote that the benefit to medical science was small compared to the trouble caused by the inquiries, and a perusal of the follow-up records supports that view, as does a reading of the reports resulting from the records which reached very limited conclusions indeed.[124]

What is unclear from the records is whether the sense of stigma arose more often from a belief in the hereditary nature of the disease or its infectiousness; it appears to be a combination of both. Marcus Paterson received a letter in 1909 from an ex-patient whose wife and parents-in-law wanted a divorce because they believed that tuberculosis was hereditary.[125] The *Tubercle* reported the case of an annulment of a marriage in America in 1919 for eugenic reasons when one of the partners had failed to reveal a history of tuberculosis before the marriage.[126] Sir Robert Philip wrote in 1933 of the more or less daily statements of his patients on being diagnosed as tuberculous that the disease was 'not in the family'.[127] In 1936 the Press reported 'the tragic case of Mrs Swann, who killed her child fearing it had inherited tuberculosis'.[128] K. Coltart, head of the almoner's department at the Brompton Hospital from 1943, wrote of the common response of patients on hearing they had tuberculosis, that it had never been in the family.[129] A 1952 survey revealed that 55 per cent of those surveyed considered tuberculosis definitely hereditary, 20 per cent thought it ran in the family in some other way, and 5 per cent did not know.[130]

The role of heredity, which had been played down by British tuberculosis specialists earlier in the century with their focus on infection, was gaining medical support by the 1930s in the form of

---

[121] Frimley Follow-up Records, 1923, i. 97.
[122] Brompton Hospital Records 11, 1942, *Tubercle*, 24 (1943), 110.
[123] Frimley Sanatorium Follow-up Records, 1925, ii. 275.
[124] Ibid., 1922, i. 59; Brompton Hospital Records 4, 1935, *Tubercle*, 17 (1936), 319.
[125] Marcus Paterson Collection Va 606, W. Willcock to Paterson, 14 May 1909.
[126] *Tubercle*, 1 (1920), 480.
[127] *19 NAPT 1933*, pp. 35–43.
[128] NAPT Council Minutes, Report of Publicity Sub-committee, 20 Apr. 1936, p. 248.
[129] M. Coltart, H. Raine, and E. Harrison, *Social Work in Tuberculosis* (London 1959), 17.
[130] *Tubercle*, 33 (1952), 83.

'tuberculous diathesis'. John Guy wrote in 1935 that 'There is today a general belief among physicians as to the existence of an hereditary tuberculous diathesis,' although they were still equivocal—he added that it had been demonstrated that, if a child born into an infected home was removed from such source of infection, it became 'a healthy and vigorous child in no wise differing from the child born of healthy stock'.[131] A medical textbook published in 1947 referred to such an inherited tendency to tuberculosis.[132] G. S. Erwin, medical superintendent of the Liverpool Sanatorium, wrote in 1944 that heredity was said to play a part in resistance. In 1946 he addressed the question of why the disease ever affected the rich if it were a disease of poverty, and maintained that hereditary weakness may be so marked as to overcome the counteracting influence of good environment. In his opinion, individual susceptibility could not be estimated in advance, except when there was a family history of tuberculosis.[133] Dubos wrote in 1953 of the past belief in the tendency of tuberculosis to run in families: 'It is now realized that familial occurrence is, to a large extent, the result of a common source of infection in the household; but it is also probable that the manner in which the body responds to infection is conditioned by certain inborn traits that are hereditary, and that often bind several members of a family to a common destiny of disease.'[134] A textbook on tuberculosis published in 1979, however, belittled the importance of any hereditary tendency or resistance: 'It is becoming increasingly clear that much, probably most, of what has been called natural resistance to tuberculosis is due to acquired immunity.'[135] Nevertheless, Geoffrey Beven, who managed Ealing Chest Clinic, London, in the 1940s, believed that a tuberculosis tendency ran in families, and that this was the main cause of the secrecy surrounding the disease.[136]

While belief in the hereditary nature of tuberculosis caused personal problems, the knowledge of the infectiousness of the disease caused even greater problems socially and professionally. The tuberculous

---

[131] J. Guy, in C. W. Hutt and H. H. Thomson (eds.), *Principles and Practice of Preventive Medicine*, (London, 1935), i. 331.

[132] F. W. Price (ed.), *A Textbook of the Practice of Medicine*, 7th edn. (Oxford, 1947), 36.

[133] Erwin, *A Guide for the Tuberculous Patient*, p. 8; ibid., 2nd edn. (London, 1946), 99; Erwin, *Tuberculosis and Chest Diseases for Nurses*, p. 140.

[134] R. and J. Dubos, *The White Plague: Tuberculosis, Man and Society* (London, 1953), 188.

[135] G. P. Youmans, *Tuberculosis* (Philadelphia, 1979), 205.

[136] Geoffrey Beven, interview, 27 Sept. 1984.

were either likened to lepers or strongly feared that this would be the case. Coltart considered that this was the patient's main fear, and wrote of the 'leper complex' which sensitive patients often developed on being told that they had tuberculosis.[137] H. Bannister, lecturer in experimental psychology at Cambridge University, concluded from a psychological study of adult male tuberculous patients, that no specific psychoses or psychoneuroses were connected with tuberculosis as a direct consequence of the disease. The abnormalities which arose were expressions of maladjustment and not least the feeling of being an outcast.[138]

Doctors working with tuberculous patients recognized this stigma as very real. Bardswell said in 1911 that the opening of windows was enough to excite suspicion, and quoted a letter from an ex-patient: 'It is depressing to find how frightened people are becoming of us. I am being turned out of my rooms, and this will make my fourth move in this particular town.'[139] There was some indication that the fear of tuberculous patients was increasing in the early twentieth century, possibly partly related to the intensive efforts of the NAPT to publicize the infectiousness of the disease. Harold Vallow, TO for Bradford, claimed in 1915 that in his experience, a large number of employers and fellow workers of a consumptive would not have such a person working for or with them, and that the unfortunate patient was treated as a 'human leper'. Patients had told him that they had not let their employers and fellow employees know that they had been treated for consumption, and that they dared not take a sputum flask with them to their work, because immediately it was produced and seen they would lose their employment.[140] Clive Rivière similarly believed that in the public view the tuberculous person was 'a pariah and outcast'.[141] F. Rufenacht Walters wrote in 1924 of the dread of infection which prevented ex-patients from gaining employment even if they had completely recovered.[142] Bardswell addressed a conference in Oxford in 1935 on the subject of rehousing of tuberculous ex-patients in council housing estates, and was surprised at the amount of opposition the proposal aroused. Public health workers apparently expressed

[137] Coltart *et al.*, *Social Work in Tuberculosis*, pp. 32, 50.
[138] *Lancet*, 1 (1930), 784.
[139] King Edward VII Sanatorium, Midhurst, Annual Report 1910–11, p. 43.
[140] H. Vallow, *The Inevitable Complement: The Care and After-care of Consumptives* (London, 1915), 44–5.
[141] C. Rivière, *Tuberculosis and How to Avoid It* (London, 1917), 6.
[142] F. R. Walters, *Domiciliary Treatment of Tuberculosis*, 2nd edn. (London, 1924), 250.

horror at the suggestion that 'their nice new municipal cottages should be contaminated by the tuberculous' and a recommendation in support of the proposal was carried by the narrowest margin.[143]

When local authorities allocated houses on their estates to families with a tuberculous patient, they did so singly and not in colonies in order not to excite suspicion. J. E. Chapman of the Ministry of Health did not think that the addition of balconies to the houses for open-air treatment was a good idea as it would label them.[144]

The extent of the infectiousness of the disease is still unknown. What is clear, however, is that the effect on sufferers of the widespread belief in the infectiousness of the disease was considerable, for they could not be isolated for a short period as were smallpox patients because of the chronicity of the disease and therefore had to bear the stigma for life. Nor does the stigma appear to have lessened over time; if anything it seemed to increase until the 1950s when tuberculosis was finally believed to be under control in the Western world. The increasing difficulty of staffing institutions was partly attributed to a growing fear of infection. Esther Carling maintained in 1937 that 'lately even outside painters [were] afraid'.[145] Joan McCarthy referred to the problem of coping with 'the distancing or the "social" withdrawal of former acquaintances' following treatment in a sanatorium.[146]

In a newspaper article, written in 1938 under the heading 'Public must learn that tuberculosis does not mean taboo,' one patient with pulmonary tuberculosis voiced his anxieties:

. . . the world regards the 'lunger' as an outcast . . . Filled with an exaggerated dread of any word ending in 'osis', unthinking people recoil from anyone who has 'had it' . . . Every week scores of 'lungers' are released from clinics, hospitals and sanatoria . . . Each patient goes his own way. Yet each one finds himself up against the same problem . . . He is not wanted; he is avoided; he is feared—and then, alack! forgotten . . . You need not run from him as from some foul, contaminating influence, flee as to escape pollution . . . His own relatives are afraid to have him in the house . . . Jobs are out of reach . . . Two kinds of sufferings have attended me through the battle [to get well in the sanatorium]. One was the distressful horror of the disease itself. The other is the mental agony born of the knowledge that when I emerge from the fight . . . I am taboo to my fellowmen.[147]

[143] *Tubercle*, 17 (1936), 292; *Oxford Times*, 4 Oct. 1935 (Churchill Hospital, Oxford).
[144] PRO MH55/1125, A. J. Moore, 13 Apr. 1938.   [145] *Tubercle*, 18 (1937), 456.
[146] McCarthy, '"Tuberculosis" Before and After Waksman', p. 44.
[147] *Western Mail*, 5 Nov. 1938 (PRO MH96/1031).

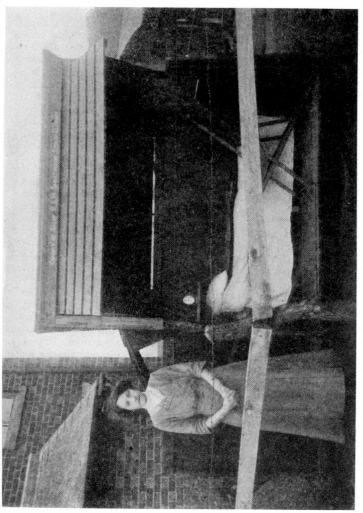

Plate 6. The stigma of tuberculosis: an ex-patient standing by her open-air shelter lent by a local sanatorium. *Source*: NAPT Annual Report of Council 1913, p. 45.

Nor was the statement about not being allowed in the house a total exaggeration, for shelters were a common phenomenon among tuberculous patients returning home, often lent out by local councils or after-care committees (see Plate 6).

Thus, the overwhelming impression is of a stigma attached to having tuberculosis in the twentieth century. Describing the stigmatization of herpetics, Alan Brandt pointed out that the whole notion of a noun which identified the infected individual by the disease itself contributed to the stigma that the infection carried. Few other diseases had generated such words and almost all of those which had, were stigmatized in particular ways: diabetic, epileptic, syphilitic, schizophrenic; the patient was the disease.[148] To this list of terms one could add 'the tuberculous' or 'lunger', which had the added repulsive connotation of being infectious through casual contact. As with venereal disease, the social construction of the disease was often more severe in its consequences than the disease itself.

[148] A. M. Brandt, *No Magic Bullet: A Social History of Venereal Disease in the US since 1880* (New York, 1985), 181–2; see also E. Goffman, *Stigma: Notes on the Management of Spoiled Identity* (New York, 1974).

8

Tuberculosis and the State, 1939 and Beyond

THE Second World War was a turning point in the administration of tuberculosis services in Britain. During the war, mass radiography was introduced to discover early cases, national allowances for tuberculous patients and their families were introduced foreshadowing other post-war welfare measures, national rehabilitation schemes were started, and BCG and pasteurization as preventive measures were considered seriously for the first time. The war also created a crisis in the administration of the services, related to the problem of staff recruitment, at a time of increasing demands for beds as new cases were discovered through the use of mass radiography. Following the war, the tuberculosis services were reorganized along with health and medical services in general under the new National Health Service. This chapter discusses the nature of these changes, the role played by the war itself, and the effect of chemotherapy introduced in the late 1940s.

(1) ALLOWANCES, REHABILITATION, AND MASS RADIOGRAPHY

It has been argued that the Second World War did not create a new demand for social reform, so much as give those who had been committed to social reform before the war a chance to publicize their views.[1] This was certainly true in relation to tuberculosis. Many tuberculosis specialists and others were advocating State intervention in the 'after-care' of tuberculous patients before the war, but it was the war itself which created the opportunity for the problem to be presented as particularly urgent. P. D'Arcy Hart, director of the tuberculosis work of the MRC and member of the Socialist Medical Association, argued in 1942: 'The present time, when production is of paramount importance, the demand for labour acute, makes it urgently

---

[1] P. Thane, *The Foundations of the Welfare State* (London, 1982), 223, 237.

necessary to arrive at a solution [to the tuberculosis problem]. We cannot afford to have unhealthy workers, nor can we permit the unnecessary spread of infection.' The experiences of the First World War were invoked as a warning of the potential dangers of warfare: 'If a repetition of the serious increase in tuberculosis during the last war is to be avoided in this—and some increase has already taken place— speedy action must be taken to minimise the effect of war stresses on industrial workers.' Hart outlined the factors which he thought would be likely to lead to an increase in tuberculosis, especially among young adults. These included food shortages, increased overcrowding as a result of a lack of fuel, lessened ventilation entailed by blackout precautions, and greater involvement in industry by young women in particular.[2]

The first two years of war had indeed seen some increases in tuberculosis incidence and mortality. The pulmonary tuberculosis death-rate in London in 1941 was 100 per 100,000 population, a 72 per cent increase over 1938; non-pulmonary rates had also increased by 67 per cent. The increases for England and Wales between 1938–9 and 1941 for pulmonary and non-pulmonary tuberculosis were 10 and 21 per cent respectively. The increase in non-pulmonary forms was mainly due to tuberculous meningitis. In Scotland, there was an 18 per cent rise in pulmonary and 28 per cent in non-pulmonary tuberculosis deaths in this period.[3]

Moreover, tuberculosis services were disrupted at the start of the war, adding to fears of the spread of the disease. In the period of anticipated bombing at the beginning of the war, dispensary work was curtailed as tuberculosis officers were involved with air raid preparation work. Many sanatoria were converted into war hospitals, operative treatment of tuberculosis patients was temporarily brought to a standstill, in some cases before a many-staged procedure had been

---

[2] 'The War, Tuberculosis and the Worker: A Report Prepared by a Committee of the Socialist Medical Association of Great Britain' (P. D'Arcy Hart and M. Daniels), pamphlet issued by the Socialist Medical Association, 2nd edn. (May 1942), printed in *Medicine Today and Tomorrow*, 3/2, (1941), 7; see also *Lancet*, 1 (1940), 835, and *BMJ* 1 (1940), 361, 786; G. P. Wright and P. D'Arcy Hart, *The American Review of Tuberculosis*, 43/3 (1941), 362; *Hospital* (Nov. 1942), 277; *Tubercle*, 22 (1941), 212.

[3] *Medical Officer* (22 May 1943), 162; *BMJ* 2 (1942), 419: it was pointed out that London had particularly excessive rates not only because of war conditions, but also because those with tuberculosis were excluded from the Forces and, as they were sick, were often reluctant to be evacuated and for the same reason (as well as the fact that in many cases their economic status was low) they would have difficulty in finding accommodation in reception areas.

completed, and care committees' work largely ceased. Open-air schools were disbanded and the children billeted in the country, thereby arousing the qualms of householders who feared contact with children presumed to be tuberculous.[4] The event which caused the greatest alarm in the early war period was the evacuation of tuberculosis institutions, involving the discharge of approximately 8,000 tuberculosis patients, some believed to be in a highly infectious state (representing 30 per cent of all those receiving residential treatment at the time). In Wales, approximately 60 per cent of all tuberculous patients were bundled home within 24 hours.[5] One eminent surgeon contributed to the general scare of infection by his statement that 'every tuberculous person turned forth is like a bomb thrown among the public'.[6] A letter to *The Times* by Lady Titchfield, chairman of the NAPT, Sir Percival Horton-Smith Hartley, and J. Harley Williams, stressed the urgency of the situation, reiterating the bomb analogy.[7] To discuss tuberculosis administration in wartime, the Minister of Health, Walter Elliot, summoned a deputation in October 1939 representing the NAPT, the JTC, and the TA, who presented him with a memorandum:

. . . tuberculosis is likely to show an increase in the civil population and among members of the Forces, and further, that this expected increase may not be confined to the generation primarily affected by the war. We believe, therefore, that the maintenance and it may be the extension, of tuberculosis schemes, so far as war necessities permit, is an essential part of National Defence.[8]

The Minister replied to the deputation that if, through some misunderstanding, infectious cases had been discharged, they should be sought out and brought back for treatment.[9]

As a result of the deputation, a Standing Advisory Committee on Tuberculosis was formed to assist the Ministry of Health, with Hartley as chairman, and Williams as secretary. The committee consisted of representatives of the NAPT, the JTC, the TA, the TG SMOH, the

---

[4] F. R. G. Heaf and N. L. Rusby, *Tubercle*, 21 (1940), Suppl., 18.
[5] R. M. Titmuss, in J. W. K. Hancock (ed.), *Problems of Social Policy: History of the Second World War (UK) Civil Series*, (London, 1950), 193–4.
[6] Quoted in a letter to the editor by S. L. Cummins, *BMJ* 2 (1939), 621 and ibid., 2 (1941), 632.
[7] *The Times*, 20 Oct. 1939. The bomb analogy was widely repeated, e.g., *Hospital* (Nov. 1942), 277–8.
[8] *Tubercle*, 21 (1939), 26.
[9] *Medical Officer* (27 Oct. 1939), 180; ibid., (Nov. 1939), 188.

LCC, as well as the Ministry of Health and the Department of Health for Scotland.

The Ministry of Health had arranged for approximately 6,000 beds to be added to tuberculosis institutions to receive air-raid casualties. As the anticipated bombing of London did not occur, the Standing Advisory Committee persuaded the Ministry to release some of these beds for the treatment of tuberculosis. Another initial preoccupation of the Advisory Committee related to the nutritional problems of tuberculous patients in wartime, and the Committee was responsible for the introduction of a two-pint-a-day milk priority for them, and later for prolonging the validity of the milk certificate from one month to three months.[10] It was decided, contrary to former (and some current) medical belief, that tuberculous patients did not have any special dietary needs apart from milk.[11]

A heightened concern about tuberculosis during the war was also manifested when a Committee for the Study of Social Medicine aproached the NAPT in 1942 to form a joint committee to inquire into the income and food expenditure of tuberculous households in wartime. The committee concluded that 31 per cent of the 1,346 families investigated did not have sufficient money to reach the League of Nations' nutritional standard (which, they pointed out, was based on the requirements of healthy persons and did not take into account any additional nutritional needs of the tuberculous).[12] The survey showed a change of emphasis in the NAPT from notions of self-responsibility to a greater social awareness. Disregarding their former stress on self-help and voluntary aid, the NAPT issued a manifesto in 1942: 'More careful application will have to be given by the Government and Local Authorities to the provision of economic security for the tuberculous family, as part of a national scheme of social welfare and rehabilitation.'[13]

At the request of the Ministry of Health, the MRC set up the Committee on Tuberculosis in War-time in 1941 with Lord Dawson of Penn as chairman and D'Arcy Hart as secretary, 'To assist in

---

[10] PRO MH55/1183, TSAC (The committee sat until 1949, with Sir Robert Young as chairman from 1944, holding 51 meetings and many more sub-committee meetings: Jameson to Young, 13 Jan. 1949); *Tubercle*, 23 (1942), 127.

[11] MRC, *Medical Research in War, Report of the MRC for the Years 1939–45*, Cmd. 7335 (1947), 121.

[12] NAPT and Committee for the Study of Social Medicine, *Report of Joint Committee set up to Enquire into the Income and Food Expenditure of Tuberculosis Households in War-time*, Chairman: G. Lissant Cox, (London, 1944), 4.

[13] *Tubercle*, 23 (1942), 56.

promoting an investigation of the extent and causes of the war-time increase in the incidence of tuberculosis, particularly among young women, and also to advise the Council regarding possible preventive measures.'[14]

The report issued by the committee was strongly influenced by D'Arcy Hart, who had anticipated its conclusions in an earlier publication. In a pamphlet issued by the Socialist Medical Association in 1941, Hart and Marc Daniels (Prophit Research Scholar, and employed by the MRC from 1946), advocated the use of the newly developed miniature X-rays, in order to 'forestall the dangerous possibilities of war-time increase of the disease'. They believed that this would 'revolutionize the outlook for tuberculosis by securing really early diagnosis and consequently more frequent care'.[15]

Miniature radiography, capable of taking 100 1½-inch chest photographs per hour, had been developed in the decade before the war, with Germany, USA, the Netherlands, and Britain all contributing various inventions to the technique. It was first used in Britain by Hart and others at University College Hospital in 1940 from which—with other studies—it was estimated that 1–2 per cent healthy adults would be shown to have tuberculous lesions.[16] It was advocated at the beginning of the war as a means of preventing the absorption of tuberculosis sufferers into the armed services. Despite regulations which required tuberculosis officers to send lists of tuberculosis sufferers to the recruiting agencies (disregarding the confidentiality of notification) and which required recruits to sign a declaration that they had not had tuberculosis, it was found that early cases of tuberculosis slipped through. Their condition was aggravated by war service, which was 'dangerous to the individual and costly to the community'.[17] When miniature (or 'mass') radiography was first used in the Navy, it revealed an active case-rate among new recruits of 3.2 per thousand.[18] It was subsequently advocated for the civilian population, in particular those in war-related industries. However, Dr Hyacinth Morgan,

[14] MRC, *Report of the Committee on Tuberculosis in War-time*, (SRS 246; London, 1942).

[15] Hart and Daniels, *Medicine Today and Tomorrow*, 3/2 (1941), 6.

[16] Heaf and Rusby, *Tubercle*, 21 (1940), Suppl., 20.

[17] Hart and Daniels, *Medicine Today and Tomorrow*, 3/4 (1941), 1.

[18] Heaf and Rusby, *Tubercle*, 23 (1942), 112; PRO MH55/1135, Tuberculosis and Recruiting, Public Health (Tuberculosis) Regulations, 1940; PRO MH55/1184, Marchbank to N. F. Smith, 6 Jan. 1941; see also V. Z. Cope (ed.), *History of the Second World War, Medicine and Pathology*, (London, 1952), 319, 328.

medical adviser to the Trades Union Congress (also MP and member of the Socialist Medical Association), had misgivings concerning the economic consequences of such a scheme for the cases so discovered.[19] As Hart and Daniels also pointed out,

> Unless the fall in the standard of living which the tuberculous worker suffers can be alleviated, no scheme for early diagnosis by mass radiography can be expected to succeed; for, since the cases discovered will be frequently accompanied by few or no feelings of illness, it will be difficult to persuade a worker to face economic disaster on the assurance of ultimate benefit to his health.[20]

The MRC committee recommended the use of mass radiography among selected groups of supposedly healthy people in order to detect early cases of pulmonary tuberculosis, as well as a system of allowances and rehabilitation to ensure the success of the radiography scheme. These recommendations led to the issuing of Memo 266/T by the Ministry of Health outlining a scheme of mass radiography and the payment of allowances to early cases of pulmonary tuberculosis in order to induce them to give up work and undertake treatment at a time when their disease was still 'curable'. The allowances consisted of a standard rate of maintenance payable without inquiry into means (beyond current wages and National Health Insurance benefits), corresponding to the maintenance rates payable by the Unemployment Assistance Board (excluding the rent element in that rate but including 10s. 6d., and with slightly more generous rates for dependants until the Assistance Board rates were revised in December 1943). Additional payments could be given at the discretion of the authorities and after need had been established. The assessment lasted 13 weeks, during which time the recipient was to declare any changes in financial circumstances.

The system of allowances, which became known as Memo 266/T, commenced in September 1943 and was received with great enthusiasm. The *NAPT Bulletin* described it as a 'bold, imaginative, and comprehensive scheme', and the *Tubercle*, as 'a revolution in the tuberculosis world'.[21] Heaf believed it to be 'epoch making', and according to a medical group set up to consider post-war reorganization of the medical services, the Medical Planning Research, 'this official

[19] H. C. Morgan, *Lancet*, 2 (1940), 246–7; ibid., 2 (1940), 605.
[20] Hart and Daniels, *Medicine Today and Tomorrow*, 3/2 (1941), 9.
[21] *NAPT Bulletin*, 5/3 (1943), 4; *Tubercle*, 24 (1943), 89.

recognition of the importance of the economic factor in the tuberculosis problem will stand as a landmark in the fight against the disease'.[22] But before long, the allowances were subject to severe criticism, first because they were pitched so low, in fact no higher than Public Assistance, and second because they excluded non-pulmonary and advanced pulmonary cases of tuberculosis, resulting in the qualification of only approximately 10 per cent of those on the tuberculosis registers.[23]

The level of the allowances was decided by a committee chaired by T. Lindsay, Principal Assistant Secretary of the Ministry of Health. The continuing adherence to the principle of 'less eligibility' in the formulation of social policies ensured that general standards were kept low by the fear of providing disincentives to work.[24] Ironically the tuberculosis allowances were initially designed *as* a disincentive to work, but the committee argued that 'The financial help should not be so great that the patient has no incentive to achieve his financial independence . . . It should not, on the other hand, be so small that the patient is driven to exertion for which he is not yet fit.'[25] Peter Edwards of the Cheshire Joint Sanatorium feared that payments might provide a disincentive to work in tuberculosis colonies.[26] However, according to the JTC, the payments were not adequate to relieve patients with families of such anxieties and thus did not attain the object of securing willing prolonged treatment.[27] The NAPT also doubted whether the assessments bore any relation to 'current prices of food and other normal needs of a civilised home'.[28] An important reason to keep the allowances low despite the severe criticism was the reluctance of the Government to admit to a minimum desirable rate and thereby set a precedent before the post-war welfare legislation was formulated. Ernest Brown, Minister of Health from 1941 to 1943, argued that the main value of the allowances lay in the avoidance of the stigma of Public Assistance. When family allowances were introduced in 1946, tuberculosis allowances were reduced according to the amount

---

[22] *NAPT Bulletin*, 5/4 (1943), 3; *Tubercle*, 24 (1943), 175.
[23] PRO MH55/1288, Lindsay Committee, Conference with Local Authority Representatives, 13 Jan. 1944.
[24] See Thane, *The Foundations of the Welfare State*, p. 217.
[25] PRO MH55/1288, Lindsay Committee meeting, 12 Dec. 1942.
[26] PRO MH55/1288, P. Edwards to N. F. Smith, Ministry of Health, 3 Mar. 1943.
[27] PRO MH55/1145, Interim Report of JTC on Ministry of Health Memo 266/T, 21 July 1945, p. 5.
[28] *NAPT Bulletin*, 9/1 (1947), 20–1.

received from family allowances, which was strongly objected to by the SMOH as well as many local councils.[29] The Ministry of Health was accused by some of basing its policies on eugenics, discouraging the tuberculous from having families. In fact, there is no evidence to suggest that this was a consideration; it was merely an attempt to keep the rates of payment to a minimum. The reduction also applied to other allowances, such as the widows' and orphans' pensions, public assistance allowances and unemployment assistance allowances—those, according to one commentator, 'unorganised in trade unions owing to the death, ill-health, or unemployment of the breadwinner'.[30] The Ministry of Health argued, however, that if a family received both payments each child would be paid for twice.[31]

The other criticism of the allowances was that they were limited to 'curable' cases of pulmonary tuberculosis. Responding to complaints that non-pulmonary cases were excluded, Ernest Brown pointed out that they were not infectious in the same way as pulmonary cases. However, if infection were an important consideration, then why were advanced pulmonary cases excluded, the most infectious of all? Brown reiterated that the scheme was designed to encourage early cases to give up work and undergo treatment, as a wartime national emergency measure, and that any extension of the allowances would require fresh legislation.[32] The scheme was clearly based on old COS principles, as the after-care schemes before the war had been—only those who could eventually be made self-reliant were to be helped. The Lindsay Committee maintained

> There will also be cases in which it becomes apparent that even prolonged treatment (or, if the expression is preferred, prolonged employment under supervision) will never restore full working capacity. Such a decision should not lightly be reached but if it is clear that disability will be permanent we feel that the justification for the special tuberculosis allowances cannot be longer maintained.[33]

Tuberculosis officers complained that the termination of allowances was equivalent to passing a death sentence on the patient which was

[29] PRO MH55/1287, Tuberculosis Allowances, Effects of Family Allowances Act 1945, Circular 114/46, 20 June 1946; SMOH to Ministry of Health, 31 Oct. 1946 (also many other letters in file).

[30] PRO MH55/1287, A. T. Collis, Stepney Pacifist Service Unit, 13 Aug. 1946.

[31] *Hansard*, 5th Series, 1945–6, 426 (1946), 213–14.

[32] *Hansard*, 5th Series, 1942–3, 393 (1943), 865; *National Insurance Gazette*, 3 June 1943; *NAPT Bulletin*, 5/4 (1943), 1.

[33] PRO MH55/1288, Lindsay Committee, 12 Dec. 1942.

cruel and psychologically injurious.[34] The TG SMOH resolved 'that ultimate fitness for work should not be the criterion for eligibility for allowances under Memo 266/T, but that all cases of pulmonary tuberculosis who conform with the instructions of the Tuberculosis Officer should be eligible to receive allowances'.[35] The Cumberland CC similarly sent representations to the Ministry of Health that the allowances should be expanded to provide financial assistance for the advanced cases and their families conditional on their complying with such instructions as to mode of life as might be laid down by the local authority dispensing the allowances.[36] Tuberculosis officers regarded the allowances essentially as an opportunity to increase medical supervision of tuberculous patients. This was indeed an important element in the scheme, for patients who did not comply with the tuberculosis officer's instructions (apart from undergoing a major operation) could be deprived of the allowances.[37]

Ferguson and Fitzgerald evaluated the tuberculosis allowance scheme as among the less successful aspects of wartime policy: 'Can it take a worthy place among such developments as the widening school meals and milk service, the national milk and vitamin food schemes, the increased old age pensions, the abolition of the household means test from social service payments . . .?'[38] It could not in fact do so, and the reason lies in the different conception and objectives of the tuberculosis allowances scheme compared with the other welfare measures. It was not concerned with minimum levels but was essentially regarded as a medical measure for a specific and limited group, an attempt to restore working power, justified in the interests of national efficiency.

Some local authorities extended the allowances to include all cases of tuberculosis without differentiation, paying for those not covered by the scheme out of local rates. Northamptonshire, Caernarvonshire, and Monmouthshire were among the first to do so in 1944.[39] While the allowances had been estimated by the Treasury to cost £3 million a

---

[34] PRO MH55/1145, Interim Report of JTC on Memo 266/T, p. 9. *Hansard*, 5th Series, 1942–3, 393 (1943), 865; ibid., 1945–6, 414 (1945), 2175.
[35] *Tubercle*, 25 (1943), 191.
[36] Ibid., 28 (1947), 102.
[37] PRO MH55/1288, Lindsay Committee, Conference with Local Authority Representatives, 13 Nov. 1942.
[38] S. Ferguson and H. Fitzgerald, *Studies in the Social Service*, in W. K. Hancock (ed.), *History of the Second World War (UK) Civil Series*, (London, 1954), 283. See also Titmuss, *Problems of Social Policy*, p. 515.
[39] *Medical Officer* (2 Dec. 1944); PRO MH96/1077.

year in 1943, the actual cost for the year ending 31 March 1945 was £650,000. In the following years the cost continued to be less than a quarter of the original estimates, which, according to the NAPT, was evidence of the glaring parsimony of the tuberculosis allowances scheme.[40]

The MRC Committee on Tuberculosis in War-time also recommended that rehabilitation should be considered an essential part of the treatment of tuberculous patients, and that arrangements should be made for their gradual return to industry in part-time or modified work. During the period of rehabilitation, a supplement to wages should be provided, so that an adequate standard of living could be maintained. This would ensure the success of the mass radiography scheme. The TA argued that 'it would hardly seem a reasonable procedure to adopt mass examination without at the same time making provision for the future employment of the patients so discovered'.[41]

Rehabilitation of tuberculous patients must be seen in the context of rehabilitation of the disabled in general, which was given a sense of urgency owing to the wartime need to maximize manpower resources, and an increased awareness of the problems of the disabled arising from the large number of war casualties. Titmuss maintained that the creation of a framework for a national rehabilitation scheme might be recorded as one of the chief successes of the Government's Emergency Medical Service.[42] Ernest Bevin, becoming Minister of Labour in 1940, had been urging legislation for the disabled before 1939, but the war gave him the opportunity to act.[43] In 1941 the Ministry of Labour and National Service introduced an interim scheme for the training and resettlement of disabled persons. A Ministry of Health circular pointed out that the scheme was applicable to quiescent (sputum-negative) cases of tuberculosis who could be reintroduced into whole-time employment under ordinary industrial conditions. While this in fact only applied to a few cases, the NAPT believed that it was significant in recognizing the need for rehabilitation, and they hoped that it would be extended after the war.[44]

[40] *NAPT Bulletin*, 9/1 (1947), 21; PRO MH55/1179, E. Brown, 26 NAPT Conference, 28 July 1943 (unpublished); PRO MH55/1145, Interim Report of JTC on Memo 266/T, p. 5.
[41] MRC, *Tuberculosis in War-time*, pp. 24, 30; *BMJ* 1 (1942), 197; *Tubercle*, 23 (1942), 136.   [42] Titmuss, *Problems of Social Policy*, p. 480.
[43] H. Bolderson, 'The Origins of the Disabled Persons Employment Quota and its Symbolic Significance', *Journal of Social Policy*, 9 (1980), 169–86.
[44] *NAPT Bulletin*, 4/3 (1942), 15; See also MRC, *Tuberculosis in War-time*, p. 23;

An Inter-departmental Committee set up in 1941 under George Tomlinson, Parliamentary Secretary to the Ministry of Labour, to consider employment for the disabled, recommended in 1943 that firms employ a definite quota of disabled people on their staff. Like the MRC Committee on Tuberculosis in War-time, it also recognized the need for rehabilitation schemes and subsidized wages for the disabled. The concern of the committee was for disabled persons generally, but Tomlinson told an NAPT meeting that in making the recommendations, he had chiefly in mind bronchial and tuberculous cases. The Disabled Persons (Employment) Act of 1944, which followed the Report, was described by the NAPT as 'more constructive than the mere monetary compensation of Health Insurance and 266/T', and as 'a fresh principle in health legislation'.[45]

Under the Act, a National Advisory Committee on the Employment of Disabled Persons was set up with Viscount Ridley as chairman. Industrial rehabilitation and vocational training courses were organized by the Ministry of Labour and National Service, and employers were obliged to take a quota of disabled. The Disabled Persons Employment Corporation Limited, or 'Remploy', was also established under a board of directors chaired by Lord Portal, and was to organize special industrial concerns for the disabled. For the purposes of the scheme, a disablement register was started and disablement resettlement officers appointed.

The NAPT pointed out that although tuberculosis was not specifically mentioned in the clauses of the Act, repeated assurances had been given that the tuberculous person was in the same position in respect to the Act as the miner with the broken back, the limbless soldier, the blind, and the sufferer from neurosis. Nevertheless, the NAPT was disappointed that there were no tuberculosis specialists on the National Advisory Committee.[46] As far as the disablement quota of the 1944 Act was concerned, it was reported in 1947 that neither public nor private businesses were as yet showing signs of including tuberculosis sufferers in their quota of physically disabled workers.[47] Moreover, tuberculous patients were said to be reluctant to register as

PRO MH96/1118, Interim Scheme for Training and Resettlement of Disabled Persons, Ministry of Labour and National Service, London, Oct. 1941, PL 93/1941.

[45] *NAPT Bulletin*, 6/1 (1944), 1; ibid., 7/1 (1945), 2; *Tubercle*, 27 (1946),97.

[46] PRO MH96/1118, Ministry of Health Circular 52/46, 1944 Disabled Persons (Employment) Act and Tuberculosis, 15 May 1946; *NAPT Bulletin*, 7/1 (1945), 14.

[47] C. Hendrick-Duchaine, 'L'évolution des lois sociales en Grande-Bretagne et la tuberculose', *Revue Belge de la Tuberculose* (1947), 2.

disabled, which was essential to gain employment. In some places it was discovered that the disablement resettlement officers were declining to register people with tuberculosis who, although infectious (sputum-positive), were pronounced fit by their doctors for work in sheltered employment, and, in other places, doctors were discouraging their patients from registering because facilities were limited. The NAPT urged patients to register so that the need for more facilities would be recognized.[48]

By 1947 Remploy had established twelve factories, but only one for workers suffering from tuberculosis. However, by 1952 seven 'Special' factories for those with tuberculosis had been opened—in London (the Spero factories) and at Birmingham, Bristol, Hull, Leeds, Portsmouth, and Sheffield, with a total employment capacity of 565. At the end of 1951 they were employing approximately 450 people, and 490 by 1955.[49] The main work at the factories was general woodwork, light engineering, packaging, and cardboard-box making. The factory medical officers were usually the local tuberculosis officers (now 'chest physicians') or members of their staff, who visited regularly. It was normal practice to work 44 hours a week in Remploy factories, but in the 'Special' factories arrangements were sometimes made in consultation with the factory medical officer for workers to start on a shortened working week.

With allowances and rehabilitation measures to encourage workers' co-operation, mass radiography among the civilian population was introduced in 1943 by the MRC. Initially 23,000 people were X-rayed from two factories, a large office group, and a mental hospital in Greater London. Significant tuberculous lesions were discovered in approximately 1 per cent of the apparently normal persons examined. Treatment was considered necessary for 3–4 per 1,000, half of whom had tubercle bacilli in their sputum.[50] According to E. R. Boland, Dean of the Medical and Dental Schools of Guy's Hospital, these were terrifying figures, for if this distribution were equal throughout the 41 million inhabitants of England and Wales, it would mean that there were over 100,000 as yet undiagnosed cases of tuberculosis in need of treatment, of which about a half were a source of infection for

[48] *NAPT Bulletin*, 8/5 (1946), 149; ibid., 9/6 (1947), 157.
[49] *NAPT Handbook*, 14th edn. (1952), 285; ibid., 15th edn. (1957), 212.
[50] MRC, K. C. Clark, P. D'Arcy Hart, P. Kerley and B. C. Thompson, *Mass Miniature Radiography of Civilians for the Detection of Pulmonary Tuberculosis (Guide to Administration and Technique with a Mobile Apparatus using 35-mm Film and Results of a Survey)*, (SRS, 251; London, 1945), Preface and p. 88.

their fellows. Indeed, a JTC Rehabilitation Committee set up during the war had already estimated in 1942 that there were 77,000 infectious cases of tuberculosis in England alone.[51]

In December 1942 the Ministry of Health announced that mobile miniature radiography sets were available for the use of a limited number of local authorities. Lancashire was the first local authority to take up the offer. From 1943 to 1945, 19,240 X-rays were taken in Lancashire, and 69 cases of active tuberculosis found (3.6 per 1,000), with 31 sputum-positive cases.[52] By 1945, 13 local authorities had introduced mass radiography schemes, and by 1948, 36. Over 3 million people had been X-rayed by 1948, among whom 4 per 1,000 cases of previously unsuspected active pulmonary tuberculosis were discovered.[53]

(2) CRISIS IN HOSPITAL ADMINISTRATION

These new cases discovered by mass radiography created additional pressures on institutional accommodation. According to the MRC Committee on Tuberculosis in War-time, the greatest difficulty at that time confronting the tuberculosis service was the lack of usable in-patient accommodation largely because of a shortage of nursing and domestic staff. In Wales, for example, 150 out of 1,952 beds were empty for this reason. It was estimated that 600 more nurses were needed to supplement the 2,600 nurses in tuberculosis institutions in England and Wales, and that another 600 were required to nurse tuberculous patients in the emergency hospitals. It was also estimated that an additional 900 domestic servants were needed to supplement the 4,800 domestics in tuberculosis institutions.[54]

H. G. Trayer (medical superintendent of Baguley Sanatorium) investigated the nursing and domestic arrangements of 109 sanatoria in England in 1941, and concluded that 70 per cent would possibly have to close down as a result of a shortage of nursing and domestic staff.[55] Among the principal reasons for the shortage, according to a

---

[51] *BMJ* 2 (1948), 17; *Tubercle*, 23 (1942), 30–1.
[52] Lancashire CC, *30th Annual Report of Central Tuberculosis Officer 1945* (1946), 11; *Tubercle*, 26 (1945), 165.
[53] *Ministry of Health Annual Report 1947–8* (1948), 77.
[54] MRC, *Tuberculosis in War-time*, p. 18.
[55] PRO MH55/1183, TSAC, 8 Aug. 1941: Appendix 1, Report by H. G. Trayer, 2 July 1941, p. 14.

deputation representing the various tuberculosis organizations to the Ministry of Health in 1942, was that nurses thought it more glamorous to nurse wounded soldiers than tuberculous patients. Working in a sanatorium in the peaceful surroundings of the countryside apparently had no connection with real national service and therefore was not attractive.[56] However, the poor recruitment of nurses was not a new problem, but preceded the war, as already discussed.

An Inter-departmental Committee on Nursing Services had issued an interim report in 1939 with recommendations relating to salaries, pensions, hours of duty, holidays, and conditions of service.[57] Commenting on the report, the WNMA asserted that the complete adoption of the recommendations, with their repercussions on the remuneration and accommodation of the augmented domestic staffs, was not likely to be practicable for many years.[58] Yet repeated advertisements had failed to attract applicants, as was lamented at the North Wales Sanatorium where an attempt to recruit candidates from the Nursing Reserve had only produced one applicant.[59] William Bickle of the WBH expressed the increasingly common view among officials and administrators that 'anything short of compulsion or the drafting of personnel from the Forces is not likely to solve this problem'.[60] G. L. C. Elliston, secretary of the SMOH from 1929 to 1952, could not understand the Minister of Health's refusal to compel women to nurse in sanatoria: 'If there is any class in the community which is accustomed to discipline, and to doing any kind of work which is allotted to them, it is our hospital nurses.'[61]

The WNMA believed that its problem had not been helped by the Ministry of Health's Circular 2340, which had placed a ban on the employment of Civil Nursing Reserve personnel under 21 years of age in tuberculosis institutions, and which therefore had increased the popular prejudice against tuberculosis nursing by its implications of an added risk of contracting the disease.[62] The Ministry replied that the circular had not been widely distributed and therefore could not have

[56] PRO MH55/1140, Deputation, 22 June 1942; *Tubercle*, 23 (1942), 118.
[57] *Athlone Report* (1939). See also B. Abel-Smith, *A History of the Nursing Profession* (London, 1960), 145–7.
[58] PRO MH75/31, WNMA 28 Feb. 1939, p. 4; MH75/32, Conference, WBH, WNMA, and local authorities, 29 Mar. 1939.
[59] PRO MH75/32, D. Davies to W. Elliot, 16 Mar. 1940.
[60] PRO MH96/1031, W. Bickle to H. K. Ainsworth, Ministry of Health, 18 May 1942.
[61] *Hansard*, 5th Series, 1941–2, 381 (1942), 144.
[62] PRO MH55/1146, WNMA Deputation to Minister of Health, June 1942, p. 3.

had much influence.[63] The circular did, however, reflect general public feeling about tuberculosis, a fear of infection which appeared to be increasing. Two nurses employed at Papworth in the 1920s had not thought fear of infection a consideration in taking up the work, but in 1937 Esther Carling maintained that parents were increasingly averse to allowing their daughters to take up tuberculosis nursing.[64] A nurse who started working in a sanatorium in the Second World War said she had chosen to do so because she wanted to do something just as dangerous as her brother who had joined the Air Force.[65] Considering, as we have seen, that at least one eminent surgeon thought that the discharge of a tuberculous person was just as dangerous as dropping a bomb on a centre of population, it is hardly surprising that this nurse considered her chosen career a dangerous one. Evidence suggested moreover that the fear of infection in tuberculosis institutions rested on some foundation. The work of Heimbeck in Oslo, as already noted, was widely known.

According to the WNMA, even if it were granted for the sake of argument that there was an added risk, there seemed no logical basis for such a regard for the health of young women undertaking the nursing of tuberculous patients, as compared with women undertaking general nursing in 'target' towns. The Association added that risks also accompanied the entry of young women into any of the Service organizations, into factories or munition works, and of men, who were given no option where they were sent into the Forces.[66]

The ban imposed by the Ministry of Health on the employment of Civil Nursing Reserve recruits in sanatoria was in fact shortly lifted on the grounds that it was illogical to allow young student nurses but not young members of the Reserve to work in the sanatoria. Nevertheless, a committee of the Royal College of Nursing, chaired by Lord Horder, recommended in 1943 that advanced cases in tuberculosis wards of general hospitals should not be nursed by young nurses in training.[67] The Prophit Survey, published following the war, when the problem of recruitment was still unsolved, contributed further to the fear of infection. Investigating 4,000 nurses, the survey estimated that nurses in general hospitals with tuberculosis wards were 4 times as liable to

[63] PRO MH96/1031, J. G. Jones, 6 June 1942.
[64] Mrs Goozee, Mrs Langdon, interviews, Papworth, 23 Mar. 1983; *Tubercle*, 18 (1937), 456.
[65] *NAPT Bulletin*, 6/6 (1944), 15.
[66] PRO MH55/1146, WNMA, June 1942, p. 3.
[67] *Horder Report*, Sect. 2, 1943.

contract tuberculosis as women in the general population. The publication of this report caused much annoyance among those trying to recruit nurses.[68]

A report of the Nurses' Salaries Committee, appointed by the Ministry of Health in 1941 under the chairmanship of Lord Rushcliffe, recommended in 1943 that salaries in tuberculosis institutions should be made higher to compensate for the disadvantages. While the recommended salaries for nurses in all other types of hospitals were £100–140 per annum, those for tuberculosis institutions were £110–150. The report also recommended that the salaries of matrons and assistant matrons should be as high as in hospitals approved for training by the General Nursing Council.[69] However, in their report in the same year, the Royal College of Nursing advised that the extra money involved in the Nurses' Salaries Committee recommendations to increase the pay of sanatorium nurses above the normal scale, would be better spent on additional safeguards to health.[70]

Some improvements were made in staff living conditions in the 1940s, but two major factors inhibiting recruitment, low wages and the refusal of the General Nursing Council to recognize the TA certificate, remained unchanged. Greater attention was paid, however, to the problem of infection. In 1946 it was reported that one large local authority had decided to exclude all Mantoux-negative nurses from tuberculosis wards in general and from special tuberculosis hospitals except in the case of two sanatoria taking early cases.[71] A nurse who contracted tuberculosis in a hospital was awarded compensation for the first time in 1948.[72] In 1950 on the recommendation of the Industrial Injuries Advisory Council, the Minister of National Insurance decided to insure nurses and other health workers 'in close and frequent contact with tuberculous infection' under the National Insurance (Industrial Injuries) Act.[73] This was undoubtedly related to the problem of the nursing shortage which had become even more

---

[68] R. R. Trail, *NAPT Bulletin*, 7/4 (1945), 5.

[69] *Rushcliffe Report*, Cmd. 6424 (1943), 7, 21, 31.

[70] *Horder Report*, p. 31.

[71] W. E. Snell, *NAPT Bulletin*, 8/2 (1946), 45.

[72] *NAPT Bulletin*, 11/3 (1949), 117.

[73] *BMJ* 2 (1950), 1340; Ministry of National Insurance, *Report of Industrial Injuries Advisory Council, in accordance with Section 61 of the National Insurance (Industrial Injuries) Act 1946, on the question of whether Tuberculosis and other Communicable Diseases should be prescribed under the Act in relation to Nurses and other Health Workers*, Chairman: Sir Wilfrid Garrett, Cmd. 8093 (1950).

acute in the post-war period. In 1950 it was estimated that 2,900 more nurses were required for the tuberculosis service.[74]

(3) BCG VACCINATION

The rising problem of nurse recruitment during the war was an important reason for the serious consideration given at that time to BCG vaccination. BCG was the subject of a TA conference in 1943, at which the results of its use in Scandinavia, Canada, and the USA were discussed. At the close of the meeting it was resolved to ask the Minister of Health to facilitate a regular supply of BCG in Britain, and to instigate an extended investigation of its use. A deputation was sent to the Minister of Health, led by W. H. Tytler, professor of tuberculosis at the Welsh National School of Medicine, and including representatives from the NAPT and the TA. Thus, support was growing for the introduction of BCG.[75]

Not everyone was in favour of BCG however. An opponent of some influence was G. S. (later Sir Graham) Wilson, head of the Emergency Public Health Laboratory Service, who maintained in 1944, 'On pure *a priori* grounds . . . I should doubt whether BCG vaccination is likely to form a serious contribution to the control of human tuberculosis in this country.'[76] At an international conference in 1947, the advantages and disadvantages of BCG were debated by Wilson and Arvid Wallgren who had been instrumental in introducing the vaccine into Sweden. The latter argued that Wilson was shouldering a great responsibility when he endeavoured to discourage the introduction of BCG into Britain, and urged Britain at least to undertake 'an unbiased trial' of BCG.[77] The BBC considered producing a story on BCG in 1947, but it was advised by the Ministry of Health that 'there is no big story'.[78]

In 1947 the Ministry of Health set up a committee to advise it on clinical trials of BCG. In 1948 a group of tuberculosis specialists visited Copenhagen to study the vaccine, and the first consignment of

---

[74] *NAPT Bulletin*, 11/5 (1949), 161; *BMJ* 2 (1950), 1285. (4,409 of the 27,763 beds for tuberculosis were unstaffed, while there were 11,000 patients on the waiting lists.)
[75] MRC 1319/1, Tytler to E. Mellanby, 16 May 1944.
[76] MRC 1319/1, Wilson to Mellanby, 1 June 1944.
[77] *NAPT Bulletin*, 10/5 (1948), 155; *BMJ* 1 (1948), 1128.
[78] Ministry of Health, Public Relations Officer, to BBC Chief Producer, 8 Sept. 1947 (reference supplied by Tom Wildy).

BCG arrived from Copenhagen in 1949. In the same year the Ministry issued a circular instructing local authorities to offer BCG to persons who had known contact with tuberculous infection, with hospital nurses and medical students given high priority. The circular emphasized that BCG would not be used on the whole population, or anything like it, in the first instance.[79] An article in the *BMJ* in 1950 maintained that those acquainted at first hand with the use of BCG in Scandinavian countries were 'exasperated by Britain's backwardness. Even now it is necessary to import the vaccine that is to be used to a limited extent.'[80]

The MRC launched a controlled trial of BCG and vole bacillus vaccine (discovered by A. Q. Wells at the Dunn School of Pathology, Oxford, in 1937) among adolescent boys and girls in 1950. Those found at an initial X-ray examination to be suffering from pulmonary tuberculosis and those known to have been in recent contact with a case of pulmonary tuberculosis at home, were excluded from the trial. By December 1952, approximately 56,700 children had been included in the trial. They were all in their final year at secondary modern schools in or near North London, Birmingham, and Manchester, and were nearly all between 14½ and 15 years of age. A random process was used to allocate children with a negative reaction to tuberculin to three groups—those in one group were not vaccinated, those in another received BCG vaccine, and those in a third group received vole bacillus vaccine. For the first 9 years of the trial, the participants were the subjects of a repeated cycle of examinations by MRC teams, consisting of a postal enquiry, a home visit, and a chest radiograph and tuberculin test, each cycle lasting about 14 months. The postal enquiries were continued for a further 6 years.

Reports were published in 1956, 1959, and 1963. In 1959 it was reported that the results showed that 'the two vaccines conferred substantial protection against tuberculosis for this period in a large group of adolescents living under the ordinary urban and suburban conditions prevailing in industrial communities in Britain'. BCG was found to be slightly more effective than vole bacillus vaccine. The reduction in incidence of tuberculosis in the BCG vaccinated group,

---

[79] *CMOH Annual Report 1949* (1950), 104; Ministry of Health Circular 72/49; Ministry of Health, Department of Health for Scotland, BCG Vaccination, Medical Memo 322/BCG, July 1949, p. 8.

[80] *BMJ* 2 (1950), 1384; see also PRO MH55/1163, BMA Chest Group, Nov. 1950, p. 6, and *NAPT Bulletin*, 12/2 (1950), 261.

compared with the tuberculin-negative unvaccinated group, was 87 per cent. In 1963, it was concluded that the vaccine offered 79 per cent protection for the 12½ years covered in the survey.[81]

General vaccination in schools was introduced to a limited extent in England and Wales in 1953, that is before the publication of the MRC reports, which suggests that lack of scientific evidence had not been the only or main hindrance to its introduction formerly. By the end of 1954, 250,000 persons had been vaccinated, rising to 600,000 by the end of 1956 (about half of them were school children). Vaccination in schools was more widely adopted after the 1956 MRC report. Scotland had already introduced a general vaccination policy in 1950 possibly because tuberculosis there had risen during and after the Second World War. By the end of 1956, about 200,000 persons in Scotland had been vaccinated with BCG.[82]

(4) PASTEURIZATION OF MILK

The MRC Committee on Tuberculosis in War-time also recommended an extension of pasteurization of milk throughout the country, and where this was not practicable, that all milk consumed by children should be boiled, or else dried milk provided: 'If all milk for human consumption were pasteurised in licensed plants under adequate supervision, it is no exaggeration to say that tuberculosis of bovine origin would be eliminated.'[83]

Practices of pasteurization, as already noted, varied throughout the country. One result of the wartime evacuation policy was to transfer a considerable number of children from London and other large towns, where a substantial proportion of the milk supply was pasteurized or otherwise heat-treated, to small urban and country districts where practically all of it was supplied raw, causing a heightened public concern for the problem of bovine tuberculosis. The Government's

---

[81] 'First (Progress) Report of the MRC by their Tuberculosis Vaccines Clinical Trials Committee', *BMJ* 1 (1956), 413–27; Second Report, *BMJ* 2 (1959), 379–95; Third Report, *BMJ* 1 (1963), 973–8; P. D'Arcy Hart, *BMJ* 1 (1967), 587–92; Ian Sutherland, *Tubercle*, 40 (1959), 413; Heaf, *Tubercle*, 35 (1954), 154.

[82] *Ministry of Health Annual Report 1954*, pp. 98–9; ibid., *1956*, pp. 98–9; *Department of Health for Scotland Annual Report 1956*, p. 30; see also C. Webster, *Problems of Health Care: the British National Health Service before 1957* (in press).

[83] MRC, *Tuberculosis in War-time*, p. 11; PRO MH55/1141, TSAC also passed a resolution on milk, 10 Feb. 1942, p. 4.

scheme for milk for nursing and expectant mothers and children under five years of age, as well as for school children, led to further discussion about the safety of the milk supply, since the schemes did not insist on pasteurization and were vague in regard to cleanliness requirements.[84]

In 1943 R. M. F. Picken, acting chairman of the council of the BMA, led a large deputation to the Minister of Food, Lord Woolton, to urge the need for complete and efficient pasteurization of milk. The deputation included representatives from the Royal College of Physicians and the Royal College of Surgeons, NAPT, JTC, the British Paediatric Association, and the People's League of Health. As a result, Lord Woolton asked the Milk Marketing Board to draw up practical proposals for ensuring cleanliness of the milk supply and elimination of tuberculous infection, but no immediate action was taken. Further evidence in favour of pasteurization came from a study undertaken during the war by the MRC's Emergency Public Health Laboratory Service of the relationship between the wartime rise in the non-pulmonary tuberculosis death-rates and the quality of the milk supply. A preliminary report in 1947 suggested that the nation's raw milk supply 'appears to be almost as heavily contaminated with tubercle bacilli now as it was twenty years ago'. In contrast to previous experience, the maximum incidence of infection with the bovine type of bacillus was in the 5–9 instead of the 0–4 age group. The report suggested that the greater care in infant feeding resulted in the partial protection of the pre-school child, while the introduction of the milk-in-schools scheme, without adequate measures to safeguard the purity of the milk, might have led to the increase in the proportion of bovine infection in older children. The conclusion of the report was that 'the value of this information for supporting the introduction of compulsory pasteurisation of all but TT milk needs no stressing'.[85] In 1948, E. R. Boland wrote,

It is amazing that this country, which claims, and I believe claims rightly, to be a pioneer and leader in hygiene and preventive medicine should lag behind other countries in the enforcement of this life-saving measure . . . Medical authorities, the Medical Research Council, the Royal College of Physicians, the BMA, and experts in hygiene have recommended its adoption for years . . .[86]

[84] *Public Health* (1940), 105–8.
[85] MRC, *Medical Research in War, Report 1939–45*, pp. 171–2; *Public Health* (1940), 105–8; Titmuss, *Problems of Social Policy*, p. 512.
[86] *BMJ* 2 (1948), 16.

Pasteurization was being extended in other countries at this time. In Sweden, a royal ordinance of 1937, which came into operation in 1939, made the pasteurization of all milk and cream, with the exception of adequately supervised raw milk, universal and compulsory. Pasteurization was extensively employed in larger towns in Germany by 1941. In France, a law imposing compulsory pasteurization (with some exceptions) for human consumption had been passed in 1935. Pasteurization was made compulsory in the Canadian province of Ontario in 1938 and by 1941 92 per cent of all milk in Ontario was said to be pasteurized.[87]

In Britain, by the Milk (Special Designations) Act of 1949, no milk was to be sold by retail in a given area except that which was designated under the categories 'Tuberculin-tested', 'Accredited' (for England and Wales) or 'Standard' (for Scotland), and 'Pasteurized'. 'Accredited' or 'Standard', which was only applicable when the milk came from a single herd, was to be phased out as a legal category after five years. The BMA Tuberculosis and Diseases of the Chest Group believed that when the Act was implemented it would go a long way towards solving the difficulties of bovine infection.[88] In 1960 the whole of Britain became an 'attested area' (that is with all milk pasteurized or tuberculin-tested).

(5) THE NATIONAL HEALTH SERVICE

During the Second World War, the JTC formed a committee on the reorganization of the tuberculosis services, at a time when medical and health services in general were being reviewed. In a report published in 1944, this committee stressed as important that administrators should deal with clinical work as well as with the social problems arising from tuberculosis.[89] In 1946, the committee commented on the Government's proposals to split the tuberculosis services so that public health aspects would be the responsibility of local health authorities, and clinical aspects would be managed by the regional hospital boards:

The Joint Tuberculosis Council regard the Minister's proposals as gravely

[87] G. S. Wilson, *The Pasteurization of Milk* (London, 1942), 71.
[88] PRO MH55/1163, BMA Chest Group, Nov. 1950, p. 6; *BMJ* 2 (1950), 1384; *NAPT Bulletin*, 11/4 (1949), 151.
[89] JTC Report on the Reorganization of the Tuberculosis Service, *Tubercle*, 25 (1944), 91.

inadequate and as constituting a danger to public health. They view with alarm the separation of the social, environmental and epidemiological aspects of tuberculosis from the purely clinical aspect. They hold strongly the view that the family and not the patient should be the unit. They reject the Minister's implied assumption that tuberculosis requires no differentiation from other diseases. No matter how the disease manifests itself in any individual . . . he requires prolonged special supervision of his mode of life and environment. This is essential, not merely for his own safety, but for the safety of the community. This special supervision should be the responsibility of someone with special knowledge of the disease and of each individual case.[90]

The committee believed that the best interests of the tuberculous patient and of the community would be served if the existing service were transferred intact to the new hospital organization.[91] F. Ridehalgh, Chief TO of the City of Leeds, also argued for a greater emphasis on public health work. The tuberculosis officer, in his view, was 'clinician, administrator, epidemiologist, and economist'; to his patient he was 'guide, philosopher, and friend'. He believed that there was a real danger that in concentrating on the clinical aspects of chest disease, the 'tuberculosis family' might be forgotten, and even predicted a rise in tuberculosis rates under the new service, with a return to 'the bad old days before 1912'.[92] The WNMA and the SMOH also attached great importance to keeping an integrated service.

Tuberculosis specialists were not, however, unanimous in their rejection of the proposals. Dispensaries were increasingly becoming centres for the diagnosis of diseases of the chest. Cases of non-pulmonary tuberculosis were not often referred to the tuberculosis officer, but rather to an orthopaedic or a genito-urinary surgeon, or occasionally to a skin specialist. According to the Medical Planning Research, this was the natural division of clinical medicine; specialists were more suitably divided on the basis of physiology or anatomy, rather than into departments dealing with single diseases. Not only were non-pulmonary cases rarely referred to dispensaries, but many pulmonary tuberculosis cases were regular attenders as artificial pneumothorax refills became an increasingly large part of dispensary work. Other chest conditions were also being diagnosed at the dispensaries; the proportion of new cases seen at the dispensaries of England and Wales in 1937 diagnosed as tuberculous was just over 25 per cent.[93] Thus, one favourable feature of the new scheme, in the

---

[90] *Tubercle*, 27 (1946), 120.
[91] Ibid.   [92] Ibid., 160–1.   [93] Ibid., 24 (1943), 160.

view of the editor of the *Tubercle*, was that tuberculosis officers would become chest physicians dealing with all chest conditions and would be in charge of chest clinics in hospitals.[94] The change in designation from tuberculosis officer to chest physician as well as from tuberculosis dispensary to chest clinic had been suggested before the war, and can be seen as part of the process of professionalization. In Bristol in 1937 tuberculosis dispensaries were centralized in a new health clinic with full X-ray apparatus, and at the same time, the words 'tuberculosis officer' and 'tuberculosis clinic' ('dispensary' having been previously discarded), were abandoned in favour of 'chest physician' and 'chest clinic'.[95] In 1934 the term 'dispensary' had been dropped in favour of 'tuberculosis and chest clinic' in East Ham, where Philip Ellman was not the 'tuberculosis officer' but the 'physician'. Ellman pointed out that, of those sent to the clinic as suspected cases of tuberculosis in 1933, only 28 per cent proved to be tuberculous.[96] In 1946 Ellman again argued in favour of changing the designation as well as location of dispensaries. With the existing location of the dispensaries, he claimed that tuberculosis was divorced from general medicine with the result that students had little opportunity to become familiar with the disease. Specialist chest units had been established at certain of the LCC and Emergency Medical Service hospitals during the war, and according to Ellman, closer consultation with pathologists, radiologists, thoracic and nose and throat surgeons, had proved of great advantage.[97]

The stigma attached to dispensaries was an important factor in the drive to change their names. Under the mass radiography schemes it was feared that those requiring follow-up examinations would be reluctant to attend a dispensary and would thereby jeopardize the success of the schemes. In 1942 the Standing Advisory Committee on Tuberculosis had resolved that, 'in view of the developments likely to be forthcoming from the mass radiographical examination of groups of the population, the time is appropriate for Local Authorities to be instructed to rename their centres for the diagnosis of chest diseases "chest clinics"'.[98] According to the *Tubercle*, the very name of tuberculosis officer upset prospective patients as would the name of cancer officer, if such a category of practitioner were to exist working in a cancer dispensary.[99]

[94] Ibid., 27 (1946), 120.   [95] *NAPT Bulletin*, 9/2 (1947), 40.
[96] 20 *NAPT 1934*, p. 74; *Tubercle*, 15 (1934), 375; P. Ellman, *Chest Disease in General Practice with Special Reference to Pulmonary Tuberculosis* (London, 1932), 163–6.
[97] *Tubercle*, 27 (1946), 88–9.
[98] PRO MH55/1183, TSAC, 9 Oct. 1942.   [99] *Tubercle*, 27 (1946), 120.

Under the NHS, the tuberculosis service, together with other local authority services such as the maternity and child welfare service, was disbanded. The NAPT did not greet the new service with applause. It feared that, under the service, the patient 'would drift, a homeless entity, a mere file of useless documents from one Authority to another'.[100] There were indeed several authorities involved in dealing with tuberculous patients. First were the regional hospital boards providing residential treatment; second were the local health authorities, responsible for preventive work and after-care but not allowed to provide monetary support. Third was the Ministry of National Insurance, which provided financial assistance following the termination of Memo 266/T. Fourth was the National Assistance Board, for those with special needs, and finally, the Ministry of Labour, which provided rehabilitation schemes.

The NAPT also predicted a substantial lowering in the standard of living of many tuberculous patients after July 1948 when National Insurance was introduced. It criticized the rigidity of National Insurance based on a flat rate, in contrast to the elasticity of Memo 266/T. It was maintained that Memo 266/T had not been a pension but an effective contribution towards medical treatment, that tuberculosis could not be lumped together with other diseases as it had special psychological and social consequences. The National Insurance rate was slightly less than Memo 266/T. The National Assistance Act of 1948 was designed to cater for specifically needy cases, but the NAPT believed it questionable whether patients would be likely to accept National Assistance any more readily than Public Assistance. As a consequence, according to the NAPT, after-care committees were even more important than they had been in the past. The *NAPT Bulletin* reported in 1947 that many health authorities were forming new tuberculosis care committees:

They are wise to do so, for otherwise next July may see a substantial lowering in the standard of life of many of our tuberculous patients, such as was not thought possible under Circular 266/T—much abused in its time, but now seen in the light of what is to come to be a humane and progressive charter of welfare, for so many of our tuberculous patients.[101]

With the introduction of the NHS in 1948, dispensaries became

[100] *NAPT Bulletin*, 8/6 (1946), 177.
[101] Ibid., 8/1 (1946), 22; see also ibid., 8/2, pp. 48, 50; ibid., 8/3, p. 45; ibid., 8/6, p. 22; ibid., 9/6 (1947), 146.

'chest clinics' overnight, 'whether they were in the cellars of a Town Hall or the out-patients of a General Hospital'.[102] Tuberculosis officers became chest physicians, with consultative and public health functions but with an emphasis on the former—eight-elevenths of their pay was to come from hospitals for their consultative work and three-elevenths from health authorities at a lower rate of remuneration for their public health duties. The emphasis was clearly on consultation. This did not pass without criticism. Robert Cavill Wofinden, deputy MO for Bristol, for example, argued that the 'chest physician' rather than the 'tuberculosis physician' would concern himself, in all probability, more and more with treatment and less and less with the preventive aspects of the disease, to the detriment of the services.[103] Andrew S. Semple, deputy MO for Liverpool, held that if cases were suitable for thoracic surgery, they were likely to receive it more adequately than in the past, but added that unfortunately the 'interesting cases' were the few and the more extensive or chronic cases the many. In his opinion the care of the latter, 'the social medicine of tuberculosis', had regressed.[104]

Thoracic surgery did develop in the 1940s. The Society of Thoracic Surgeons had been formed in 1938, although it did not hold its first meeting until 1946. However, facilities did not match the increased popularity of surgery, and despite the attempt to centralize thoracic surgery on a regional basis starting in 1939, there were still far too few thoracic surgeons to meet the need.[105] Artificial pneumothorax was developed more widely in the 1940s than before; Geoffrey Beven maintained that it was not until the 1940s that artificial pneumothorax really developed on a large scale in this country.[106] A possible reason for the increased use of the technique was that it did not require long periods of institutional treatment. After an initial period in an institution, patients could continue to receive the treatment by attending a dispensary. In this way, artificial pneumothorax was a contribution to the problem of the acute bed shortage. Artificial pneumothorax was also being carried out in the patients' homes to ease the accommodation problem. At one clinic, 60 out of 90 new patients were treated in their own homes by this method, enabling their applications for sanatorium accommodation to be cancelled, as well as

---

[102] *British Thoracic Association (The First Fifty Years)* (London, 1978), 43.
[103] *NAPT Bulletin*, 11/4 (1949), 143.
[104] Ibid., 12/2 (1950), 261–2; ibid., 12/3 (1950), 307–8.
[105] PRO MH55/1183, TSAC, 9 Oct. 1942.
[106] Dr G. Beven, interview, 27 Sept. 1984.

boosting their morale. Treatment in individual homes was not, however, a cheap solution.[107]

When the regional hospital boards took over the institutions in 1948 there was a waiting list of 9,000 patients and an average waiting period of 9 months. The Standing Advisory Committee on Tuberculosis recommended the use of general hospitals and isolation hospitals.[108] E. R. Boland believed that every general hospital should reserve 5 per cent of its beds for tuberculosis. He pointed out that there was no type of case for which it was so difficult to secure admission to the general hospital as the tuberculous case, largely because of the danger of infection, but also because many physicians regarded pulmonary tuberculosis as being as much outside their responsibility as syphilis.[109] G. E. Godber, Chief Medical Officer of the Ministry of Health, also noted the resistance by large general hospitals to the idea of converting 20 out of 200 beds for the use of tuberculous patients.[110] General hospitals were also possibly reluctant to have their beds occupied by chronic tuberculous patients at the expense of more 'interesting' cases.

In 1950 the BMA Tuberculosis and Diseases of the Chest Group, which had been set up after the war to deal with the medico-politics of the tuberculosis service, described the health services relating to tuberculosis as 'a national scandal'.[111] There were now 11,000 awaiting admission to the 27,000 beds provided for the treatment of the disease. The *Hospital* held that the problem of tuberculosis was among the most serious which faced the National Health Service at that time.[112] The Nursing Standing Advisory Committee recommended a scheme of secondment of student nurses to tuberculosis institutions for three months to alleviate the staffing shortage; the North West Metropolitan Board was one of the few to organize an effective secondment scheme.[113] In 1948 a special committee was set up to advise the Secretary of State for Scotland on tuberculosis in Scotland, where the crisis was particularly acute (Scotland experienced a death-rate from tuberculosis of 80 per 100,000 population at this time, compared to 55 for England and Wales). A scheme was started in 1951 to send patients from Britain to Switzerland for treatment to reduce the waiting list. The scheme originated in Scotland, and half of the £400,000 per

[107] *BMJ* 2 (1949), 151; ibid., 2 (1950), 1373.
[108] *CMOH Annual Report 1952* (1953), 99.
[109] *BMJ* 2 (1948), 18.
[110] PRO MH55/1158, G. E. Godber, 15 Aug. 1950.
[111] *BMJ* 2 (1950), 1382; *Lancet*, 2 (1950), 809; *British Thoracic Association*, p. 39.
[112] *Hospital* (1951), 47.   [113] Webster, *Problems of Health Care* (in press).

annum made available by the Exchequer for the scheme was reserved for Scottish cases. When the scheme came to an end in 1955, only 1,043 Scottish patients and 1,025 English and Welsh patients had been sent to Switzerland. The size of the scheme, and consequently its cost, was considerably less than was originally envisaged.[114]

The solution to the pressing bed shortage for cases of tuberculosis was to come, in the event, from an entirely unanticipated direction, primarily from the introduction of effective chemotherapy considerably reducing the recommended length of institutional treatment.

(6) CHEMOTHERAPY

The first effective anti-tuberculosis drug, streptomycin, was discovered in 1943 at the Department of Microbiology of the New Jersey Agricultural Experiment Station, Rutgers University, USA, by Selman A. Waksman, who was awarded a Nobel Prize for it in 1952. Laboratory and clinical experiments were immediately undertaken at the Mayo Clinic, University of Minnesota, by W. H. Feldman and H. C. Hinshaw, showing enormous success. In Britain, the MRC set up a Streptomycin Committee in September 1946. In December 1946, 50 kilograms of streptomycin were bought from America, enough to treat up to 200 cases. Domestic supplies were not fully established until 1949, by which time over 350 kilograms had been purchased from America at a cost of almost £1 million.[115]

The MRC decided to conduct a 'rigorously planned investigation with concurrent controls', because of past difficulties in assessing tuberculosis treatment (for example, sanocrysin, as previously discussed). The type of patient to be investigated was carefully defined as 'acute progressive bilateral pulmonary tuberculosis of presumably recent origin, bacteriologically proved, unsuitable for collapse therapy, aged 15 to 25 [later extended to 30]'. The selection of this type of patient was justified as a parallel series of patients would be receiving the only other available treatment for that type of patient at the time—bed-rest. It was also pointed out that there was not enough streptomycin to treat all patients in any case.

The first patients were admitted in January 1947 to the chosen

---

[114] *CMOH Annual Report 1951* (1952), 83; *CMOH Annual Report 1955* (1956), 102; *Department of Health for Scotland Annual Report 1956*, p. 30.
[115] *BMJ* 2 (1948), 276.

centres—the Brompton and Colindale Hospitals in London, and Harefield Hospital in Middlesex. After three months, when the trials committee still had not found enough patients in the London and Middlesex areas, it approached local authorities in Wales and Scotland. Also included were patients from a hospital in Leeds, and from another in London. The trial included 107 patients, 55 allocated to the streptomycin group and 52 to the control group.

Determination of whether a patient would be treated by streptomycin and bed-rest or by bed-rest alone was made by reference to a statistical series based on random sampling numbers drawn up for each sex at each centre by A. (later Sir Austin) Bradford Hill, honorary director of the MRC's Statistical Research Unit and professor of medical statistics at the London School of Hygiene and Tropical Medicine. The details of the series were unknown to any of the investigators. Patients were not told before admission that they were to get special treatment. Control patients did not know throughout their stay in hospital that they were controls in a special study. Clinicians were asked to adopt collapse therapy only if the course of the disease so changed that such therapy became indispensable and urgent—this happened in none of the streptomycin cases and in 5 of the control cases.

The trial lasted six months. The results were analysed by changes in radiographic appearances. These were assessed by a panel of three without knowledge of whether the films being viewed were those of streptomycin or control patients. The overall results left no doubt as to the beneficial effect of streptomycin. Seven per cent of the streptomycin patients died before the end of six months and 27 per cent of the controls, a statistically significant difference. Considerable improvements were noted in 51 per cent of the streptomycin cases and 8 per cent of the controls. The results were published in the *BMJ* in October 1948. It was noted that this was the first controlled investigation of its kind to be reported and quite apart from the results, would serve as a model for other such studies.[116]

Investigations were also being undertaken into tuberculous meningitis and miliary tuberculosis, organized by the MRC and the Ministry of Health, in London, Liverpool, and Glasgow. No controls were used in these investigations as no cure had previously been available.[117] Initially only children up to the age of 7 were accepted for treatment.

[116] *BMJ* 2 (1948), 769–82.
[117] *EMJ* 42 (1935), 130.

In September 1947, the MRC published preliminary results stating that, as available supplies of streptomycin permitted, patients suffering from tuberculous meningitis and miliary tuberculosis should be given the opportunity of receiving treatment with the drug. The number of beds for this treatment was extremely limited however, only 150 in 1947 rising to 200 in 1948.[118]

Early in the trials, the *BMJ* published a particularly unfavourable appraisal of the new drug:

The evidence of the trials already made in America leaves it at present quite uncertain whether streptomycin will prove, in the long run, to have greater therapeutic value in tuberculosis, and it may eventually be decided that the chief clinical uses of the drug lie in the treatment of certain other infections resistant to penicillin. The results of American and limited British tests of streptomycin in tuberculous meningitis have, in particular, been far less encouraging than was previously hoped; there seems to be a very real risk that, even if the infection is controlled (as has only very rarely happened) the patient will usually be left mentally deficient, deaf, blind, or otherwise a hopeless invalid.[119]

This pessimism was probably a response to the publicity the drug had previously been given, leading to demands for the drug, sometimes quite desperate and far exceeding supplies.[120]

Subsequent reports assumed a quite different tone. For example, in 1950, a report from a hospital in Dublin, Ireland, claimed that prior to the introduction of streptomycin, 300 cases of tuberculous meningitis had been treated in the wards in 13 years. All of these cases died in deepening coma within two or three weeks of admission. With streptomycin 1 in every 4–5 cases recovered from the disease provided that treatment was undertaken early and not abandoned too soon.[121]

However, scepticism of the new drug persisted among the medical profession. The Ministry of Health pointed out in 1950, 'There appears to be a belief prevalent among medical practitioners that streptomycin treatment does no more than prolong life or produce "recovery" as a physical and mental wreck. This is not true.' A Ministry of Health investigation had shown a 40 per cent recovery rate among cases treated early, as opposed to the previous 100 per cent

---

[118] *BMJ* 1 (1948), 131.
[119] Ibid., 2 (1946), 906; see also D. A. Mitchison, *NAPT Bulletin*, 10/2 (1948), 52, and ibid., 10/3 (1948), 83.
[120] *BMJ* 2 (1946), 906; ibid., 2 (1947), 138; ibid., 2 (1948), 276.
[121] *Tubercle*, 31 (1950), 210.

mortality. The Ministry advised medical practitioners who doubted the efficacy of the treatment to visit some of the special units treating these patients.[122]

In the treatment of pulmonary tuberculosis with streptomycin, a new problem arose which was the appearance of streptomycin-resistant strains of bacilli. This caused a general fear that those who developed streptomycin-resistant strains could become a serious public health risk by passing on the resistant strain to others. However, this problem was solved by combining streptomycin with another recently discovered drug, para-amino-salicylic acid, PAS. PAS was first shown to have a pronounced reaction on the tubercle bacillus by Jürgen Lehmann of Sweden by 1946. This discovery did not, however, at that time receive as much publicity as streptomycin. In 1948, the MRC undertook a second controlled trial to assess the new drug. The same type of case was used as in the first trial, and patients were grouped randomly for various combinations of drugs: streptomycin alone, PAS alone, or both drugs. Eleven hospitals were involved in the trials which lasted three months. It was demonstrated unequivocally that the combination of PAS and streptomycin prevented the development of streptomycin-resistant strains of the tubercle bacillus.[123] Anti-tuberculosis chemotherapy continued to develop, although surgery and sanatorium treatment remained more orthodox for tuberculosis at least until 1960.

As late as 1962 at a conference on tuberculosis treatment, two thoracic surgeons, H. D. Teare and Sir Clement Price Thomas, attempted to persuade their audience that there was still a place for surgery in the treatment of pulmonary tuberculosis. They advocated operations combined with chemotherapy as an alternative to a prolonged course of chemotherapy (the minimum length was generally six months), although J. G. Scadding (director of studies at the Institute of Diseases of the Chest, Brompton Hospital), pointed out that there was no statistical proof that surgery affected the final outcome. F. C. Edwards, thoracic surgeon for the Liverpool and Welsh Regional Hospital Boards, believed that surgery had a place in modern treatment. He worked in an industrial area with a strong Irish element: 'These patients are temperamentally undisciplined from the point of view of taking drugs, and also racially they are very susceptible to the disease . . . the intelligence of many of them, often women, who

---

[122] *Tubercle*, 31 (1950), 214; see also *EMJ* 87 (1950), 161.
[123] *BMJ* 2 (1949), 1521.

are procreating children at a vast rate, is low, and they literally have not time to take nor appetite for these drugs.'[124] Nevertheless, surgery for pulmonary tuberculosis was becoming redundant, 'to the greater comfort of the patients'.[125] Thoracic surgeons increasingly directed their attention to heart surgery. When the Final Report of the National Survey on Major Surgery for Pulmonary Tuberculosis was published in 1964, it was a final report in more senses than one. At the start of the survey in 1953, it was common to combine surgery with chemotherapy, as shown by the inclusion of over 8,000 cases in the study receiving an operation from 1953 to 1954. But by 1958, experience with more prolonged chemotherapy led to a questioning of the necessity for surgical intervention. The Report concluded that surgery was only of value in cases of difficult-patient control and drug resistance, primarily in places of 'lower standards of living and of social discipline'.[126]

(7) THE NATIONAL TUBERCULOSIS SERVICE: AN ASSESSMENT

Chemotherapy was indeed a revolution in the tuberculosis world, held largely responsible for a dramatic decline of 97 per cent in death-rates from tuberculosis—from 430 per million in 1950 in Britain to 14 per million in 1974. Yet chemotherapy was only responsible for the final dropping off in the mortality rates from tuberculosis. On Thomas McKeown's calculations it was responsible for 3.2 per cent of the total decline in the period 1848 to 1971.[127] The disease was declining throughout the twentieth century, so that the Government's White Paper on the National Health Service in 1944 could claim that the tuberculosis service had 'very tangible results to its credit over the last twenty years reflected in improvements in the rate of mortality from the disease'. Similarly, a history of the WNMA claimed, 'There were few families in Wales without reason for gratitude to the WNMA.'[128]

---

[124] *Tubercle*, 43 (1962), Suppl., 49.
[125] *British Thoracic Association*, p. 62.
[126] *Tubercle*, 45 (1964), 67–8.
[127] T. McKeown, *The Role of Medicine: Dream, Mirage or Nemesis?* (Oxford, 1979), 93. His calculation is, however, highly speculative, as it is based on the assumption that the rate of decline before 1950 would have continued unaltered into the following decades had chemotherapy not intervened.
[128] Ministry of Health, Department of Health for Scotland, *A National Health Service*,

The tuberculosis service had been created in the early twentieth century as a result of a changing direction in public health. Public health in the nineteenth century had been primarily concerned with attempts to control the environment through sanitary engineering. By the early twentieth century, the focus was beginning to shift to the health of the individual. It was the Boer War of 1899–1902 in South Africa which was largely responsible for elevating individual health to a position of national importance. The rejection of a third of the recruits for medical reasons led to some concern about the state of the physical health of the British population and its effect on national efficiency. The epidemic diseases which had ravaged Britain in the nineteenth century were disappearing or declining, yet ill-health was clearly still widespread. The heightened concern for the health of the individual in the name of 'national efficiency' was given expression in particular in three health movements: an infant welfare movement, the school medical service, and the tuberculosis service. Infants and children became an object of concern as the next generation of fighters and workers. Tuberculosis attracted attention primarily as the number one killer of adults, the most productive age group.

Much of the attention of the tuberculosis service throughout the period was devoted to providing a curative service, particularly in the case of the WNMA. There was great faith in the value of institutional treatment in the early twentieth century, which was initially responsible for attracting considerable voluntary and State aid. The president of the (American) NTA could assert in 1914, 'Scientific medicine can no longer be reproached with helplessness in combating consumption. It now places at the command of the physician an extensive armamentarium of efficient, well-tried weapons.'[129] The confidence of the period was related to the development of the science of bacteriology, supplying medical practitioners with a sound, scientific, theoretical framework for their craft. However, bacteriology did not lead to a specific cure for tuberculosis, as was increasingly realized. By the inter-war period tuberculosis was even said by some to be incurable. Yet by this time an elaborate and expensive structure of institutions for the treatment of tuberculosis had been created which supported a new profession of medical specialists. Treatment

Cmd. 6502 (1944), 60; G. R. Jones, in J. Cule (ed.), *Wales and Medicine* (London, 1975), 36–7.

[129] L. F. Flick, *Consumption: A Curable and Preventable Disease: What a Layman Should Know*, 7th edn. (London, 1914), 209.

consisted of teaching or imposing an altered mode of life, the main ingredient of which, in Britain at least, was work therapy. Work therapy was similar to moral therapy practised in nineteenth-century mental asylums, and did equally little to enhance the specialist status of its practitioners. This was an important reason for the adoption of collapse therapy, which, involving technology and special skills, brought tuberculosis treatment more into line with orthodox twentieth-century medicine. However, there is no evidence that collapse therapy had any major effect on the course of the disease.

As the strength of the tuberculosis service could not be said to lie in treatment, one must look to preventive services for its impact. Discussing the role of immunization, Winter concludes, 'Active immunization procedure dates from the pioneering work of Jenner and Pasteur, but was extended in this century for the treatment of typhoid, cholera and tuberculosis . . . few would deny the importance of the role of immunization in preventing a serious recrudescence of these killer diseases during the political and economic upheavals of this century.'[130] Yet during those upheavals—the First World War, the economic depression of the inter-war period, and even the Second World War—BCG was not used in Britain, and therefore the role of immunization in the diminishing tuberculosis rates before 1950 must be denied.

The medical historian W. H. McNeill pointed to 1921 as the date for the introduction of an effective anti-tuberculosis vaccine, ignoring the fact that in Britain at least, it was another thirty years before it was used on any scale. According to McNeill,

long before [that date], new knowledge of how the disease propagated itself, and systematic efforts to isolate sufferers from consumption in sanatoria, together with such simple methods of prophylaxis as slaughtering milk cattle found to harbour tubercle bacilli and prohibition of spitting in public places, had done a good deal to hasten the retreat of pulmonary forms of the infection from Western countries.[131]

In fact, one could argue that long after that date, such attempts had still had little impact. Tuberculosis institutions were not effective in isolating the source of infection. Eradication by isolation was recognized as impractical because of the slowness and incompleteness

[130] J. M. Winter, 'The Decline of Mortality in Britain, 1870–1950', in T. Barker and M. Drake (eds.), *Population and Society in Britain 1850–1980* (London, 1982), 111–12.
[131] W. H. McNeill, *Plagues and People* (Oxford, 1977), 283.

of diagnosis, and the chronicity of the disease meant that patients would sometimes have to be isolated for a very long time. Most institutions in any case attempted to attract early 'curable' cases rather than the chronic and more infectious cases. Local authorities did not make use of their statutory powers of isolating infectious cases compulsorily, possibly partly because this involved local authority maintenance of dependants while the patient was in the institution, but in any case they did not have the necessary accommodation. It was estimated in 1941 that there were 77,000 infectious cases of tuberculosis in England alone, for which there were 28,087 beds.[132] The ratio was even greater in earlier decades. Despite legislation relating to the slaughter of tuberculous cattle, little action was taken in this direction before the Second World War. The NAPT did have an active anti-spitting campaign in the early twentieth century. However, spitting was still relatively prevalent in the 1930s,[133] and anti-spitting warning signs in public places, especially on buses, were almost universal in cities up to around the 1960s suggesting that the habit had not been (still has not been) totally eradicated.

As in the area of infant welfare work, preventive measures for tuberculosis concentrated primarily on education, particularly the education of wives and mothers. Such work was carried out by the NAPT, the WNMA, and health visitors. The NAPT stressed above all fresh air, yet they did not become involved in the smoke pollution campaign which was thriving in the 1920s. Their attention was directed to the reformation of the personal habits of the people. It is difficult to assess the influence of such work. How seriously was the NAPT taken? Was the advice of health visitors heeded, or did they evoke the same resentment as the Frimley almoner sometimes did? One of the objections to notification was that it involved intrusion into homes by officials, indicating that such officials were not always welcomed.

Another major focus of the tuberculosis preventive campaign was 'pre-tuberculous' children. This may seem surprising at first in view of the relatively low incidence of tuberculosis among children. However, it must be seen in the context of the early twentieth-century school hygiene movement, itself related to concern for national efficiency and

---

[132] *Tubercle*, 23 (1942), 30–1.
[133] PRO MH75/15, Chalke Report, unrevised, 1931, pp. 33, 61, 87; J. Guy, in C. W. Hutt and H. H. Thomson (eds.), *Principles and Practice of Preventive Medicine*, i (London, 1935), 368.

the general health of the nation, as has been noted. Children were to be made healthy and strong to prevent disease from developing at a later stage, by being temporarily boarded out in the country and by attending open-air schools. The anti-tuberculosis campaign with its emphasis on fresh air exerted an important influence on school policy, specifically the development in the inter-war period of the pavilion-type elementary school and outdoor physical education. With children, as with their parents, the focus of the anti-tuberculosis campaign was primarily on education. Boarding out of children was generally in the hands of local voluntary after-care committees, not actually falling within the ambit of local authority tuberculosis services.

Possibly the most useful unit in the tuberculosis service was the after-care committee which provided material support for patients and their families, and acted primarily as a charitable organization despite official instructions that such committees were not to become another organ of public assistance. The number of committees in existence and their ability to provide assistance varied greatly from area to area. Support given by local authorities to this work also varied considerably. Some local authorities also sponsored housing and employment schemes for tuberculous patients, but such schemes were generally small, sporadic, and unrelated to local need. The WNMA, in particular, neglected this area in favour of providing a curative service. After-care was also relatively neglected in Scotland.

Thus, if the national tuberculosis service had any impact on declining tuberculosis rates, it was first in the very nebulous area of health education and secondly in the work of the voluntary after-care committees which received little State support. If the service did not contribute substantially to the decline in death-rates, neither did it provide adequate care for advanced cases. Possibly the most serious indictment of the service was the neglect of advanced or chronic cases who had no hope of recovering their working capacity.

As a result of a fear of an increase of tuberculosis under war conditions during the Second World War, preventive efforts were intensified. In particular, a scheme for the detection of early cases through mass radiography was launched, and national allowances and rehabilitation schemes for tuberculous patients were introduced. Yet once again the focus was on those who could be restored to working capacity; 'national efficiency' was the motivating factor. The allowances were also kept low, in keeping with the 'less eligibility' principle which underlay social policy in general in this period. Two other preventive measures which received serious consideration for the first time, were pasteurization and BCG, although their implementation was delayed until the 1950s, well after the war.

(8) EXIT TB?

Largely as a result of effective chemotherapy starting in the early 1950s, together with mass radiography through which early cases were detected, by 1955 the waiting list for tuberculosis treatment in England and Wales had dropped to below 2,500 with a considerably shortened waiting period. In the following year the waiting list was virtually eliminated. By 1955, there was a surplus of tuberculosis beds in Scotland. Yet mass radiography units continued to operate, with 70 in operation in England and Wales in 1954, and 10 in Scotland. In the Sheffield region the number of miniature X-ray examinations increased from 109,000 in 1950 to 354,000 in 1957. Increasingly the service concentrated on intensive campaigns in areas with above-average incidence, such as Liverpool and Glasgow. Mass radiography was also increasingly involved with screening for conditions other than tuberculosis, in particular industrial lung disease and lung cancer. Chest physicians gradually became diverted towards these latter conditions. Mass radiography of the general public ceased in 1969.[134]

By the early 1960s, at a time when deaths from lung cancer had begun to exceed those from pulmonary tuberculosis, many of the institutions themselves had been closed or converted to other purposes. While drug treatment required hospitalization, the period was considerably shortened and there seemed no need for special open-air treatment. Under the National Health Service, Papworth Village Settlement and Preston Hall were divided into hospitals under regional hospital boards, and industrial concerns under private ownership. In 1957, Papworth admitted disabled persons in general to the industries, and the hospital expanded to include other chest and heart conditions. The NAPT altered its constitution in 1956 to include non-tuberculous diseases of the chest and heart within its purview.[135] The TA (now BTA) similarly became involved with diseases other than tuberculosis after 1956, although the name of the Association was

---

[134] *British Thoracic Association*, p. 76; see also Webster, *Problems of Health Care* (in press).

[135] *NAPT Handbook*, 15th edn. (London, 1957), p. viii.

not changed until 1968 when it became the British Thoracic and Tuberculosis Association (becoming the British Thoracic Association in 1977).

Chemotherapy facilitated a change in the public image of the tuberculous patient, by lessening the dread of the disease. Nevertheless, as late as 1960, a JTC survey discovered attitudes of 'ostracism and prejudice' to be common. It was noted in the survey that the greatest difficulty was in getting the first job after a long absence from work and that patients were frequently rejected, on grounds of 'doubtful validity', as soon as the reason for such absence became known. Chest physicians were thought to be sometimes responsible for the difficulties experienced by ex-patients, as a result of prescribing light work or part-time work which might not be strictly necessary or attainable in the area. It was also pointed out that ex-patients were handicapped with respect to life assurance and emigration.[136]

In the 1960s, tuberculosis increasingly became a problem associated with recent arrivals to Britain from the New Commonwealth: the Indian sub-continent, the West Indies, and Africa. In 1965 it was discovered that while immigrants formed 4 per cent of the total population of Britain, they provided 16.5 per cent of the tuberculosis notifications. Incidence of tuberculosis, as shown by notifications, was among Pakistanis 26 times that of the local population, among Indians 12 times, among other Asians 6 times, and among Caribbean Islanders 3 times that of the British-born.[137] A survey in 1971 showed that while there was a decrease of 43 per cent in the number of notifications of tuberculosis in that year as compared with 1965, there was a 68 per cent increase from among those born in India, Pakistan, and New Commonwealth countries in Africa. Forming 5 per cent of the population, immigrants now accounted for 32 per cent of the tuberculosis notifications. The notifications among Pakistanis were 54 times those of the local population, among Indians 27 times, and among Africans 10 times. It was not known whether their disease was active on arrival, or whether new disease was acquired after arrival, or quiescent disease reactivated, since neither a chest radiograph nor a tuberculin test was obligatory on entering Britain.[138] Screening had been advocated since 1953 when the subject was raised by the Standing Advisory Council on Tuberculosis. X-ray apparatus was installed at Heathrow Airport, London, in 1965, but was described as only 'partly successful' and

---

[136] *Tubercle*, 41 (1960), 370–5.   [137] Ibid., 47 (1966), 145.
[138] *BMJ* 3 (1971), 362; *Tubercle*, 54 (1973), 249; Ibid., 65 (1984), 83–91.

soon abandoned as impracticable.[139] In 1978–9, notification among immigrants was 50 times higher than that among the local population.[140] Despite the fact that tuberculosis was now curable by chemotherapy, it was still responsible for 2,000 deaths annually in England and Wales by 1970. A survey of tuberculosis deaths in that year concluded that diagnostic error was responsible for 20 per cent of the deaths investigated, 'mismanagement in hospital' (mainly among the elderly) for 40 per cent, and patients were thought to be responsible for their own deaths in the remaining 40 per cent as a result of failure to seek medical advice. This study considered medical education to be deficient in the field of tuberculosis.[141]

Another study reported in 1983 by the MRC Tuberculosis and Chest Diseases Unit, found that tuberculosis notification rates were still much higher among recent arrivals from the Indian sub-continent. This report attached greater weight to socio-economic conditions than to race in its explanation of the high rates. It was noted that in general the population of Indian sub-continent ethnic origin was less well housed than the white population and was concentrated in boroughs of poorer socio-economic status. The high rates among the white ethnic groups in these boroughs, according to the study, were also more likely to be a reflection of poor socio-economic conditions than the proximity of the Indian ethnic groups.[142]

In 1986 a Vaccination Sub-committee of the Department of Health and Social Security recommended that the BCG vaccination scheme in schools be abandoned by 1990 and replaced by a more selective scheme giving BCG vaccine to the neonates of Afro-Asian parents, Afro-Asian immigrants, and those who, because of their work or residence abroad, had above-average risk of infection. This committee believed that the number of additional notifications as a result of stopping routine vaccination of school children would be small. The suggestion provoked critical response; for example, R. B. Buttery of the Cambridge Health Authority wrote of selective BCG vaccination, 'although we may have a "mind's eye" picture of the typical high risk family, the precise definition of high risk groups is extremely difficult'. He was reluctant to replace a successful scheme (with a 97 per cent

---

[139] *BMJ* 2 (1979), 189.
[140] *Tubercle*, 63 (1982), 75–88, 158–65.
[141] *BMJ* 2 (1971), 419; *Tubercle*, 52 (1971), 1.
[142] MRC, Tuberculosis and Chest Diseases Unit, *Report on the Geographical Distribution of Tuberculosis Notification in a National Survey of England and Wales in 1983* (reference supplied by J. M. McCarthy), 12–13.

takeup in schools) with some vague and undefined scheme for vaccinating high-risk groups. He pointed out that young people were often mobile, so that the problem was not restricted to areas with particular ethnic groups.[143] Two correspondents to the *BMJ* from the Royal Hospital for Sick Children, Glasgow, also reminded their readers that the indigenous population continued to be at risk from tuberculosis. They pointed out that in Britain in 1985 there were still 5,930 notified cases of tuberculosis and 492 deaths.[144]

Contrary to the confident predictions of the early twentieth century that tuberculosis would be wiped out within a generation, in the last quarter of the twentieth century the prevailing belief is that the disease is never likely to disappear entirely (with some predicting the development of drug-resistant strains).[145] However, as long as chemotherapy does remain effective, tuberculosis is not likely to re-emerge as the social problem it was before 1960 in Britain. Since the anti-tuberculosis campaign subsided, tuberculous patients have been left in peace to cope with the new regimen of drug treatment (admittedly still with problems, but of a different nature). Draughts and physical labour are no longer imposed. The stress of the anti-tuberculosis campaign on open-air work, reflecting a national near-obsession with fresh air, must have subjected some patients to much hardship. But possibly more importantly, the anti-tuberculosis propaganda in which infection figured so prominently (coupled with a deep-seated belief in hereditary predisposition) increased the fear and stigma attached to the disease and its victims. The resultant secrecy surrounding the disease, of which there is much evidence in the Frimley Sanatorium follow-up records, indicates a profound sense of shame at having contracted the disease. Tuberculosis had indeed become a crime, as in Samuel Butler's *Erewhon* (1872), as well as, in Wingfield's words, a 'life sentence'; tuberculosis was both the crime and the punishment. The social reality of tuberculosis in twentieth-century Britain differed drastically from its nineteenth-century romantic image.

[143] *BMJ* 2 (1986), 956.
[144] Ibid., 760.
[145] *Tubercle*, 63 (1982), 158–65; G. P. Youmans, *Tuberculosis* (Philadelphia, 1979), 2.

BIBLIOGRAPHY

I. UNPUBLISHED

(A) ARCHIVAL

Bodleian Library, Oxford

Addison (Christopher) Collection.
NAPT Propaganda Literature, 1930–8.
NAPT Miscellaneous Publications, 1944–58.
E. and H. Carling, 'Peppard Hospital, A Short History', 1938, followed by 'A Summary of Events, 1938–1970', 1970.

British Film Institute Archives, London

'Air and Sun' (NAPT), 1924.
'Papworth Village Settlement' (British Council), 1945.
'The Story of John M'Neil' (NAPT), 1911.

Cambridgeshire County Record Office

Cambridgeshire CC Public Health Committee Tuberculosis Sub-committee Minute Books, 1921–48.
Mr and Mrs F. W. A. Ives, 'The History of Papworth', 1958.
Winifred Janes, 'History of Papworth Everard', 1946.
Papworth Village Settlement, Annual Reports of Committee of Management, 1925, 1942–5.

Cardiothoracic Institute (associated with the National Heart and Chest Hospitals), University of London

Marcus Paterson Collection, 1905–10.

Chest, Heart and Stroke Association (formerly NAPT), London

NAPT, Council Reports, 1913–50, Minute Books, 1899–1950, and Sub-committees' Minute Books, 1931–7.
NAPT, Catalogue of Exhibits at the Tuberculosis Exhibition, Town Hall, Reading, 1911.
Transactions of NAPT Annual Conference, London, 19 July 1911.

Churchill Hospital, Headington, Oxford

Oxfordshire Branch of NAPT, Annual Reports, 1910–48, and Minute Books, 1910–53.
Press cuttings.

East Sussex Record Office, Lewes

Darvell Hall Sanatorium Medical Superintendent, Annual Reports, 1929–49.
—— Committee of Management, Minute Books, 1921–48.
—— Visiting Committee, Report Books, 1929–59.
—— Publications and photographs, including Sanatorium magazines and 'Coronation Souvenir', 1953.
East Sussex CC, 'Tuberculosis, General', 1932–8.
Eversfield Hospital, Annual Reports, 1884–1947.
—— Council of Management, Minute Books, 1884–1945.
—— 'The Jubilee of Eversfield', 1934; press cuttings, 1887–1933.
—— Patients' records, 1940–50.
Tuberculosis Care Committee for Borough of Hastings, Annual Reports, 1918–48, and Minute Books, 1918–48.

King Edward VII Hospital, Midhurst, Sussex

Annual Reports, 1906–11, 1930–9.
'A Brief History', *c.*1978.
Consulting Staff Reports, 1906–13, and Minute Books, 1906–35.
N. D. Bardswell's scrapbook on opening of King's Sanatorium, 1906.

Medical Research Council ('Committee' before 1920), London

Files relating to tuberculosis, 1913–50.

Northumberland County Record Office

Records of Stannington Hall Sanatorium.

Papworth Village Settlement Archives, Papworth Everard, Cambridgeshire

Annual Reports, 1917–43.
Press cuttings, visitors' accounts, patients' accounts, Papworth magazines, 1917–79.

Public Record Office, Kew, London

Local Authority files relating to tuberculosis, 1919–50 (MH 52).
Local Government Board files relating to tuberculosis, 1910–19 (MH55).
Ministry of Health files relating to tuberculosis, 1919–50 (MH55).
WBH and WNMA files relating to tuberculosis, 1911–50 (MH75, MH96).

Radcliffe Infirmary, Oxford

Annual Reports, 1926–39.
Committee of Management Minutes, 1917–48.
N. J. England, 'Tuberculosis in Oxfordshire and the Development of the Tuberculosis Service 1934–59' (typescript, 1960).
Scrapbook of press cuttings.

Royal Berkshire Hospital, Reading

Berks. and Bucks. Joint Sanatorium, Peppard Common, Committee Minute Books, 1943–8.

Royal British Legion Industries (Preston Hall) Incorp., Kent

Annual Reports, 1925–46.
Council of Management Minutes (including medical superintendent's monthly reports), 1925–43.

Royal Hospital of St Bartholomew, London

Papers relating to Henry Philbrick Nelson, thoracic surgeon at Papworth, 1930–6.

Wellcome Unit for the History of Medicine, Oxford

Brompton Hospital Sanatorium, Frimley, clinical records, 1906–31.
—— Patient follow-up records, 1906–59.
—— Nurses and Servants: Engagement Book 1904–51.
—— General correspondence, 1910–48.
Papers relating to H. D. Chalke.
T. E. Jones Davies, 'A Study of the Incidence and Epidemiology of Tuberculous Infection in the Elementary School Population of the County of Radnor, Report to Radnor Education Committee' (typescript, 1943).
Society of Medical Officers of Health, Tuberculosis Group, Minute Books, 1920–57, and Metropolitan Sub-group of Tuberculosis Group, Minute Books, 1922–39.

Miscellaneous

J. R. Bignall, MS notes for book, *Frimley: The a Biography of a Sanatorium* (London, 1979), 1976–8, in author's possession.
Lady Pedlar, 'The Maitland Story, A Pioneer Fight Against Tuberculosis in This Country Between 1897–1957, c.1968, in author's possession.

(B) INTERVIEWS

Mrs Suzanne Beven and Dr Geoffrey Beven, 27 Sept. 1984.
Dr J. R. Bignall, 5 July 1983.
Miss Kathleen Colgate, 1 Oct. 1984.
Miss Margaret Coltart, 9 Jan. 1984.
Mrs Goozee, 23 Mar. 1983.
Dr P. D'Arcy Hart, 20 May 1983.
Mrs Kathleen Liddall Hart, 3 July 1984.
Dr P. J. D. Heaf, 15 July 1983.
Dr John Hurford, 29 Sept. 1983.
Mr Harold and Mrs Doris Huffer, 23 Mar. 1983.
Frank Jordan, 23 Mar. 1983.
Mr Norman and Mrs Dorothy Langdon, 23 Mar. 1983.
Drs F. J. W. and S. M. Miller, 22 Feb. 1986.
Dr Walter Pagel, 6 Mar. 1983.
Lady Pedlar and Mrs F. C. Carling, 20 Mar. 1984.
Mr Charlie Stockford and Mrs Stockford, 22 June 1983.
Dr W. E. Snell, 27 June 1983.
Sir Geoffrey Todd, 25 Aug. 1983.
Sir Graham Wilson, 3 June 1986.

(C) UNPUBLISHED THESES

Bryder, L., 'The Problem of Tuberculosis in England and Wales, 1900–1950', D.Phil. thesis, Oxford, 1985.
Cairns, M., 'The History of Pulmonary Tuberculosis in the Boot and Shoe Industry and its Relation to Social Conditions', D.Phil. thesis, Oxford, 1953.
McCarthy, J. M., '"Tuberculosis" Before and After Waksman', Dissertation, BA (General) Health and Community Studies, Chester College, 1986.
McGuaign, K. M., 'The Campaign against Tuberculosis in Canada, 1900–1950', MA thesis, McGill University Montreal, 1979.

2. PUBLISHED SOURCES

(A) PERIODICALS

American Review of Tuberculosis (Baltimore).
Archives of Disease in Childhood (London).

British Journal of Social Medicine (London).
British Journal of Tuberculosis (London).
British Medical Journal (London).
Diseases of the Chest (El Paso, Texas).
Edinburgh Medical Journal (Edinburgh).
Glasgow Medical Journal (Glasgow).
Hospital (London).
Hospital Gazette (London).
Journal of Hygiene (Cambridge).
Journal of the Royal Statistical Society (London).
Journal of State Medicine (London).
Journal of Thoracic Surgery (St Louis).
Lancet (London).
Manchester Guardian (Manchester).
Medical Classics (Baltimore).
Medical Officer (London).
Medicine, Today and Tomorrow (London).
Morning Post (London).
National Association for the Prevention of Tuberculosis Bulletin (London).
National Association for the Prevention of Tuberculosis, Transactions of the Annual Conferences (London).
Practitioner (London).
Public Health (London).
South Wales Argus and Monmouthshire Daily (Newport, Monmouthshire).
The Times (London).
Tubercle (London)
Tuberculosis: Journal of the National Association for the Prevention of Tuberculosis (London).
Western Mail and South Wales News (Cardiff).

(B) OFFICIAL PUBLICATIONS (PUBLISHED BY HMSO, LONDON)

(1) *Periodical Reports (Special Reports listed separately)*

Cambridgeshire CC Medical Officer, *Annual Reports*, 1919–49.
Chief Medical Officer of the Ministry of Health, *Annual Reports*, 1919–50.
Lancashire CC, *Reports of the Central Tuberculosis Officer of the Lancashire County Council*, 1926–32.
Local Government Board Annual Reports, Supplements: *Reports of Medical Officer*, 1905–19.
Medical Research Council, *Annual Reports*, 1914–50.
Ministry of Health, *Annual Reports*, 1919–50.
Oxfordshire CC Medical Officer, *Annual Reports*, 1919–49.

Registrar-General, *Statistical Review of England and Wales, Text* and *Tables, Part I, Medical,* 1901–50.

——*Decennial Supplement, England and Wales, 1921, Part 2, Occupational Mortality, Fertility & Infant Mortality* (1927); ibid., 1931 (1938).

——*Decennial Supplement, England and Wales, 1951, Occupational Mortality,* Part 1 (1954).

Registrar-General for Scotland, *Annual Reports,* 1901–50.

Scottish Board of Health, *Annual Reports,* 1919–28; Scottish Department of Health, *Annual Reports,* 1929–45.

(2) Special Reports on Tuberculosis

Departmental Committee on Tuberculosis, Chairman Lord Astor, *Interim Report,* Cd. 6164 (1912); *Final Report,* i, Cd. 6641 (1913); ibid., ii, Cd. 6654 (1913).

Greenwood, M., 'Epidemiology of Pulmonary Tuberculosis', *Annual Report of Chief Medical Officer of the Ministry of Health, 1919–20,* Cmd. 978 (1920), Appendix 5, pp. 322–48.

Inter-departmental Committee Appointed to Consider and Report upon the Immediate Practical Steps Which Should be Taken for the Provision of Residential Treatment for Discharged Soldiers and Sailors Suffering from Pulmonary Tuberculosis and for their Re-introduction into Employment, Especially on the Land, Final Report, Chairman: Lord Astor, Vice-chairman who presided: Sir Montague Barlow, Cmd. 317 (1919).

International Congress on Tuberculosis 1905: Report of C. Theodore Williams and H. Timbrell Bulstrode, the Delegates of His Majesty's Government to the International Congress on Tuberculosis held at Paris 2–7 October 1905, Cd. 2898 (1906).

International Congress on Tuberculosis 1908: Report of the British Delegates to the International Congress on Tuberculosis held at Washington, 21 September–3 October 1908 (A. Newsholme, J. P. MacDougall, T. J. Stafford), Cd. 4508 (1909).

List of Institutions Approved by the Welsh Insurance Commissioners under the National Insurance Acts, 1911 to 1913, for the Treatment of Persons Suffering from Tuberculosis and Resident in Wales (Including Monmouthshire), Cd. 7804 (1915).

Local Government Board, *List of Sanatoria and Other Residential Institutions Approved by the Local Government Board under the National Insurance Act, 1911, for the Treatment of Persons Suffering from Tuberculosis, and Resident in England (excluding Monmouthshire), with the Names of the Administrative Counties and County Boroughs in which the Institutions are Situate, and the Date on Which the Approval Expires in Each Case* (1918).

Local Government Board, H. Timbrell Bulstrode, *35th Annual Report 1905–6, Supplement in Continuation of the Report of the Medical Officer for 1905–6, On*

Sanatoria for Consumption, and Certain Other Aspects of the Tuberculosis Question, Cd. 3657 (1908).

Ministry of Health, *A Memorandum on Bovine Tuberculosis in Man with Special Reference to Infection by Milk* (Reports on Public Health and Medical Subjects, 63; 1931).

—— *Report of the Committee of Inquiry into the Anti-tuberculosis Service in Wales and Monmouthshire*, Chairman: Clement Davies (1939).

—— A. S. MacNalty, *A Report on Tuberculosis, Including an Examination of the Results of Sanatorium Treatment* (Reports on Public Health and Medical Subjects, 64; 1932).

—— T. W. Wade, *A Report of an Investigation into the Alleged High Mortality Rate from Tuberculosis of the Respiratory System among Slate Quarrymen and Slate Workers in the Gwyrfai Rural District* (Reports in Public Health and Medical Subjects, 38; 1927).

Ministry of National Insurance, *Report of the Industrial Injuries Advisory Council in accordance with Section 61 of the National Insurance (Industrial Injuries) Act, 1946, on the Question of Whether Tuberculosis and Other Communicable Diseases Should be Prescribed under the Act in Relation to Nurses and Other Health Workers*, Chairman: Sir Wilfrid Garrett, Cmd. 8093 (1950).

Oxfordshire CC, *Annual Report of the County Health Service*, Part II, Report by the CMO (H. C. Jennings), 'An Inquiry into Some Factors Affecting the Incidence of Tuberculosis in the County of Oxford' (1933).

Royal Commission Appointed to Inquire into the Relations of Human and Animal Tuberculosis, Part 1, Final Report, Cd. 5761 (1911).

(3) *Other Reports and Official Publications*

Hancock, W. K. (ed.), *History of the Second World War (UK) Civil Series:*
Titmuss, R. M., *Problems of Social Policy* (1950).
Ferguson, S. and Fitzgerald, H., *Studies in the Social Services* (1954).

Inter-departmental Committee on Nursing Services Interim Report, Chairman: Earl of Athlone (1939).

Inter-departmental Committee on Physical Deterioration, Report, vol. i, Cd. 2175 (1904).

MacNalty, A. S., *History of the Second World War (UK) Medical Series:*
Cope, V. Z. (ed.), *Medicine and Pathology* (1952).
Dunn, C. L. (ed.), *The Emergency Medical Services*, i and ii (1952 and 1953).
Green, F. H. K. and Covell, G. (ed.), *Medical Research* (1953).
MacNalty, A. S. (ed.), *Civilian Health and Medical Services* (1953).

Macpherson, W. G., Leishman, W. B., and Cummins, S. L. (eds.), *History of the Great War: Medical Services: Pathology* (1923).

Mines Department, Sutherland, C. H. and Bryson, S., *Report of an Inquiry into the Occurrence of Disease of the Lungs from Dust Inhalation in the Slate Industry in the Gwyrfai District* (1930).

Ministry of Agriculture and Fisheries, *Report of the Reorganisation Commission on Milk*, Chairman: Sir Edward Grigg, (Economic Series 38, 1933).

Ministry of Food, *Report of the Committee on Milk Distribution*, Cmd. 7414 (1948).

Ministry of Health, Department of Health for Scotland, *A National Health Service*, Cmd. 6502 (1944).

—— Department of Health for Scotland and Ministry of Labour and National Service, *Report of the Working Party on the Recruitment and Training of Nurses*, Chairman: Sir Robert Wood (1947).

—— *First Report of Nurses' Salaries Committee: Salaries and Emoluments of Female Nurses in Hospitals*, Chairman: Lord Rushcliffe, Cmd. 6424 (1943).

—— Newman, G., *An Outline of the Practice of Preventive Medicine, a Memorandum to the Minister of Health* (1926).

Ministry of Works, *The Welsh Slate Industry, Report by a Committee appointed by the Ministry of Works*, Chairman: Sir F. Rees (1947).

Report of the Royal Commission on the Poor Laws and Relief of Distress, Cd. 4499 (1909).

Webster, C., *Problems of Health Care: The British National Health Service before 1957* (in press).

(4) *Medical Research Council (Committee 1913–20) Special Report Series:*

Bardswell, N. D. and Thompson, J. H. R., *Pulmonary Tuberculosis: Mortality after Sanatorium Treatment*, 33 (1919).

Bentley, F. J., *Artificial Pneumothorax: Experience of the London County Council*, 215 (1936).

Blacklock, J. W. S., *Tuberculous Disease in Children: its Pathology and Bacteriology*, 172 (1932).

Brownlee, J., *An Investigation into the Epidemiology of Phthisis in Great Britain and Ireland*, Parts 1 and 2, 18 (1917), Part 3, 46 (1920).

Burrell, L. S. T. and MacNalty, A. S., *Report on Artificial Pneumothorax*, 67 (1922).

Buxton, J. B. and MacNalty, A. S., *The Intradermal Tuberculin Test in Cattle: Collected Results of Experience*, 122 (1928).

Clark, K. C., Hart, P. D'Arcy, Kerley, P. and Thompson, B. C., *Mass Miniature Radiography of Civilians for the Detection of Pulmonary Tuberculosis (Guide to Administration and Technique with a Mobile Apparatus using 35-mm Film, and Results of a Survey)*, 251 (1945).

Dawson of Penn, Viscount, (chairman), Hart, P. D'Arcy (secretary), *Report of the Committee on Tuberculosis in War-time*, 246 (1942).

First Report of the Special Investigation Committee upon the Incidence of Phthisis in Relation to Occupations: The Boot and Shoe Industry, 1 (1915).

Greenwood, M. and Tebb, A. E., *An Inquiry into the Prevalence and Aetiology of*

Tuberculosis among Industrial Workers, with Special Reference to Female Munition Workers, 22 (1918).

Griffith, A. S., *Studies of Proection against Tuberculosis: Results with BCG Vaccine in Monkeys*, 152 (1931).

Hart, P. D'Arcy, *The Value of Tuberculin Tests in Man, with Special Reference to the Intracutaneous Test*, 164 (1932).

Hart, P. D'Arcy and Aslett, E. A. with contributions by D. Hicks and R. Yates, *Chronic Pulmonary Disease in South Wales Coalminers, Part 1, Medical Studies, (B) Medical Survey*, 243, part 1 (1942).

Hartley, P. H.-S., Wingfield, R. C., and Thompson, J. H. R., *An Inquiry into the After-histories of Patients Treated at the Brompton Hospital Sanatorium at Frimley, During the Years 1905–14*, 85 (1924).

Hill, A. B., *An Investigation into the Sickness Experience of Printers (with special reference to the incidence of Tuberculosis)*, MRC with Industrial Fatigue Research Board, 54 (1929).

Hill, L. E., *The Science of Ventilation and Open-air Treatment*, Part 1, 32 (1919), Part 2, 52 (1920).

Jordan, L., *The Eradication of Bovine Tuberculosis*, 184 (1933).

Scott, H. H., *Tuberculosis in Man and Lower Animals*, 149 (1930).

Tuberculin Committee, *Tuberculin Tests in Cattle, with Special Reference to the Intradermal Test*, 94 (1925).

Vallow, H., *Tuberculosis in Insured Persons Accepted for Treatment by the City of Bradford Health Committee*, 76 (1924).

Wilson, G. S., *Tuberculous Bacillaemia: A Review*, 182 (1933).

(C) BOOKS AND ARTICLES

ABEL-SMITH, B., *A History of the Nursing Profession* (London, 1960).
—— *The Hospitals* (London, 1964).

ALLSOP, J., *Health Policy and the National Health Service* (London, 1984).

AYERS, G. M., *England's First State Hospitals and the Metropolitan Asylums Board 1867–1930* (London, 1971).

BARDSWELL, N. D., *The Consumptive Working Man: What Can Sanatoria Do for Him?* (London, 1906).
—— (ed.), *The Tuberculosis Clinic* (London, 1922).
—— *Urban Work Centres for the Tuberculous: The Experience of the Spero Firewood Factory, London* (London, 1930).
—— and CHAPMAN, J. E., *Diets in Tuberculosis: Principles and Economics* (London, 1908).

BENTLEY, F. J., GRZYBOWSKI, S., and BENJAMIN, B., *Tuberculosis in Childhood and Adolescence, with Special Reference to the Pulmonary Form of the Disease* (London, 1954).

BIGNALL, J. R., 'A Century of Treating Tuberculosis', *Tubercle*, 63 (1982), 19–22.

—— *Frimley: The Biography of a Sanatorium* (London, 1979).

—— 'Treating Tuberculosis in 1905: The First Patients at the Brompton Hospital Sanatorium', *Tubercle*, 58 (1977), 43–52.

BISHOP, P. J., 'Some Curiosities of the Literature of Tuberculosis', *Tubercle*, 55 (1974), 153–62.

—— 'Some Recent Papers on the History of Tuberculosis', *Tubercle*, 46 (1965), 301–7.

—— 'The History of the Brompton Hospital', *Transactions and Studies of the College of Physicians, Philadelphia* (Medical and History Series V, 3; 1979), 171–82.

—— 'The Marcus Paterson Collection', *Tubercle*, 48 (1967), 63–74.

BODINGTON, G., *An Essay on the Treatment and Cure of Pulmonary Consumption: On Principles Natural, Rational and Successful, with Suggestions for an Improved Plan of Treatment of the Disease among the Lower Classes of Society; and a Relation of Several Successive Cases Restored from the Last Stage of Consumption to a Good State of Health* (London, 1840); repr. with Preface by A. E. Bodington (Lichfield, 1906).

BOLDERSON, H., 'The Origins of the Disabled Persons Employment Quota and its Symbolic Significance', *Journal of Social Policy*, 9 (1980), 169–86.

BRADBURY, F. C. S., *Causal Factors in Tuberculosis* (London, 1932).

BRANDT, A. M., *No Magic Bullet: A Social History of Venereal Disease in the US since 1880* (New York, 1985).

BREND, W. A, *Health and the State* (London, 1917).

BRIEGER, E. M., *The Papworth Families, a Twenty-Five Years' Survey* (London, 1944).

British Congress on Tuberculosis 1901, *Transactions*, 4 vols. (London, 1902).

British Thoracic Association (The First Fifty Years) (London, 1978).

BROCKINGTON, C. F., *A Short History of Public Health*, 2nd edn. (London, 1966).

BROWN, L., *The Story of Clinical Tuberculosis* (Baltimore, 1941).

BRYDER, L., 'Papworth Village Settlement: a Unique Experiment in the Treatment and Care of the Tuberculous?', *Medical History*, 28 (1984), 372–90.

—— 'Occupational therapy and tuberculosis', *SSHM Bulletin* 40 (1987), 64–6.

—— 'The First World War: Healthy or Hungry?', *History Workshop Journal* 24 (1987), 141–57.

—— 'The King Edward VII Welsh National Memorial Association and its Policy towards Tuberculosis in Wales, 1910–48', *The Welsh History Review*, 13/2 (1986), 194–216.

—— 'Tuberculosis and the Medical Research Council, 1911–39', *SSHM Bulletin*, 37 (1985), 68–72.

—— 'Tuberculosis as a Romantic Disease: Sontag and Others', *SSHM Bulletin*, 38 (1986), 84.

—— 'Tuberculosis, Silicosis and the North Wales Slate Industry', in P. Weindling (ed.), *The Social History of Occupational Health* (London, 1986).

BUNYAN, J., *The Life and Death of Mr Badman* (London, 1680), ed. John Brown (Cambridge, 1905).

BURN, J. L., *Recent Advances in Public Health* (London, 1947); 2nd edn. (1959).

BURNET, M. and WHITE, D. O., *Natural History of Infectious Disease*, 4th edn. (Cambridge, 1972).

BURRELL, L. S. T., *Artificial Pneumothorax* (London, 1932); 3rd edn. (London, 1937).

—— *Recent Advances in Pulmonary Tuberculosis* (London, 1929); 2nd edn. (London, 1931).

BURTON-FANNING, F. W., *The Open-air treatment of Pulmonary Tuberculosis* (London, 1905); 2nd edn. (London, 1909).

CAMERON, V. and LONG, E. R., *Tuberculosis Medical Research, The National Tuberculosis Association 1904–55* (New York, 1959).

CARR-SAUNDERS, A. M., JONES, D. CARADOG, and MOSER, C. A., *A Survey of Social Conditions in England and Wales* (Oxford, 1958).

CARTWRIGHT, F. F., *A Social History of Medicine* (London, 1977).

CHADWICK, H. D. and POPE, A. S., *The Modern Attack on Tuberculosis* (New York, 1942).

CHALKE, H. D., 'The Impact of Tuberculosis in Literature, History and Art', *Medical History*, 6 (1962), 301–18.

CLARK, H., *The Dispensary Treatment of Pulmonary Tuberculosis* (London, 1915).

CLARKE, B. R., *The Causes and Prevention of Tuberculosis* (Edinburgh, 1952).

COBBETT, L., *The Causes of Tuberculosis, Together with Some Account of the Prevalence and Distribution of the Disease* (Cambridge, 1917).

COLE, G. D. H. and M. I., *The Condition of Britain* (London, 1937).

COLEBROOK, L., *Almroth Wright: Provocative Doctor and Thinker* (London, 1954).

COLLINS, J. J., 'The Contribution of Medical Measures to the Decline of Mortality from Respiratory Tuberculosis: an Age–Period–Cohort Model', *Demography*, 19/3 (1982), 409–27.

COLTART, M., RAINE, H., and HARRISON, E., *Social Work in Tuberculosis* (London, 1959).

COOK, G. A., *A Hackney Memory Chest* (London, 1983).

COOTER, R., *The Making of Modern Orthopaedics: A Social History 1881–1945* (forthcoming).

COPE, V. Z., *Almroth Wright: Founder of Modern Vaccine-Therapy* (London, 1966).

CRONJÉ, G., 'Tuberculosis and mortality decline in England and Wales, 1851–1910', in R. Woods and R. Woodward (eds.), *Urban Disease and Mortality in Nineteenth-Century England* (London, 1984).

CROWTHER, M. A., *The Workhouse System 1834–1929: The History of an English Social Institution* (London, 1981).

CUMMINS, S. L., *Tuberculosis in History from the Seventeenth Century to our own Times* (London, 1949).

DANIELS, M., RIDEHALGH, F., SPRINGETT, V. H., and HALL, I. M., *Tuberculosis in Young Adults, Report on the Prophit Tuberculosis Survey 1935–1944*, Royal College of Physicians (London, 1948).

DAVIDSON, M., *A Practical Manual of Diseases of the Chest*, 2nd edn. (London, 1941); 3rd edn. (London, 1948); 4th edn. (London, 1954).

DAVIES, C., *Rewriting Nursing History* (London, 1980).

DAVIES, H. M., *Pulmonary Tuberculosis: Medical and Surgical Treatment* (London, 1933).

DAVIN, A., 'Imperialism and Motherhood', *History Workshop Journal* 5 (1978), 9–65.

DICK, A., *A Walking Miracle* (London, 1942).

DRUMMOND, J. C. and WILBRAHAM, A., *The Englishman's Food: A History of Five Centuries of Diet* (London, 1939), revised edn. (London, 1957).

DUBOS, R. and J., *The White Plague: Tuberculosis, Man and Society* (London, 1953).

DWORK, D., 'The Milk Option: An Aspect of the History of the Infant Welfare Movement in England 1898–1908', *Medical History*, 31 (1987), 51–69.

—— *War is Good for Babies and other Young Children: A History of the Infant and Child Welfare Movement in England 1898–1918* (London, 1987).

DYHOUSE, C., 'Working-class Mothers and Infant Mortality in England, 1895–1914', *Journal of Social History*, 12 (1978), 248–67.

ELLIS, A. E., *The Rack* (Harmondsworth, 1958).

ELLMAN, P., *Chest Disease in General Practice with Special Reference to Pulmonary Tuberculosis* (London, 1932).

ERWIN, G. S., *A Guide for the Tuberculous Patient* (London, 1944), 2nd revised edn. (London, 1946).

—— *Tuberculosis and Chest Diseases for Nurses* (London, 1946).

EYRE, J. G., *Tuberculosis Nursing* (London, 1949); 2nd edn. (London, 1957).

FLAVELL, G., *An Introduction to Chest Surgery* (London, 1957).

FLICK, L. F., *Consumption: A Curable and Preventable Disease: What a Layman Should Know*, 7th edn. (London, 1914).

—— *Development of Our Knowledge of Tuberculosis* (Philadelphia, 1925).

FLINN, M. W. (ed.), *Scottish Population History from the Nineteenth Century to the 1930s* (Cambridge, 1977).

FOSTER, W. D., *A History of Medical Bacteriology and Immunology* (London, 1970).

FOSTER-CARTER, G. S., MYERS, M., GODDARD, D. F. H., YOUNG, F. H., and BENJAMIN, B., *The Results of Collapse and Conservative Therapy in Pulmonary Tuberculosis: A Statistical Survey with Special Reference to Artificial Pneumothorax, by the Research Department of the Brompton Hospital* (London, 1946).

FOWLER, J. K., *Arrested Pulmonary Tuberculosis* (London, 1892).
—— *Problems in Tuberculosis* (London, 1923).
—— *Pulmonary Tuberculosis* (London, 1921).
—— and GODLEE, R. J., *The Diseases of the Lungs* (London, 1898).
FRASER, D., *The Evolution of the British Welfare State* (London, 1973).
FRAZER, W. M., *History of English Public Health* (London, 1950).
FRIED, A. and ELMAN, R. M. (eds.), *Charles Booth's London* (London, 1969).
GAFFNEY, R., 'Poor Law Hospitals 1845–1914', in O. Checkland and M. Lamb (eds.), *Health Care as Social History: the Glasgow Case* (Aberdeen, 1982).
GARLAND, C. H. and LISTER, T. D., *Sanatoria for the People: The State Campaign against Consumption* (London, 1911).
GIBBON, G. and BELL, R. W., *History of the London County Council 1889–1939* (London, 1939).
GILBERT, B. B., *British Social Policy 1914–1939* (London, 1970).
—— *The Evolution of National Insurance in Great Britain. The Origins of the Welfare State* (London, 1966).
GLOVER, J. R. *et al.*, 'Effects of Exposure to Slate Dust in North Wales', *British Journal of Industrial Medicine* 37 (1980), 152–62.
GLOYNE, S. R., *Social Aspects of Tuberculosis* (London, 1944).
GOFFMAN, E., *Asylums: Essays on the Social Situation of Mental Patients and Other Inmates* (Harmondsworth, 1961).
—— *Stigma: Notes on the Management of Spoiled Identity* (New York, 1974).
GRACEY, D. R. and ADDINGTON, W. W., *Tuberculosis (Discussions in Patient Management)* (New York, 1979).
GRANGE, J. M. and BISHOP, P. J., '"Über Tuberkulose": A Tribute to Robert Koch's Discovery of the Tubercle Bacillus, 1882', *Tubercle*, 63 (1982), 3–17.
GREENWOOD, M., *Epidemics and Crowd-diseases: An Introduction to the Study of Epidemiology* (London, 1935).
HARDY, A., 'Diagnosis, Death and Diet; The Case of London, 1750–1909', *Journal of Interdisciplinary History* (1987, in press).
HARRIS, J. *Unemployment and Politics: A Study in English Social Policy 1886–1914* (Oxford, 1972).
HART, P. D'ARCY and WRIGHT, G. P., *Tuberculosis and Social Conditions in England with Special Reference to Young Adults, a Statistical Study* (London, 1939).
HEAF, F. R. G. (ed.), *Symposium of Tuberculosis* (London, 1957).
—— and RUSBY, N. L., *Modern Advances in Pulmonary Tuberculosis*, 4th edn. (London, 1948).
HEWINS, A, *Mary, After the Queen: Memories of a Working Girl* (Oxford, 1986).
HOLTBY, W., *The Land of Green Ginger* (London, 1927).
HONIGSBAUM, F., *The Division of British Medicine: A History of the Separation of General Practice from Hospital Care 1911–1968* (London, 1979).

HOUGHTON, L. E. and SELLORS, T. H., *Aids to Tuberculosis Nursing: A Complete Textbook for the Nurse*, 1st edn. (London, 1945); 3rd edn. (London, 1949).

HOWARD, E., *Garden Cities of Tomorrow*, 2nd edn. (London, 1902).

HOWE, G. M., *Man, Environment and Disease in Britain: A Medical Geography through the Ages* (New York, 1972).

HUTT, C. W. and THOMSON, H. H. (ed.), *Principles and Practice of Preventive Medicine*, i and ii (London, 1935).

IGNATIEFF, M., 'Total Institutions and Working Classes, A Review Essay', *History Workshop Journal*, 15 (1983), 107.

IRVINE, K. N., *BCG and Vole Vaccination: a Practical Handbook*, 1st edn. (London, 1954), 2nd edn. (London, 1957).

—— *BCG Vaccination in Theory and Practice* (London, 1949).

—— *BCG Vaccine* (London, 1934).

JONES, G. R., 'The King Edward VII Welsh National Memorial Association, 1912–48', in J. Cule (ed.), *Wales and Medicine* (London, 1975), 30–41.

KAYNE, G. G., *The Control of Tuberculosis in England: Past and Present* (Oxford, 1937).

—— PAGEL, W., and O'SHAUGHNESSY, L., *Pulmonary Tuberculosis* (London, 1939).

KEERS, R. Y., *Pulmonary Tuberculosis: A Journey down the Centuries* (London, 1978).

KELYNACK, T. N., *The Sanatorium Treatment of Consumption* (London, 1904).

—— (ed.), *Tuberculosis in Infancy and Childhood: Its Pathology, Prevention and Treatment* (London, 1908).

—— (ed.), *Tuberculosis Yearbook and Sanatoria Annual* i, *1913–14* (London, 1914).

KENNEDY, I., *The Unmasking of Medicine: A Searching Look at Health Care Today* (London, 1981).

KING, L. S., *Medical Thinking: A Historical Preface* (Princeton, 1982).

Lancet, The, *Commission on Nursing, Final Report* (London, 1932).

LARGE, S. E., *King Edward VII Hospital Midhurst 1901–1986* (Chichester, 1986).

LATHAM, A. and GARLAND, C. H., *The Conquest of Consumption* (London, 1910).

—— in association with A. W. West, *The Prize Essay on the Erection of the King Edward VII Sanatorium for Consumption* (London, 1903).

LEWIS, J., 'The Peckham Health Centre, "An Inquiry into the Nature of Living"', *SSHM Bulletin, 30–1* (1982), 39–43.,

—— *The Politics of Motherhood* (London, 1980).

—— and BROOKES, B., 'The Peckham Health Centre, "PEP", and the Concept of General Practice during the 1930s and 1940s', *Medical History*, 27 (1983), 151–61.

LEFF, S., *Social Medicine* (London, 1953).

LOGAN, W. P. D., 'Mortality in England and Wales from 1848–1947', *Population Studies* (1950), 132–78.

LOWE, R. A., 'The Medical Profession and School Designs in England, 1902–14', *Paedagogica Historica*, 13/2 (1973), 425–44.

LUCKIN, B., 'Towards a Social History of Institutionalization', *Social History*, 8/1 (1983), 87–94.

MACASSEY, L. and SALEEBY, C. W. (ed.), *Spahlinger 'contra' Tuberculosis 1908–1934: An International Tribute* (London, 1934).

McBRIDE, D., 'The Henry Phipps Institute, 1903–1937: Pioneering Tuberculosis Work with an Urban Minority', *Bulletin of the History of Medicine*, 61 (1987), 78–97.

MACDONALD, B., *The Plague and I*, 3rd impr. (London, 1949).

McDOUGALL, J. B., *Tuberculosis, a Global Study in Social Pathology* (Edinburgh, 1949).

MACGREGOR, A., *Public Health in Glasgow 1905–1946* (Edinburgh and London, 1967).

McKEOWN, T., *The Modern Rise of Population* (London, 1976).

—— *The Role of Medicine: Dream, Mirage or Nemesis?* (Oxford, 1979).

McLACHLAN, G. and McKEOWN, T. (eds.), *Medical History and Medical Care: A Symposium of Perspectives* (London, 1971).

McNALLY, C. E., *Public Ill Health* (London, 1935).

McNEILL, W. H., *Plagues and People* (Oxford, 1977).

MACNICOL, J., *The Movement for Family Allowances 1918–1945: A Study in Social Policy Development* (London, 1980).

MANN, T., *The Magic Mountain*, trans. H. T. Lowe-Porter, 2 vols. (London, 1927; repr. 1979).

MARSHALL, J. D. assisted by M. E. McClintock, *The History of the Lancashire County Council, 1889–1974* (London, 1977).

MEACHEN, G. N., *A Short History of Tuberculosis* (London, 1936, repr. 1978).

MEADE, G. M., 'Edward Livingstone Trudeau', *Tubercle*, 53 (1972), 229–50.

MESS, H. A., *Industrial Tyneside: A Social Survey made for the Bureau of Social Research for Tyneside* (London, 1928).

M'GONIGLE, G. C. M. and KIRBY, J., *Poverty and Public Health* (London, 1936).

MITCHELL, M., 'The Effects of Unemployment on the Social Condition of Women and Children in the 1930s', *History Workshop Journal*, 19 (1985), 105–27.

MOORE, D. F., 'The History and Development of the BCG', *The Practitioner*, 227 (1983), 317.

MORRIS, R. O., *Tuberculosis*, and A. E. Cummins, *Home Visiting, Red Cross Society 7A* (London, 1922).

MURRAY, W. A, *A Life Worth Living, Fifty Years in Medicine* (Haddington, 1981).

MYERS, J. A., 'Eighty Years after the First Glimpse of the Tubercle Bacillus', *Diseases of the Chest*, 51 (1967), 500–19.

—— *Man's Greatest Victory over Tuberculosis* (Springfield, Ill. and Baltimore 1940).

National Association for the Prevention of Tuberculosis, *Chemotherapy in the Treatment of Tuberculosis, Papers of a Post-graduate Course for Doctors held by the Tuberculosis Educational Institute, Cambridge 1953* (London, 1954).

—— *Handbook of Tuberculosis Schemes in Great Britain and Ireland*, 2nd edn. (London, 1919); 5th edn. (London, 1927, 6th edn. (London, 1931); 7th edn. (London, 1933); 8th edn. (London, 1935); 10th edn. (London, 1939); 15th edn. (London, 1957).

—— *Historical Sketch 1898–1926* (London, 1926).

—— *Statistical Charts 1919–1923* (London, 1925).

—— *Tuberculosis in Industry, by the Tuberculosis Educational Institute* (London, 1951).

—— and Committee for the Study of Social Medicine, *Report of the Joint Committee set up to Enquire into the Income and Food Expenditure of Tuberculous Households in War-time*, Chairman: Lissant Cox (London, 1944).

NEWMAN, G., *Bacteriology and the Public Health*, 3rd edn. (London, 1904).

—— *The Building of a Nation's Health* (London, 1939).

—— *The Health of the State, Social Service Handbook* 2 (London, 1907).

NEWSHOLME, A., *Fifty Years of Public Health: A Personal Narrative with Comments* (London, 1935).

—— *Health Problems in Organized Society: Studies in the Social Aspect of Public Health* (London, 1927).

—— *Medicine and the State: The Relation between the Private and Official Practice of Medicine with Special Reference to Public Health* (London, 1932).

OAKLEY, A., *The Captured Womb: A History of the Medical Care of Pregnant Women* (Oxford, 1984).

ODDY, D. J., 'The health of the people', in T. Barker and M. Drake (eds.), *Population and Society in Britain 1850–1980* (London, 1982), 121–39.

OSWALD, N., 'In My Own Time: Tuberculosis', *British Medical Journal*, 1 (1979), 188–9.

PAGEL, W., SIMMONDS, R. A. H., MACDONALD, N., and NASSAU, E., *Pulmonary Tuberculosis, Bacteriology, Pathology, Diagnosis, Management, Epidemiology and Prevention*, 1st edn. (London, 1939); 4th edn. (London, 1964).

PARISH, H. J., *A History of Immunization* (London and Edinburgh, 1965).

PARKER, R., *On the Road: The Papworth Story* (Cambridge, 1977).

PARRY, N. and McNAIR, D. (eds.), *The Fitness of the Nation: Physical and Health Education in the Nineteenth and Twentieth Centuries: History of Education Society Conference Papers 1982* (Leicester, 1983).

PATERSON, M. S., *Auto-inoculation in Pulmonary Tuberculosis* (London, 1911).

—— *The Shibboleths of Tuberculosis* (London, 1920).

PATTISON, H. A., *Rehabilitation of the Tuberculous*, 3rd edn. (New York, 1949).

PEARSON, K., *Department of Applied Mathematics, University College, University of London, Drapers' Company Research Memoirs, Studies in National Deterioration II, A First Study of the Statistics of Pulmonary Tuberculosis* (London, 1907).

PEARSON, S. V., *Men, Medicine and Myself* (London, 1946).

—— *The State Provision of Sanatoriums* (Cambridge, 1913).

PENNINGTON, C., 'Tuberculosis', in O. Checkland and M. Lamb (eds.), *Health Care as Social History: the Glasgow Case* (Aberdeen, 1982).

PHILIP, R., *Collected Papers on Tuberculosis* (Oxford, 1937).

PINKER, R., *English Hospital Statistics* (London, 1966).

Political and Economic Planning, *Report on the British Health Services* (London, 1937).

—— *Report on the British Social Services*, (London, 1937).

POSNER, E., 'Half a Century after the Magic Mountain', *History of Medicine*, 7/1 and 2 (1976), 55.

POWELL, R. D., *On Diseases of the Lungs and Pleurae, including Consumption*, 3rd edn. (London, 1886); 4th edn. (London, 1893); 5th edn. with P. H.-S. Hartley (London, 1911); 6th edn. with P. H.-S. Hartley (London, 1921).

POWLES, J., 'On the Limitations of Modern Medicine', *Science, Medicine and Man*, 1 (1973), 1–30.

PRICE, F. W., *A Textbook of the Practice of Medicine*, 7th edn. (Oxford, 1947).

QUIGLEY, H. and GOLDIE, I., *Housing and Slum Clearance in London* (London, 1934).

RAW, N., *The Control of Bovine Tuberculosis in Man* (London, 1937).

RICE, M. S., *Working-class Wives* (London, 1939).

RIVIÈRE, C., *The Early Diagnosis of Tubercle* (London, 1914); 2nd edn. (London, 1919); 3rd edn. (London, 1921).

—— *The Pneumothorax Treatment of Pulmonary Tuberculosis* (London, 1917); 2nd edn. (1927).

—— and MORLAND, E., *Tuberculin Treatment* (London, 1912); 2nd edn. (London, 1913).

—— *Tuberculosis and How to Avoid It* (London, 1917).

ROBSON, W. A., *The Development of Local Government*, 2nd edn. (London, 1948).

ROLLESTON, H. (ed.), *After-Care and Rehabilitation* (London, 1943).

—— *The Right Honourable Sir Thomas Clifford Albutt, A Memoir* (London, 1929).

ROLLIER, A., *The Healer: 'How to Fight Tuberculosis'*, trans. A. E. Gloyn and M. Yearsley, People's League of Health (London, 1925).

ROSENKRANTZ, B. G., 'The Trouble with Bovine Tuberculosis', *Bulletin of the History of Medicine*, 59 (1985), 155–75.

ROSENTHAL, S. R. (ed.), *BCG Vaccine: Tuberculosis–Cancer*, 2nd edn. (Littleton, Mass., 1980).

ROWNTREE, B. S., *Poverty and Progress: A Second Social Survey of York* (London, 1941).

Royal College of Nursing, *Nursing Reconstruction Committee Report*, Chairman: Lord Horder (London, 1943).

SAVAGE, W. G., *The Prevention of Human Tuberculosis of Bovine Origin* (London, 1929).

SCOTT, R. B. (ed.), *Price's Textbook of the Practice of Medicine*, 12th edn. (Oxford, 1978).

SCULL, A. (ed.), *Madhouses, Mad-doctors and Madmen: The Social History of Psychiatry in the Victorian Era* (London, 1981).

SEABORNE, M. and LOWE, R., *The English School—its Architecture and Organization* ii, *1870–1970* (London, 1977).

SHYROCK, R. H., *American Medical Research: Past and Present* (New York, 1947).

—— *The Development of Modern Medicine: An Interpretation of the Social and Scientific Factors Involved* (London, 1936; repr. 1979).

—— *The History of Nursing: An Interpretation of the Social and Scientific Factors Involved* (Philadelphia, 1959).

—— *Medicine in America, Historical Essays* (Baltimore, 1966).

SINGER, C. and UNDERWOOD, E. A., *A Short History of Medicine*, 2nd edn. (Oxford, 1962).

SMITH, F. B., 'Gullible's Travails: Tuberculosis and Quackery 1890–1930', *Journal of Contemporary History*, 20 (1985), 733–56.

—— *The People's Health 1830–1910* (London, 1979).

SONTAG, S., *Illness as Metaphor* (New York, 1977).

SPRIGGS, E. A., 'Rest and Exercise in Pulmonary Tuberculosis: A Study of Fashions in Treatment', *Tubercle*, 41 (1960), 455–62.

STARR, P., *The Social Transformation of American Medicine. The Rise of a Sovereign Profession and the Making of a Vast Industry* (New York, 1982).

SUTCLIFFE, A. (ed.), *British Town Planning: The Formative Years* (Leicester, 1981).

SUTHERLAND, H. G. (ed.), *The Control and Eradication of Tuberculosis: A Series of International Studies* (Edinburgh, 1911).

—— *The Tuberculin Handbook* (Oxford, 1936).

SWAN, P., 'History of Tuberculosis. The Romantics' Death', *Nursing Times*, (13–19 March 1985), 47.

TAYLOR, R., *Medicine Out of Control: The Anatomy of a Malignant Technology* (Sydney, 1979).

TAYLOR, R., *Saranac: America's Magic Mountain* (Boston, 1985).

TAYLOR, S., *Battle for Health: A Primer of Social Medicine* (London, 1944).

THANE, P., *The Foundations of the Welfare State* (London, 1982).

THOMSON, A. L., *Half a Century of Medical Research*, i, *Origins and Policy of the Medical Research Council (UK)* (London, 1973).

—— ii, *The Programme of the Medical Research Council (UK)* (London, 1975).

THOMSON, H. H., *Consumption, Its Prevention and Home Treatment: A Guide for the Use of Patients* (London, 1910); 2nd edn. (London, 1921); 3rd edn. (London, 1928).

—— *Consumption in General Practice*, 2nd edn. (London, 1912).

—— *Pulmonary Phthisis: Its Diagnosis, Prognosis, and Treatment* (London, 1906).

—— *Tuberculosis and National Health* (London, 1939).

—— *Tuberculosis and Public Health* (London, 1920).

—— and FORD, A. P., *Tuberculosis of the Lungs: A Practical Guide for General Practitioners* (London, 1927).

TITMUSS, R. M., *Poverty and Population: A Factual Study of Contemporary Social Waste* (London, 1938).

TORCHIA, M. M., 'Tuberculosis among American Negroes: Medical Research on a Racial Disease, 1830–1950', *Journal of the History of Medicine and Allied Sciences*, 32 (1977), 252–79.

TRUDEAU, E. L., *An Autobiography* (Philadelphia, 1916).

TURNER, D. A., 'The Open-air School Movement in Sheffield', *History of Education*, 1 (1972), 58–78.

UNDERWOOD, E. A., *A Manual of Tuberculosis*, 3rd edn. (Edinburgh, 1945).

VALLOW, H., *The Inevitable Complement: The Care and After-care of Consumptives* (London, 1915).

VARRIER-JONES, P. J., *Papers of a Pioneer*, collected by P. Fraser (London, 1943).

VERNON, H. M., *Health in Relation to Occupation* (London, 1939).

WAKSMAN, S. A., *The Conquest of Tuberculosis* (London, 1965).

—— (ed.), *Streptomycin, Nature and Practical Application* (London, 1949).

WALKER, J. H., *A Book for Every Woman. Part 1, The Management of Children in Health and out of Health* (London, 1895).

—— *Open-air Treatment of Consumption, Seven Years' Experience in England* (London, 1899).

—— *The Modern Nursing of Consumption* (London, 1904); 2nd edn. (London, 1924).

WALTERS, F. R., *Domiciliary Treatment of Tuberculosis* (London, 1921); 2nd edn. (London, 1924).

—— *The Open-air or Sanatorium Treatment of Pulmonary Tuberculosis* (London, 1909).

—— *Sanatoria for Consumptives in Various Parts of the World (France, Germany, Norway, Russia, Switzerland, the United States and the British Possessions), A Critical and Detailed Description together with an Exposition of the Open-air or Hygienic Treatment of Phthisis* (London, 1899); 2nd edn. (London, 1901); 3rd edn. (London, 1905); 4th edn. (London, 1913).

WEBB, G. B., *Clio Medica: Tuberculosis* (New York, 1936).

WEBB, S. and B., *The Break-up of the Poor Law, The Minority Report of the Poor Law Commission, Part 1* (London, 1909).

WEBSTER, C., 'Healthy or Hungry Thirties?', *History Workshop Journal*, 13 (1982), 110–29.

WILKINSON, E., *The Town that was Murdered. The Life-history of Jarrow* (London, 1939).

WILKINSON, W. C., *The Principles of Immunity in Tuberculosis* (London, 1926).

—— *The Tuberculin Dispensary for the Poor* (London, 1923).

—— *Tuberculin in the Diagnosis and Treatment of Tuberculosis (Weber-Parkes Prize Essay, 1909, with additions)* (London, 1912).

—— *Tuberculin: Its Vindication by Technique* (London, 1933).

—— *Treatment of Consumption* (London, 1908).

WILLIAMS, J. H., *Between Life and Death* (London, 1951).

—— *A Century of Public Health in Britain 1832–1929* (London, 1932).

—— *The Conquest of Fear* (London, 1952).

—— *Requiem for a Great Killer: The Story of Tuberculosis* (London, 1973).

—— (ed.), *Sir Robert Philip, 1857–1939: Memories of his Friends and Pupils* (Edinburgh, 1955).

—— and HARBERT, I., *Social Work for the Tuberculous—A Practical Guide* (London, 1945).

WILSON, G. S., *The Pasteurization of Milk* (London, 1942).

WINGFIELD, R. C., *Modern Methods in the Diagnosis and Treatment of Pulmonary Tuberculosis* (London, 1924).

—— *Pulmonary Tuberculosis in Practice* (London, 1937).

—— *A Textbook of Pulmonary Tuberculosis for Students* (London, 1929).

WINTER, J. M., 'The decline of mortality in Britain 1870–1950', in T. Barker and M. Drake (eds.), *Population and Society in Britain 1850–1980* (London, 1982), 100–20.

—— *The Great War and the British People* (London, 1986).

WITTKOWER, E., *A Psychiatrist Looks at Tuberculosis* (London, 1949).

WOHL, A., *Endangered Lives: Public Health in Victorian Britain* (London, 1983).

WOODCOCK, H. DE C., *The Doctor and the People* (London, 1912).

WOODHEAD, G. S. and VARRIER-JONES, P. C., *Industrial Colonies and Village Settlements for the Consumptive* (Cambridge, 1920).

——, ALLBUTT, C., and VARRIER-JONES, P. C., *Papworth: Administrative and Economic Problems in Tuberculosis* (Cambridge, 1925).

WOODWARD, J. and RICHARDS, D., *Health Care and Popular Medicine in Nineteenth-Century England* (London, 1977).

WRIGHT, P. and TREACHER, A. (eds.), *The Problem of Medical Knowledge: Examining the Social Construction of Medicine* (Edinburgh, 1982).

YOUMANS, G. P., *Tuberculosis* (Philadelphia, 1979).

INDEX